PEDIATRICS, CHILD AND ADOLESCENT HEALTH

PEDIATRIC AND ADOLESCENT DERMATOLOGY

SOME CURRENT ISSUES

PEDIATRICS, CHILD AND ADOLESCENT HEALTH

JOAV MERRICK – SERIES EDITOR –

NATIONAL INSTITUTE OF CHILD HEALTH AND HUMAN DEVELOPMENT, MINISTRY OF SOCIAL AFFAIRS, JERUSALEM, ISRAEL

Positive Youth Development: Theory, Research and Application
Daniel TL Shek, Rachel CF Sun and Joav Merrick (Editors)
2012. ISBN: 978-1-62081-305-8
(Hardcover)

Tropical Pediatrics: A Public Health Concern of International Proportions
Richard R Roach, Donald E Greydanus, Dilip R Patel, Douglas N Homnick and Joav Merrick (Editors)
2012. ISBN: 978-1-61942-831-7
(Hardcover)

Positive Youth Development: A New School Curriculum to Tackle Adolescent Developmental Issues
Hing Keung Ma, Daniel TL Shek and Joav Merrick (Editors)
2012. ISBN: 978-1-62081-384-3
(Hardcover)

Understanding Autism Spectrum Disorder: Current Research Aspects
Ditza A Zachor and Joav Merrick (Editors)
2012. ISBN: 978-1-62081-353-9
(Hardcover)

Transition from Pediatric to Adult Medical Care
David Wood, John G. Reiss, Maria E. Ferris, Linda R. Edwards and Joav Merrick (Editors)
2012. ISBN: 978-1-62081-409-3
(Hardcover)

Child and Adolescent Health Yearbook 2012
Joav Merrick (Editor)
2012. ISBN: 978-1-61942-788-4
(Hardcover)

Child Health and Human Development Yearbook 2011
Joav Merrick (Editor)
2012. ISBN: 978-1-61942-969-7
(Hardcover)

Child and Adolescent Health Yearbook 2011
Joav Merrick (Editor)
2013. ISBN: 978-1-61942-782-2
(Hardcover)

Child Health and Human Development Yearbook 2012
Joav Merrick (Editor)
2013. ISBN: 978-1-61942-978-9
(Hardcover)

Developmental Issues in Chinese Adolescents
Daniel TL Shek, Rachel CF Sun and Joav Merrick (Editors)
2012. ISBN: 978-1-62081-262-4
(Hardcover)

Guidelines for the Healthy Integration of the Ill Child in the Educational System: Experience from Israel
Yosefa Isenberg
2013. ISBN: 978-1-62808-350-7
(Hardcover)

Chinese Adolescent Development: Economic Disadvantages, Parents and Intrapersonal Development
Daniel T.L. Shek, Rachel C.F. Sun and Joav Merrick (Editors)
2013. ISBN: 978-1-62618-622-4
(Hardcover)

University and College Students: Health and Development Issues for the Leaders of Tomorrow
Daniel TL Shek, Rachel CF Sun and Joav Merrick (Editors)
2013. ISBN: 978-1-62618-586-9
(Hardcover)

Adolescence and Behavior Issues in a Chinese Context
Daniel T.L. Shek, Rachel C.F. Sun and Joav Merrick (Editors)
2013. ISBN: 978-1-62618-614-9
(Hardcover)

Advances in Preterm Infant Research
Jing Sun, Nicholas Buys and Joav Merrick
2013. ISBN: 978-1-62618-696-5
(Hardcover)

Promotion of Holistic Development of Young People in Hong Kong
Daniel T.L . Shek, Tak Yan Lee and Joav Merrick (Editors)
2013. ISBN: 978-1-62808-019-3
(Hardcover)

Internet Addiction: A Public Health Concern in Adolescence
Artemis Tsitsika, Mari Janikian, Donald E. Greydanus, Hatim A. Omar and Joav Merrick (Editors)
2013. ISBN: 978-1-62618-925-6
(Hardcover)

Human Developmental Research: Experience from Research in Hong Kong
Daniel T.L . Shek, Cecilia Ma, Yu Lu and Joav Merrick (Editors)
2013. ISBN: 978-1-62808-166-4
(Hardcover)

Chronic Disease and Disability in Childhood
Joav Merrick (Editor)
2013. ISBN: 978-1-62808-865-6
(Hardcover)

Break the Cycle of Environmental Health Disparities: Maternal and Child Health Aspects
Leslie Rubin and Joav Merrick (Editors)
2013. ISBN: 978-1-62948-107-4
(Hardcover)

Environmental Health Disparities in Children: Asthma, Obesity and Food
Leslie Rubin and Joav Merrick (Editors)
2013. ISBN: 978-1-62948-122-7
(Hardcover)

Environmental Health: Home, School and Community
Leslie Rubin and Joav Merrick (Editors)
2013. ISBN: 978-1-62948-155-5
(Hardcover)

Child Health and Human Development: Social, Economic and Environmental Factors
Leslie Rubin and Joav Merrick (Editors)
2013. ISBN: 978-1-62948-166-1
(Hardcover)

Children, Violence and Bullying: International Perspectives
Joav Merrick, Isack Kandel and Hatim A. Omar (Editors)
2013. ISBN: 978-1-62948-342-9

Playing with Fire: Children, Adolescents and Firesetting
Hatim A. Omar, Carrie Howell Bowling and Joav Merrick (Editors)
2013. ISBN: 978-1-62948-471-6
(Softcover)

School, Adolescence and Health Issues
Joav Merrick, Ariel Tenenbaum and Hatim A. Omar (Editors)
2014. ISBN: 978-1-62948-702-1
(Hardcover)

Adolescence and Sexuality: International Perspectives
Joav Merrick, Ariel Tenenbaum and Hatim A. Omar (Editors)
2014. ISBN: 978-1-62948-711-3
(Hardcover)

Child and Adolescent Health Yearbook 2013
Joav Merrick (Editor)
2014. ISBN: 978-1-63117-658-6
(Hardcover)

Adoption: The Search for a New Parenthood
Gary Diamond and Eva Arbel
2014. ISBN: 978-1-63117-710-1
(Hardcover)

Adolescence: Places and Spaces
Myra Taylor, Julie Ann Pooley and Joav Merrick (Editors)
2014. ISBN: 978-1-63117-847-4
(Hardcover)

Pain Management Yearbook 2013
Joav Merrick (Editor)
2014. ISBN: 978-1-63117-944-0
(Hardcover)

Child Health and Human Development Yearbook 2013
Joav Merrick (Editor)
2014. ISBN: 978-1-63117-939-6
(Hardcover)

Born into this World: Health Issues
Donald E. Greydanus, Arthur N. Feinberg and Joav Merrick (Editors)
2014. ISBN: 978-1-63321-667-9
(Hardcover)

Caring for the Newborn: A Comprehensive Guide for the Clinician
Donald E. Greydanus, Arthur N. Feinberg and Joav Merrick (Editors)
2014.ISBN: 978-1-63321-760-7
(Hardcover)

Environment and Hope: Improving Health, Reducing AIDS and Promoting Food Security in the World
I. Leslie Rubin and Joav Merrick (Editors)
2014. ISBN: 978-1-63321-772-0
(Hardcover)

Pediatric and Adolescent Dermatology: Some Current Issues
Donald E Greydanus, Arthur N Feinberg and Joav Merrick (Editors)
2014. ISBN: 978-1-63321-853-6 (Hardcover)

PEDIATRICS, CHILD AND ADOLESCENT HEALTH

PEDIATRIC AND ADOLESCENT DERMATOLOGY

SOME CURRENT ISSUES

DONALD E GREYDANUS
ARTHUR N FEINBERG
AND
JOAV MERRICK
EDITORS

New York

Library of Congress Cataloging-in-Publication Data

ISBN: 978-1-63321-853-6

Library of Congress Control Number: 2014948646

Published by Nova Science Publishers, Inc. † New York

Contents

Introduction

In: Pediatric and Adolescent Dermatology
Editors: D Greydanus, A Feinberg and J Merrick
ISBN: 978-1-63321-853-6

Chapter 1

Lessons from the Fin de siècle century that have influenced pediatric dermatology in the 21st Century

Arthur N Feinberg, MD*[*1], Donald E Greydanus, MD, DrHC (Athens)[1] and Joav Merrick, MD, MMedSc, DMSc[2,3,4,5,6]

[1]Department of Pediatric and Adolescent Medicine,
Western Michigan University Homer Stryker MD School of Medicine,
Kalamazoo, Michigan, United States
[2]National Institute of Child Health and Human Development, Jerusalem Israel
[3]Office of the Medical Director, Health Services,
Division for Intellectual and Developmental Disabilities,
Ministry of Social Affairs and Social Services, Jerusalem, Israel
[4]Division of Pediatrics, Hadassah Hebrew University Medical Center,
Mt Scopus Campus, Jerusalem, Israel, [5]Kentucky Children's Hospital,
University of Kentucky College of Medicine, Lexington, Kentucky, United States
[6]Center for Healthy Development, School of Public Health, Georgia State University,
Atlanta, Georgia, United States of America

Introduction

It is fascinating to take a trip through various textbooks over generations to compare their treatment of the subject of pediatric skin disorders. Eberle on children, published in 1833 consists of 538 pages and contains one chapter consisting of six pages on induration of the skin (1). John Eberle, MD (1787-1838) is listed in his book as Professor of the Theory and Practice of Medicine in the Medical College of Ohio, member of the American Philosophical

* Correspondence: Professor Arthur N Feinberg, MD, Department of Pediatric and Adolescent Medicine, Western Michigan University Homer Stryker M.D. School of Medicine, Oakland Drive Campus, 1000 Oakland Drive, D48G, Kalamazoo, MI 49008-1284, United States. E-mail: Arthur.feinberg@ med.wmich.edu

Society, member of the Academy of Sciences of Philadelphia, and Corresponding member of the Medico-Chirurgical Society of Berlin and in Prussia. The writing is mostly descriptive and includes induration as the common element and elucidates several varieties including red, blue, yellow moist dry warm, cold. About 25% of the cases resulted in death. There were three other brief chapters describing "modified small-pox" subdivided into vaccination-associated rashes and varicella, measles and scarlet fever.

Forsythe Meigs' textbook, 3rd edition, published in 1858 consists of 715 pages (2). John Forsyth Meigs, MD (1818-1882) was listed in his book as Fellow of the College of Physicians of Philadelphia, member of the American Philosophical Society, and the Academy of Natural Sciences of Philadelphia (Pennsylvania). In his book he sought to use "details of his own experience... aimed to make this work more methodical and precise than those heretofore published..." The book was dedicated to George B. Wood, MD (1797-1879), President of the College of Physicians of Philadelphia, Professor in the Practice of Medicine in the University of Pennsylvania—dedicated "as a tribute of respect for his high professional attainments and eminent private virtues and as a mark of gratitude for his valuable instructions by his former pupil." This dedication was written in the true spirit of the Hippocratic oath that many graduating physicians take which states they will "consider dear to me, as my parents, him who taught me this art....." (3-5).

The book is divided up into classes of illness, respiratory organs, digestive organs, nervous system, eruptive fevers, diseases of the skin and worms in the alimentary canal. Eruptive fevers and diseases of the skin comprise 195 of these pages, much more allotment than in 1833. It is mostly descriptive covering all the material cited in Eberle (1), but also reflects further descriptive knowledge of vesicles, bullae, pustules, papules, squamae and ringworms.

Lewis Smith's "A treatise on the diseases of infancy and childhood", published in 1881 contains similar descriptive material and occupies 220 of 836 pages (5). J Lewis Smith, MD (1827-1897) was listed in his book as Clinical Professor of Diseases of Children in Bellevue Hospital Medical College, physician to Charity Hospital, physician to the New York Foundling Asylum, consulting physician to the New York Infant Asylum, consulting physician to the class of children's diseases—Bureau for the relief of the Outdoor Poor, Bellevue. The writer noted that this edition was expanded and written for the medical student and physician "in his daily practice." He also avoided discussion of theories of diseases except "as they influence practice."

It is interesting that one of the most revered old textbooks of pediatrics by L Emmett Holt, 5th edition published in 1910 contains sections on exanthems, but devotes nothing to other skin conditions (6). Luther Emmett Holt, MDE, ScD, LLD (1855-1924) is listed in his book at Professor of Diseases of Children in the College of Physicians and Surgeons (Columbia University), New York; attending physician to the Babies and Foundling Hospital, New York; Corresponding member of the Gesellschaft für innere Medizin under Kinderheilkunde, Vienna; and honorary member of the Gesellschaft für Kinderheilkunde, Germany—indicating the great influence medicine in Europe had on physicians in America in the 18th and 19th centuries. The book was written "for the use of students and practitioners of medicine."

Fast-forward to modern days. The most recent edition of Nelson's textbook of pediatrics, 19th edition, 2011 actually acknowledges dermatologic manifestations of multisystem disorders as well as multisystem medication reactions, but, in a nod to online emphasis in the

21st century, refers the reader to their website for further elaboration after having devoted only one paragraph to each subject (7). This famous modern textbook of pediatrics traces its origins back to 1919 and is named after Waldo E Nelson, MD (1898-1997), who had origins in common with the older book editors cited--- Dr. Nelson's birthplace was Ohio and his work as Chair of Pediatrics was at Temple University in Philadelphia. Recently literature in pediatric dermatology that has accumulated over the eons of physician observation also links the human central nervous system and the skin in the etiology of numerous dermatological and psychiatric disorders that are intertwined throughout life (8).

The integument is the largest organ system of the human body and is often described as the gatekeeper to every other system. Its integrity will not only determine the admission or rejection of many foreign invaders (bacteria, viruses, fungi, etc.), but also plays a significant role in providing the milieu for the immune system to do battle with these invaders. It is typically the first view of an examiner and often yields very important clues to seemingly non-dermatologic issues. This book takes us one step further, devoting chapters to the interplay between integument and heretofore generally unnoted strongly related psychosocial issues.

> "If I have seen further, it has been by standing on the shoulders of giants"
> (Sir Issac Newton, 1643-1727)

References

[1] Eberle J. Treatise on the diseases and physical education of children. Philadelphia, PA: Corey Fairbank, 1833.

[2] Meigs JF. Practical treatise on the diseases of children, 3rd ed. Philadelphia, PA: Lindsay Blakiston, 1858.

[3] Guthrie AD. The Hippocratic oath. Int Rec Med Gen Pract Clin 1957;170(9):473-8.

[4] Catto G. The Hippocratic oath: back to the future? Med Educ 2014;48(1):4-5

[5] Smith JL. A treatice on the diseases of infancy and childhood, 5th ed. Philadelphia, PA: Henry C.Lea's Son, 1881.

[6] Holt LM. The diseases of infancy and childhood, 5th ed. New York: D Appleton, 1910.

[7] Kliegman RM, Stanton BMD, Geme JS, Schor N, Behrman RE, eds. Nelson textbook of pediatrics, 19th ed. Philadelphia, PA: Elsevier, 2011.

[8] Tareen S, Greydanus DE, Jaffernay M, Patel DR, Merrick J, eds. Pediatric psychodermatology. A clinical manual of child and adolescent psychocutaneous disorders. Berlin: De Greuter, 2013.

Section One: Some dermatology themes

In: Pediatric and Adolescent Dermatology
Editors: D Greydanus, A Feinberg and J Merrick
ISBN: 978-1-63321-853-6

Chapter 2

Dermatology issues in the newborn period

Therdpong Tempark, MD and Tor Shwayder, MD*
Pediatric Dermatology, Henry Ford Hospital, Detroit, Michigan,
United States of America

Neonatal skin manifests itself as a clinical spectrum from transient changes, normal variants due to developmental anomalies, outright abnormalities, infections and life-threatening conditions. We review and provide updates and photographs categorizing neonatal skin conditions into six groups including i) transient physiologic changes and benign conditions ii) birthmarks (pigmented, vascular et.al iii) developmental anomalies iv) vesiculopustular and bullous diseases v) iatrogenic and vi) others.

Introduction

Neonatal skin development, structure, biochemistry and function are all distinct from the adult skin. This in turn affects the different clinical presentations. A variety of neonatal skin problems presents during the neonatal period (post-partum to less than 1 month) and/or in infancy (after 1 month to 1 year). The skin manifestations range from uncommon to common, transient to permanent, treatable to untreatable, and are necessary to recognize. This article reviews aspects of pathogenesis, clinical presentation with variants, differential diagnosis, associated conditions, treatment options and prognosis.

* Correspondence: Tor A Shwayder MD, Director, Pediatric Dermatology, Henry Ford Hospital, 3031 Grand Boulevard, Detroit, Michigan 48202, United States. E-mail: tshwayd1@hfhs.org

Transient physiologic change and benign lesions

Vernix caseosa is a grayish-white, greasy material covering the term infant skin to lubricate and facilitate delivery through the vaginal canal. This substance is increasing and thicker with gestational age of term infant and decreases in post term infants.

The major constituent of vernix is water, whereas the total amount of lipid is approximately 10% including cholesterol, triglyceride, free fatty acid, phospholipid and ceramide. The rest is composed of shed epithelial cells, shed lanugo hair and sebaceous secretions (1).

This substance provides lubrication in the birth canal and also supports the development of epidermis in utero. Vernix caseosa increases hydration of the infant skin after birth partly due to the large water content of the corneocytes that are shed into the vernix caseosa. Vernix caseosa is an aid in wound healing, has an antioxidant effect due to alpha-tocopherol (vitamin E) and melanin, as well as antibacterial and antifungal properties. The color and smell of vernix caseosa often reflects intrauterine problems such as discoloration from meconium staining and intrauterine infection.

Sebaceous gland hyperplasia

Sebaceous gland hyperplasia is a consequence of the effect of maternal androgen on the pilosebaceous follicles during the final month of gestation. It is common and occurs in more than 50% of term infants. Sebaceous hyperplasia occurs less often in preterm infants and is without sex predilection.

This condition characteristically presents with multiple yellow to flesh-colored tiny papules on the nose, cheek, upper lip, and forehead that are the openings of the pilosebaceous follicles (see figure 1). They are found at birth and spontaneously resolve in several weeks (2).

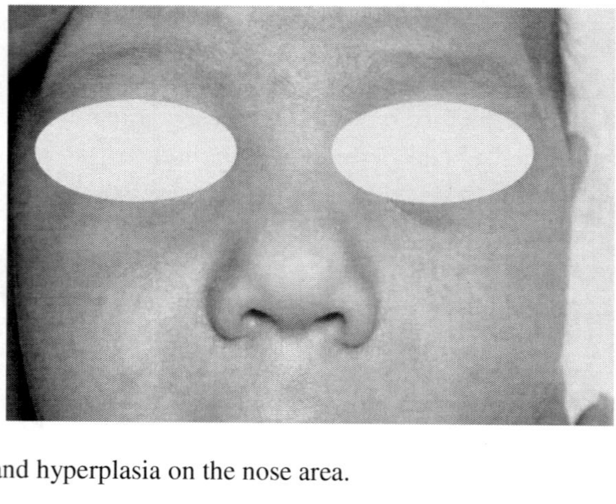

Figure 1. Sebaceous gland hyperplasia on the nose area.

Cutis marmorata

Cutis marmorata is a transient reticulated, mottled bluish to purplish discoloration of the skin, frequently found both in term and in preterm infants. The possible cause is exaggerated vasomotor response to hypothermia which increases sympathetic tone and vasoconstriction.

Physiologic cutis marmorata should be differentiated from cutis marmorata telangiectatica congenita (CMTC) which is a persistent, reticulated, mottled purplish discoloration (see figure 2). Although physiologic cutis marmorata can resolve after warming the skin, CMTC does not.

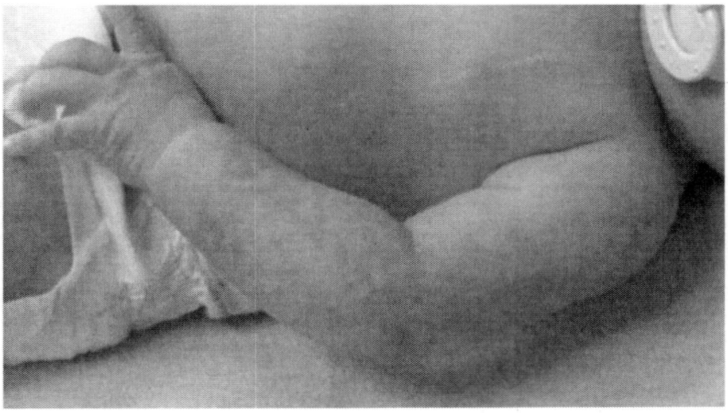

Figure 2. Cutis marmorata telangiectatica congenita (CMTC) on the left arm.

Persistent cutis marmorata had been reported in Down syndrome, trisomy 18, Cornelia de Lange syndrome, congenital hypothyroidism and El-Shanti syndrome. CMTC is a diagnostic criterion for multiple syndromes such as macrocephaly-cutis marmorata telangiectatica congenita (macrocephaly-CMTC syndrome). There are few reports of associated ipsilateral limb hypotrophy, skin atrophy and defect of soft tissue growth. Other possible associated findings include telangiectasia, phlebectasia, atrophy and ulceration. Delayed development has also been reported.

Although they may persist for several weeks to months, no specific treatment is required in physiologic cutis marmorata. The appropriate management is controlling the core, body and environmental temperature. Persistent cutis marmorata and CMTC should be evaluated for other unusual conditions as mentioned above (3).

Sucking blisters

This benign self-limited lesion is the result of sucking in utero. The typical lesions are non-inflammatory, tense vesicles or bullae, usually located on the dorsal aspect of fingers, wrists, tip or radial aspect of forearms at birth and are more commonly found as a single lesion (see figures 3 a,b). The child often puts an area of the arm into the mouth postnatally, making clear to the thoughtful observer the cause of the bulla. Spontaneous resolution occurs within a few days to weeks.

The differential diagnosis is vesiculobullous diseases including infectious causes (e.g. herpes simplex infection, bullous impetigo neonatorum), non-infectious causes (e.g. epidermolysis bullosa, friction) and inflammatory causes (e.g. bullous mastocytosis). Supportive treatment is appropriate (4).

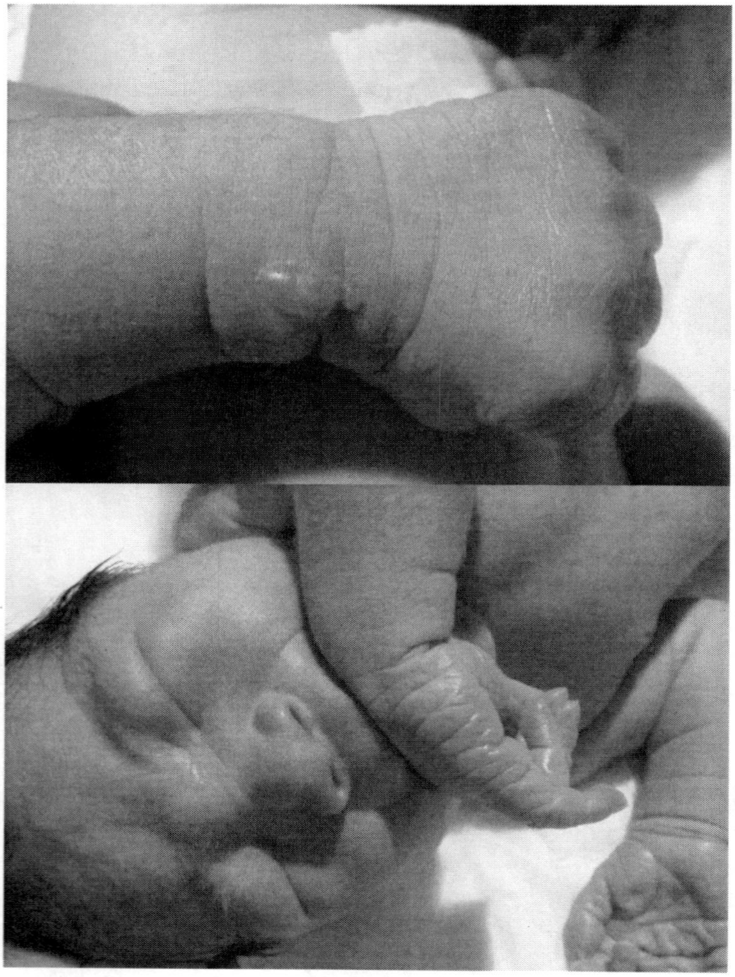

Figure 3 a,b. Sucking blister on the left wrist Note non-inflamed bulla in exact location of the child's sucking behavior.

Epstein's pearl

Epstein's pearl or a congenital epidermal inclusion cyst is a transient benign neonatal lesion in the oral cavity. They are more common in full term neonates and associated with increased birth weight. The characteristic presentations are asymptomatic, multiple discrete, whitish or yellowish cystic lesions locating along the midpalatine raphe, particularly at the junction of the hard and soft palate. They can vary in size from 2 to 3 mm. These lesions rupture spontaneously within first few weeks to months of life. Neonates with congenital milia may also have Epstein's pearls (5).

Natal and neonatal teeth

Natal teeth are present right at birth. This is distinct from neonatal teeth that occur in the first few months of life. The incidence of these conditions varies from 1:1,000 to 1:30,000 depending on method of the studies. Natal teeth are found three times more frequently than neonatal teeth. These teeth may be found both in term and in preterm infants. The exact etiology of this condition is unclear.

Natal teeth typically present in pairs (61-76%) on the sites of the central mandibular incisors (85%), maxillary incisor (11%), mandibular canine or molar (3%) and maxillary canine or molar (1%), respectively.

Natal and neonatal teeth are more frequently found in children with cleft lip and cleft palate. Multiple syndromes are associated with natal teeth including pachyonychia congenita, Ellis-van Creveld syndrome, Hallerman-Streiff syndrome and epidermolysis bullosa simplex.

The treatment depends upon the location, morphology, root development and tooth mobility. If the neonatal tooth persists in the jaw, its presence will disturb the development of the normal teeth. Therefore extraction is usually recommended, with special attention to remove the root (6).

Milia

Milia, minute epidermal inclusion cysts, usually present with white, pearly 1-2 mm. papules on the nose, cheek, chin, forehead and other parts of the body. They result from retention of keratin within the dermis.

Milia usually occur in normal healthy infants. Multiple, persistent and widespread lesions may be seen in several conditions. Berk et al (7) reviewed and classified milia as primary and secondary, and as isolated to few to multiple lesions. They then associated these with other findings and conditions. Primary milia occur spontaneously (e.g. congenital milia, milia en plaque, nodular grouped milia and multiple eruptive milia). Secondary milia are associated with multiple conditions, categorized into four groups including:

- Diseases (e.g. Stevens-Johnsons syndrome, Staphylococcal Scalded Skin Syndrome (SSSS), lichen planus, herpes zoster, Sweet syndrome and epidermolysis bullosa)
- Syndromes (e.g. Brooke-Spiegler syndrome, atrichia with papular lesion, basal cell nevus syndrome and pachyonychia congentia type II)
- Trauma (e.g. burn, skin grafts, ablative laser therapy and dermabrasion)
- Medication (e.g. topical corticosteroid, cyclosporine and penicillamine).

The differential diagnosis includes calcinosis cutis/calcified heel stick nodules, syringoma, sebaceous gland hyperplasia and folliculitis. No treatment is necessary. Simple incision and drainage can be performed if the parents desire (7).

Birthmarks

Nevus depigmentosus is a congenital, non-heritable, non-progressive hypopigmented patch or swirled macules, most commonly presenting at birth. The lesion may be single, multiple, swirled and/or in a segmental.

The pathogenesis of nevus depigmentosus is a developmental defect of the melanocytes, most likely resulting from a defect in the transferring of melanosomes from melanocytes to the keratinocytes.

Histopathological features reveal a significant decrease in the amount of melanin in the epidermal layers. However, the number of melanocytes in affected skin remains controversial.

This condition is usually solitary, well-defined border, round to oval hypopigmented macules or patches on the trunk and extremities. The trunk is the most common site of lesion. Face, neck, arm, leg are also been reported.

Coupe set up the diagnostic criteria for nevus depigmentosus in 1976 including:

- Leukoderma present at birth or early onset in life
- No alteration in distribution of leukoderma throughout life
- No alteration in the texture or change of sensation in the affected area
- No hyperpigmented border around the achromic area

The differential diagnoses of this disorder are hypopigmented lesion of tuberous sclerosis, nevus anemicus and vitiligo. The onset of clinical presentation, physical examination and Wood's lamp examination may be used to distinguish these conditions. Nevus depigmentosus usually reveals off-white accentuation without fluorescence, whereas vitiligo reveals chalky-white accentuation with obvious fluorescence in Wood's lamp examination.

This condition tends to remain stable both in size and in distribution throughout life. The treatment is unnecessary (8).

Hypopigmented macules of tuberous sclerosis (TS)

The clinical presentation characteristically reveals solitary to multiple, lance-oval-shaped hypopigmented macules (Ash leaf spot) or patches on the trunk, mostly presenting at birth. Guttate (drop-like) and linear patterns may be found. They are variable in size and location but most commonly occur on the trunk (see figure 4).

Pathogenesis is due to hypofunction of melanocytes. Although this hypopigmented lesion is not a pathognomonic sign of (TS), it should be differentiated from the other conditions (e.g. nevus depigmentosus and vitiligo). Early detection of TS is preferred for proper management.

This hypopigmented lesion usually presents in 95% of affected patients either at birth or shortly thereafter Wood's lamp may be used to detect subtle lesions in individuals with light skin color.

If the child has three or more ash leaf spots in the neonatal period and/or an isolated macule with other suspicious signs, symptoms or family history of tuberous sclerosis, they should be evaluated for diagnosis with appropriate imaging.

The additional clinical clues for diagnosis are frequently found in neonatal period, including cardiac rhabdomyoma and large fibrotic collagenous plaques (collagenoma) on the forehead. The other cutaneous signs such as adenoma sebaceum (angiofibroma) and connective tissue nevus (Shagreen patches) usually become evident in early to late childhood.

The ash leaf spot basically remains the same shape and size through life. The treatment of this hypopigmented lesion is unnecessary (9).

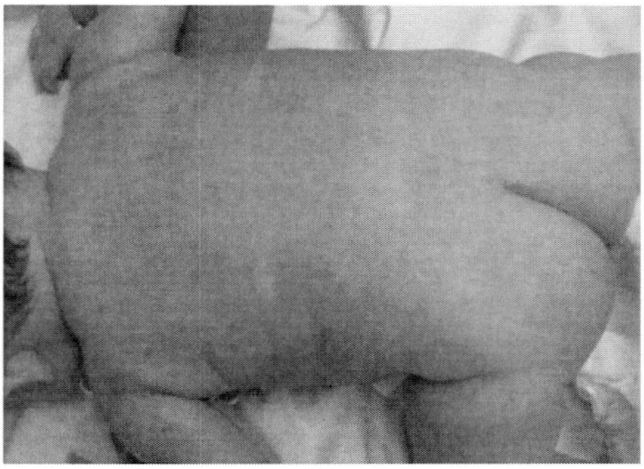

Figure 4. Hypopigmented macules of tuberous sclerosis (Ash leaf spots).

Dermal melanosis (DM)

Dermal melanosis (Mongolian spot) characteristically shows an ill-defined border, homogeneous pigmented blue gray-colored macules or patches and is generally located over the lumbosacral area and buttocks (see figure 5). Presentations are variable in racial groups with the prevalence in African-Americans 90-96%, Asians 81-86%, Hispanics 46-70%, Middle East 11-71% and Caucasian infants 10%.

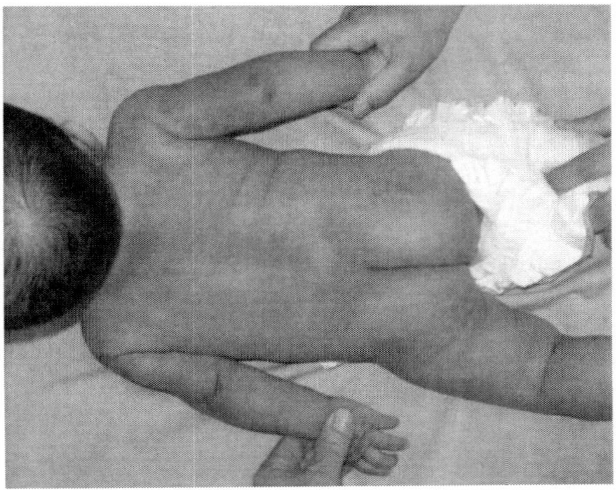

Figure 5. Mongolian spot on 6 month Indian male.

The size, location, shade of color and fading time are also variable. The most common locations of lesion are sacrogluteal area, shoulder and extensor surface of the upper extremities. The abdomen and chest are rarely affected.

The presumptive pathogenesis of this condition is incomplete migration of melanocytes from the neural crest to dermoepidermal junction during the 11th and 14th weeks of gestation. The melanocytes maintain at lower half of the dermal layer of the skin but there is no explanation why the Mongolian spot is predominanly in the sacrogluteal region.They tend to fade probably due to migration of the dermal melanocytes to the epidermis and/or are eradicated by macrophage ingestion. The fading color can be used to distinguish Mongolian spots from persistent color of nevocellular nevi.

The differential diagnoses are blue nevi, nevus of Ota, nevus of Ito and ecchymosis, due to accidental or child abuse. It behooves the pediatrician to recognize these as they may frequently be called for opinions regarding child abuse. This condition resolves spontaneously in the first few years of life without consequences. No treatment is necessary. An unusual variant "superimposed Mongolian spots", revealing pigmented Mongolian spots on top of another Mongolian spot has been reported in four Chinese infants (10).

Multiple diseases/syndromes may present with extensive, numerous and/or persistent DM, especially inborn errors of metabolism groups of lysosomal storage diseases including GM gangliosidosis type I, Hunter syndrome, Hurler syndrome, mucolipoidosis type II and Sjögren Larsson syndrome (10).

Cafe-au-lait macules (CALMs)

CALMs typically present as tan-brown, round or oval, well circumscribed macules or patches. The incidence is up to 33% in normal children. The size ranges from 0.2 to 4 cm. in diameter and enlarges proportionately with the baby's growth without regression (see figure 6). The reports of prevalence in newborn period are variable with different ethnicities (range from 0.3 to 2.7%). The most common site of lesion is the buttock area, whereas the trunk is the most common site in older children. It is not uncommon to acquire more CALMs with age.

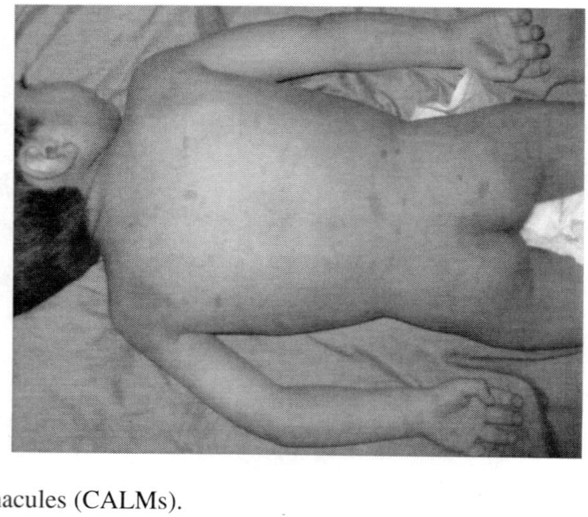

Figure 6. Café-au-lait macules (CALMs).

The acceptable numbers of CALMs in normal children varies. Previous studies of the prevalence of multiple CALMS in "normal" population revealed less than or equal to two macules in newborn period and 2-3 macules in school age children. CALMs are active melanocytes so the spots would darken with sun exposure in the summer and lighten in the winter.

Histopathological features reveal increasing melanin content in melanocytes and basal keratinocytes without melanocytic proliferation. The differential diagnoses of CALMs include nevus spilus, lentigenes, nevocellular nevus and segmental pigmentation disorders.

Although, most of children with CALMs do not have other abnormalities, many and large lesions may be a sign of multiple organ syndromes such as neurofibromatosis, McCune Albright syndrome, Russell-Silver syndrome, LEOPARD syndrome, ataxia telangiectasia, tuberous sclerosis, Bloom syndrome, Turner syndrome and Cowden's syndrome.

Treatment of this condition is unnecessary. Observation of these children with multiple CALMs during the first 5-6 years of life is recommended. The associated abnormalities will usually present in this period (e.g. learning disabilities in NF and short stature in Russell-Silver or Turner syndrome) (11).

Congenital melanocytic nevus

Congenital melanocytic nevus (CMN) is a benign melanocytic proliferation in the skin, usually presenting at birth. The melanocyte originates in the neural crest and migrates to the skin in early fetal life. The migratory arrest of melanocytes can be assumed in multiple hyperpigmented conditions including melanocytic nevus, dermal melanosis, blue nevus, nevi of Ota and Ito.

CMN have been commonly categorized in three groups according to the size of the lesion. Giant CMN is defined as bigger than 6 cm. in diameter on the body or more than 9 cm. in diameter on the head of neonates. In adults criteria are: small <1.5 cm, medium 1.5 cm-20cm and large, >20cm. Malignant potential increases with the size of lesions.

The characteristic histopathology demonstrates extension of the nevus cells in the deep dermis and subcutaneous tissue between the collagen bundles, appendages, nerves and blood vessels.

Clinical presentation of small CMN reveals solitary or multiple, brownish, well demarcated macules or papules on the body. They are variable in size, location, number, texture and color. The lesions can acquire dark hair and the nevus can darken with advanced age (see figure 7).

Giant CMN characteristically reveals irregular, brownish, well-demarcated patches or plaques with verrucous surfaces with significant background pigmentary variation. The addition of multiple small satellite nevi often accompanies the giant lesions. The acquired dark hair and darker lesions are also found in this condition, particularly at puberty (see figure 8).

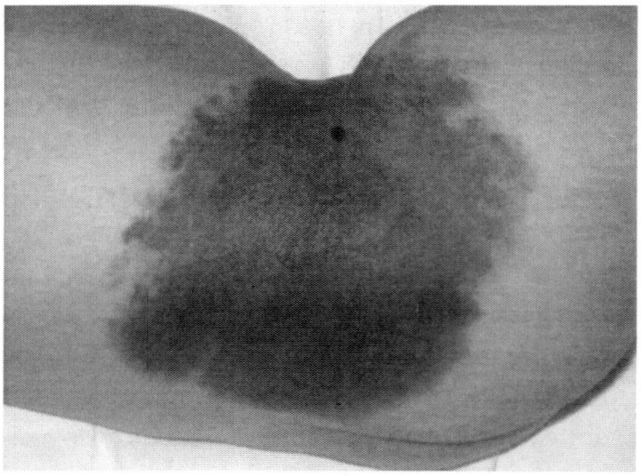

Figure 7. Congenital melanocytic nevus.

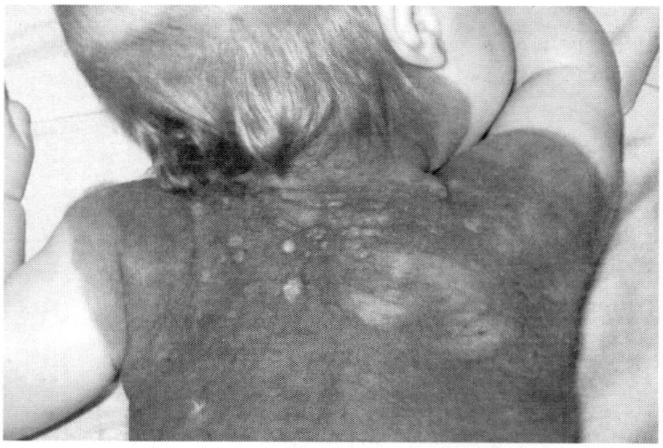

Figure 8. Giant congenital melanocytic nevus with discrete papules representing clonal proliferations of melanocytes. It takes a skilled dermatopathologist to distinguish these from melanoma on H & E. Because of the location and extent of this particular nevus, this child has higher risk of leptomeningeal melanocytosis (NCM).

The most common site of giant CMN is posterior trunk, presenting as a "garment nevus" or "bathing trunk nevus". They are variable in surface texture, color, distribution and hypertrichosis.

The main issue in congenital melanocytic nevi is cosmetic. One of the most common concerning complications of CMN is malignant transformation to melanoma. According to a systematic review of 14 large studies of CMN patients for 39 years (1966 to 2005), the overall risk of melanoma is 0.7%. The median age of melanoma diagnosis was 7 years old.

There is risk of melanoma transformation in all sizes of CMN with higher risk associated with larger size. Giant CMN risk is about 2.3-2.9 %. Satellite lesions have also been reported with transformation, but it is exceptionally rare. If melanoma occurs from giant CMN, it usually does in the first five years of life (50% of the cases).

The confounding factors that possibly increase risk of transformation include atypical clinical features (rapid growth, irregular border and pigmentation), family history of melanoma and phenotype of the nevus.

Neurocutaneous melanosis (NCM) represents intracerebral melanocytic proliferations which have a potential of developing primary leptomeningeal melanoma. The morbidity and mortality of NCM from Giant CMN on the trunk are higher in lesions on the head or extremities. Moreover, > 20 satellite lesions are associated with a five-fold increase the risk of NCM.

The proliferation of nevus cells in the central nervous system causes neurologic symptoms from increased intracranial pressure, spinal cord compression (irritability, headache, recurrent vomiting, stiff neck and papilledema), seizures and leptomeningeal melanoma transformation. These symptoms frequently present during the first 3 years of life.

The patients who have giant CMN on the posterior trunk with numerous satellite lesions should be monitored for neurological signs and symptoms and should be evaluated with an MRI scan of the brain to rule out NCM.

The management of CMN is based on a joint decision involving the parents, child and physician. The important issues include size, location, symptoms, age, cosmetics, the risk of melanoma transformation, risk of operative procedure and risk of complication after surgery.

Increased incidence of melanoma with CMN and sun exposure is not established. However it is prudent to advise parents/patients to protect the patient with CMN from sun exposure (12,13).

Vascular birthmarks

Nevus simplex is an extremely common benign superficial capillary malformation in infancy. This condition usually presents with an irregular border, pink to red macules on nape of the neck, glabella, forehead, upper eyelids (see figure 9). The nose, upper lip, occipital or parietal scalp have these lesions as well, although less frequently. The lower lip, upper back and lumbosacral region can also be involved.

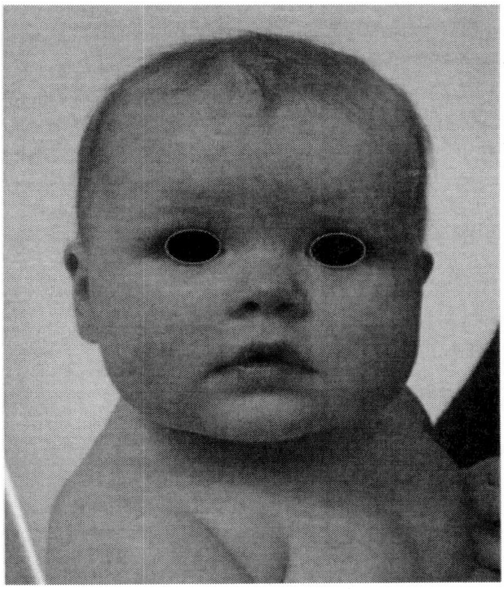

Figure 9. Nevus simplex / Salmon patch / Stork's bite.

They are usually blanchable and become more prominent during episodes of crying, breath holding, vigorous activity, physical exertion and change in ambient temperature.

Most nevus simplex spontaneously fades and disappears within 1-2 years. Parents should be reassured with this information and treatment is unnecessary. The nape of the neck tends to persistent with lesions longer than other areas. Sometimes a seborrheic-liked scale, persisting over the nevus simplex at the nape of the neck, could be misdiagnosed for tinea capitis. Pulsed Dye Laser (PDL) may be helpful in treatment of persistent salmon patches.

The natural course of nevus simplex tends toward spontaneous resolution. Nevertheless, persistent lesions may be found in conditions such as Beckwith-Wiedermann syndrome, macrocephaly-capillary malformation syndrome, Nova syndrome and odontodysplasia (14,15).

Port wine stain (PWS)/Nevus flammeus

Port wine stain (PWS) is a capillary malformation noted in infancy. They are irregularly bordered, unilateral or segmental, non-palpable, erythematous patches on any part of the body (see figure 10). Most of these are unilateral (85 %) and cover over more than one dermatome (68 %).

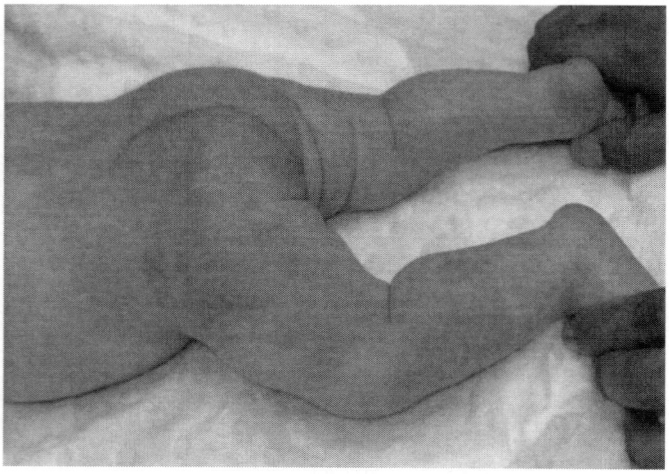

Figure 10. Port wine stain on the left leg. It would be appropriate to check for leg circumference and length discrepancies.

They are usually present at birth and maintain their color in the first decade of life. Lightening in first few months of life is sometimes seen due to physiologic anemia in early infancy. PWS tend to darken and thicken in advanced age. Histopathology shows a change of the numbers of ectatic mature capillaries in the superficial dermis and dilated and increased number of these capillaries in the deep dermis and subcutaneous tissue. The exact cause of this change is unclear. The presumptive mechanisms are impairment of neural control of vascular elements and neural regulation of blood flow in the PWS.

PWS in the midline location over the spine or scalp may be a marker for occult spinal dysraphism. This is especially true if dimples, tracks, hair tufts or asymmetric subcutaneous masses are detected. Thickening and secondary nodules of pyogenic granuloma in PWS lesions often develop in facial PWS more than in other areas.

PWS can be found either as an isolated cutaneous lesion or with associated syndromes such syndromes as Sturge-Weber, Klippel-Trenaunay, Parkes-Weber, Proteus, Wyburn-Masson syndrome and Phakomatosis pigmentovascularis.

Reasons for treatment include preventing the thickening and nodularity occurring with age, cosmetics, and psychosocial issues. Treating the superficial stain does not alter the underlying associated anomalies or syndromes.

The Pulsed Dye Laser (PDL) is the principal treatment of choice for PWS. Multiple treatments, every 4-8 weeks, are required for best results. Most of the patients accomplish lightened skin rather than complete clearance. The response rate relies on the size of lesions, location (central face has less response) and age of treatment onset (early age is better). The relative physiologic anemia of infancy can possibly be misconstrued as fading color. Anesthetic risk in young infants should also be considered. The most appropriate time to initiate treatment, anesthetic procedure, laser parameters, and the frequency of treatments are still questionable and requires additional study.

Re-darkening of PWS at 10 years after PDL treatment had been reported. Retreatment with PDL may be required to correct this condition. The fact that it takes many treatments and the risk of lightening and re-darkening should be stated to parents prior to treatments (16).

Hemangioma

Infantile hemangioma (IH) is the most common benign vascular tumor of infancy. The study from a large population based sample reveals the occurrence in 1-4% of Caucasian infants. This benign tumor possibly presents at birth as congenital hemangioma or develops shortly after birth in the neonatal period. Most of hemangiomas occur within the first few weeks of life.

Several factors are associated with increased risk of hemangioma including Caucasian race, female gender, prematurity, advanced maternal age, multiple gestational pregnancy, manipulation during pregnancy (e.g. chorionic villus sampling, amniocentesis) and low birth weight.

Clinical presentation of IH depends on timing and type and is variable in size and locations. The lesions usually begin with small erythematous patches and plaques, followed by nodules and increases in size (see figure 11). IH usually distributes in a local or segmental pattern with varying degrees of organ involvement. They may present as sole cutaneous lesions and may be associated with organ malformations and syndromes.

In the past IH had been categorized to three groups according to the depth of lesion involvement. Superficial or strawberry hemangioma, involving the epidermis and upper dermis, usually presents as bright-red nodule, mass and plaque. Deep hemangioma involves the deep dermis and subcutaneous tissue. Because of the normal thickness of epidermis, the color of the skin may be bluish or normal. Telangiectasia is also present. The combination of superficial and deep hemangioma may involve both epidermis and subcutaneous tissue. It is accepted that IH at any level of the skin represents the same physiologic process, and therefore some consider depth classifications unnecessary.

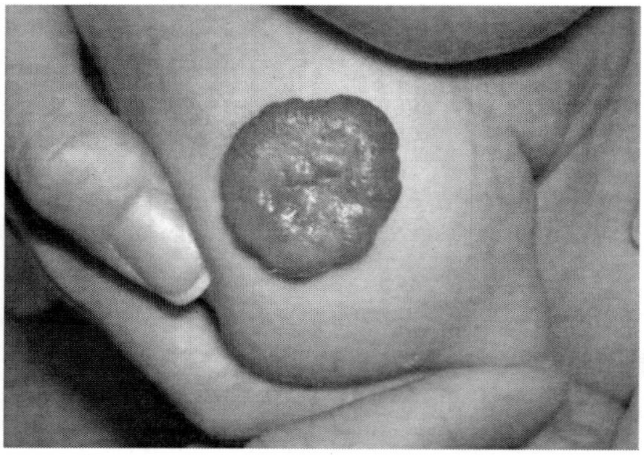

Figure 11. Hemangioma on the shoulder of this infant.

The natural history of IH growth includes three phases, proliferative, plateau and involution. The majority of superficial IH is first noticed at 2 to 3 weeks of life then grows rapidly in the first 3-5 months of life and then resolves. Eighty percent of the cases completely proliferate by 5 months of age. The growth phase may be as short as a few weeks or as long as 1-2 years of age. The involution phase typically begins by 1 year of age, occasionally earlier. The recovery rate is approximately 10% per year. IH usually leaves behind minimal skin changes e.g. telangiectasia, atrophic wrinkles, texture and pigmentary changes, redundant fibro-fatty tissues and rarely scarring.

The exact pathogenesis of the proliferative phase of IH is not understood. The endothelial cells are involved with vasculogenesis and angiogenesis. Several cellular markers of angiogenesis include basic fibroblast-growth factor (FGF), vascular endothelial growth factor (VEGF), proliferating-cell nuclear antigen and E-selectin all increase in IH. Positive glucose transporter 1 (GLUT-1), merosin and Lewis Y antigen stains are detected in both placental and endothelial cell histologic preparations.

Another recent hypothesis states that hypoxia relates to the development of hemangiomas and it has been proposed that hypoxia induces the increase of progenitor cell mediators e.g. hypoxia inducible factor 1A: HIF-1 α in IH. Similarly, the pathogenesis of the involution phase is still not verified. Programmed cell death is one proposed mechanism of this phase.

Several complications occur in IH, especially during the proliferative phase, including ulceration, bleeding, infection, and vital organ compromise (airway, eye and hepatic hemangioma). Of particular note is the sequestration of platelets or erythrocytes in large tufted hemangiomas or Kaposiform hemangioendotheliomas causing thrombocytopenia and subsequent bleeding, consumptive coagulopathy or microangiopathic anemia (Kasabach-Merritt syndrome).

The liver is the most common extracutaneous site of involvement for IH. The infant who has more than five cutaneous hemangiomas lesions should be evaluated by liver ultrasonography to rule out this possibility. Hypothyroidism is a potential complication of hepatic hemangioma, possibly by producing type 3 iodothyronine deiodinase. Some authors recommend checking thyroid function test in all cases of hepatic hemangioma.

Management should be approached on a case-by-case basis. Many factors determine which therapies to be used, including age of onset, number of lesions, age group, size, location, phenotype, phase of lesion, ulceration, infection, pain, blockage of crucial external organs, underlying disease/syndrome and internal organ involvement. Hemangiomas located around the eye should be treated early in order to prevent strabismus or blockage of the lachrymal system.

Treatments include systemic corticosteroids, intralesional corticosteroids, oral or topical propranolol, systemic anti-proliferative agents (vincristine, vinblastine), recombinant interferon alpha, laser ablation (Pulsed Dye Laser) and surgical excision.

For cases of infected ulcerated hemangioma treatment includes local wound care, pain control medication and/or antibiotics. Parents should be provided with the requisite education about the natural history, treatment options, acute and long-term management and psychological support (17).

Vascular malformation

Vascular malformations are congenital aberrant blood vessels and/or lymphatic malformations of the skin. They are most likely caused by dysfunction in pathways that regulate vascular embryogenesis. Vascular malformation almost always presents at birth and enlarges proportionately with the growth of the child. They are variable in size and location at presentation.

Vascular malformations are classified as slow-flow, fast-flow and complex. Slow-flow malformations are capillary, venous or lymphatic. Fast-flow malformations include arterial, arteriovenous malformation (AVM) and arteriovenous fistula (AVF). Complex malformations are combinations of the tissue types. Blood vessel types determine the flow characteristics, whereas the location, depth, volume and hemoglobin concentration determine the clinical features.

Vascular malformations may possibly present as an abnormal cutaneous lesion alone and/or as one part of a systemic condition or syndrome. They persist throughout life without spontaneous regression. The clinical presentations characteristically reveal bluish to purplish nodules/masses (see figure 12).

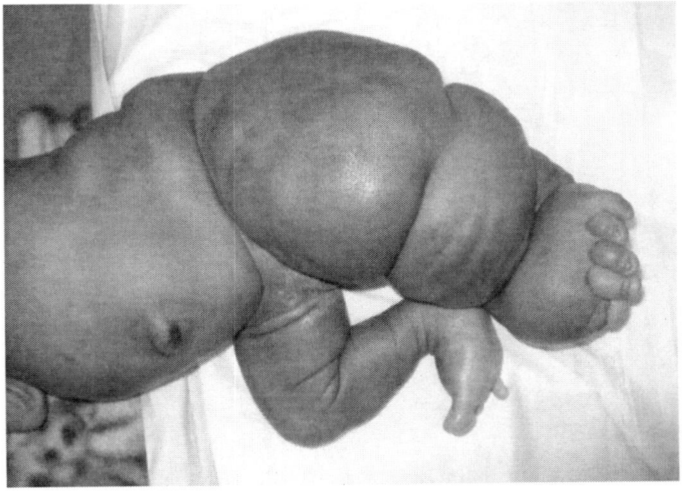

Figure 12. Vascular malformation left leg. MRI revealed a complex lesion of arterial, venous and lymphatic components. This child died of complications due to the vascular malformation.

Enlarged superifical veins and calcified phleboliths may occur. Small vascular malformations tend to be asymptomatic. However, the larger vascular malformations may induce pain from stasis, intravascular coagulopathy, thrombosis or bleeding secondary to consumption of clotting factors.

The treatment modalities vary due to type, size, location, underlying disease and associated features. One option is surgical removal, especially if there is underlying organ involvement. Embolization by percutaneous sclerotherapy is used in cases of a localized form with extracutaneous feeding vessels. Potential complications and recurrence should be considered.

Supportive treatment with pressure garments (e.g. elastic stockings) often brings pain relief and decreases the risk of coagulopathy. Low-dose aspirin therapy is appropriate with patients at risk for thrombogenic problems from the lesions (18).

Nevus sebaceous of Jadassohn

Nevus sebaceous of Jadassohn is a common congenital hamartoma of sebaceous glands. In addition to sebaceous glands, one also sees abortive hair follicles and ectopic apocrine glands in the skin. They characteristically present with solitary, thickened, hairless, yellowish, well-demarcated plaques, most commonly located on the scalp and face area but there is a variety of sizes and locations. They are often more red than yellow and thicker in the first few months of life due to the stimulation of the sebaceous elements of this hamartoma by maternal hormones. The lesion will flatten and fade in color after 3 months age. The color, surface and thickness start to grow again in puberty due to sex hormone effects (see figure 13).

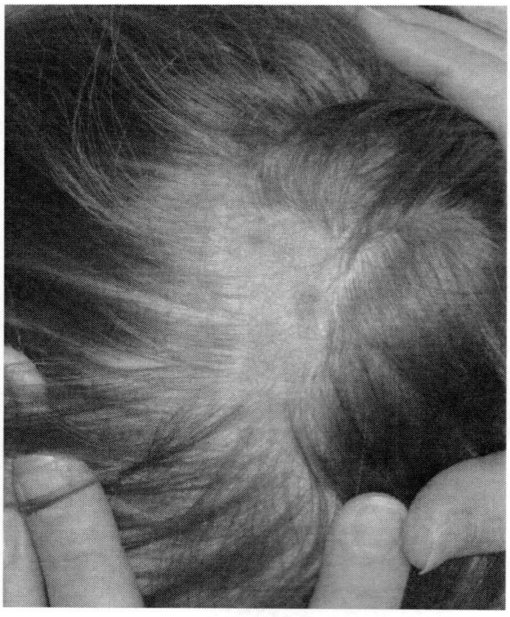

Figure 13. Nevus sebaceous in the scalp of a 5 year old WM. This one is clearly demarcated and yellow with little to no hair within it. These lesions can be red and flat before they are yellow and bumpy.

The lesions enlarge proportionate with growth of the infant. The extensive, multiple and centrofacial lesions are rarely associated with cerebral, ocular and skeletal abnormalities as in Schimmelpenning syndrome.

There is a minimal risk of secondary appendageal neoplasm (e.g. syringocystadenoma papilliferum, trichoblastoma, spiradenoma) and malignant potential (basal cell carcinoma) from the lesions.

Rosen et al (19) reviewed and reported 631 cases of nevus sebaceous in an 18 year-follow up. The overall risk of malignant transformation to basal cell carcinoma is 0.8 %. All of basal cell carcinoma lesions were located on the scalp or face. The transformation can occur even before puberty (mean age 12.5 years, range 9.7-17.4 years). The overall risk of benign neoplasm with syringocystadenoma papilliferum is 1.1 % (mean age 8.8 years, range 1.7-16.9 years).

Factors to consider before removal include the minimal risk of malignant transformation, size, location of the lesions, cosmetic/psychological issues for the child and scar formation. The parents and patient should be informed the risks and benefits prior to making any decisions. The prophylactic removal and optimal excision time of this condition remain controversial. If treatment is requested, the best recommendation is surgical removal. Laser treatment has demonstrated failure of total removal and high rate of recurrence.

Many experts would delay removal until the child wishes to have it done and if possible under local anesthesia, which minimizes risk. This usually would occur around puberty.

Developmental anomalies

Preauricular pits and/or sinuses result from an imperfect fusion of the tubercles of the first two branchial arches. They slowly progress to a palpable mass or draining sinus in the pre-auricular area with or without hearing defects. The opening of the pit into the middle ear cavity may cause recurrent otitis media (see figure 14).

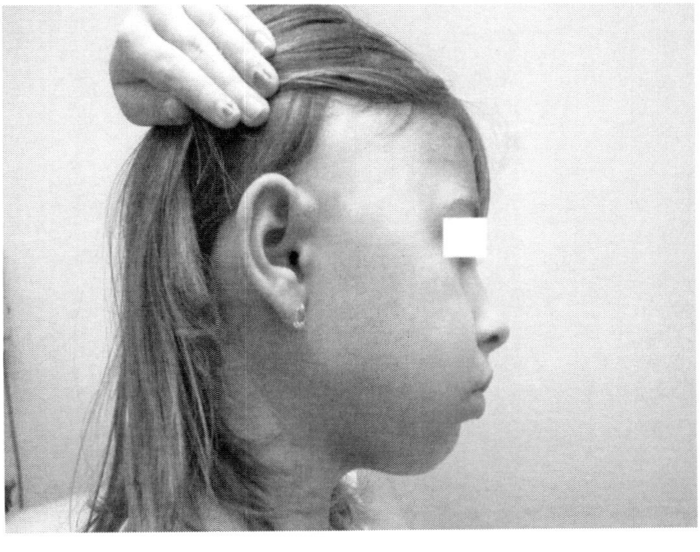

Figure 14. Pre-auricular sinus.

There is an unusual and difficult to diagnose variation of a sinus presenting in the postauricular area. The pit is seen behind the tragus usually in the sulcus where the ear attaches to the scalp. If one extends a line from the tragus over the conchal bowl to the anti-tragus, the pit is present in the corresponding area behind the auricle.

Preauricular skin tag or accessory tragus is more common than the preauricular pit. This skin tag is also developed from the dorsal portion of the first branchial arch. It presents as a soft to firm flesh-colored nodule at the preauricular area with or without a cartilaginous component. It may be single or multiple, unilateral or bilateral. Multiple tragi may be found in complex syndromes such as oculo-auriculo-vertebral syndrome (Goldenhar syndrome) and the CHARGE association syndrome. The treatment is excision of the whole extra tragus cartilage down to the deep portion of the lesion (20).

There has been a question of increased incidence of urinary tract abnormalities in children with preauricular tags and pits with prevalence between 1.1 and 8.6%. However, Kugelman et al (20) in 2002 compared 92 infants with pre-auricular tags or pits to normal controls with incidence of renal abnormalities of 2.2% in the affected group and 3.1% in the control group. The prevalence of renal anomalies and hearing impairment in patients with preauricular pits and tags was 2.7% equal in both affected and control groups (1/36, 1/36). The authors concluded that it was unnecessary to screen the kidneys or hearing in patients with preauricular pit or/and tag, who do not have associated syndromes or family history of hearing loss (20).

Thyroglossal duct cyst

A thyroglossal duct cyst is derived from the failure of obliteration of the embryonic thyroglossal duct. They occasionally contain ectopic thyroid tissues. The incidence of ectopic thyroid in thyroglossal duct cyst had been reported as 1-2%. The clinical presentation is of a small cyst midline neck between the hyoid bone and thyroid gland. The cyst moves up and down with swallowing or protrusion of the tongue (see figure 15).

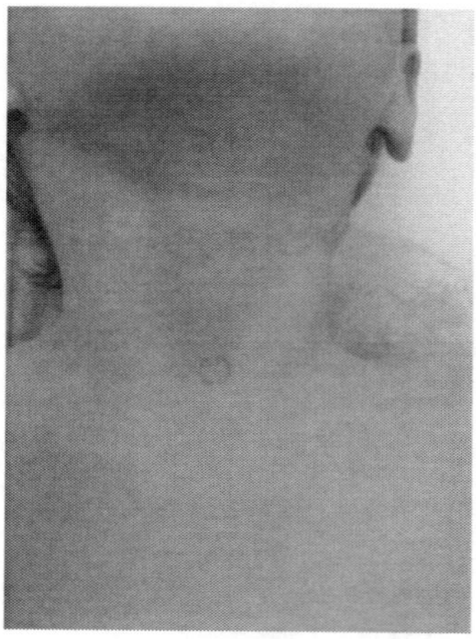

Figure 15. Thyroglossal duct cyst.

These cysts are rarely associated with the surrounding structures including larynx or tongue. They can cause complications such as compromised airway obstruction with hoarseness, dyspnea, stridor, dysphagia and sudden infant death. This complication can occur as early as a few weeks of age without palpable neck mass. The size, type and location of the cyst affect the various clinical symptoms. The differential diagnoses include ectopic thyroid gland, dermoid cyst and bronchogenic cyst.

Treatment of choice is complete surgical excision. Confirming the diagnosis and pre-operative evaluation by ultrasonography or CT scan prior to surgery should be done to prevent removal of the entire ectopic gland if this the sole source of the patient's thyroid tissue.

Bronchogenic cyst

A bronchogenic cyst develops from abnormal fusion of the primitive foregut in the fifth or sixth week of gestational age. This cyst may be of intrathoracic or extrathoracic origin. Almost half of bronchogenic cysts are found in an extrathoracic location, frequently in the mediastinum. Boys are four times more frequently affected than girls. The most common location of cutaneous bronchogenic cyst is the suprasternal notch, followed by the pre-sternal area, neck and scapula. The typical cutaneous presentation is solitary asymptomatic nodules on the supra sternal notch or over the upper part of the sternum (see figure 16).

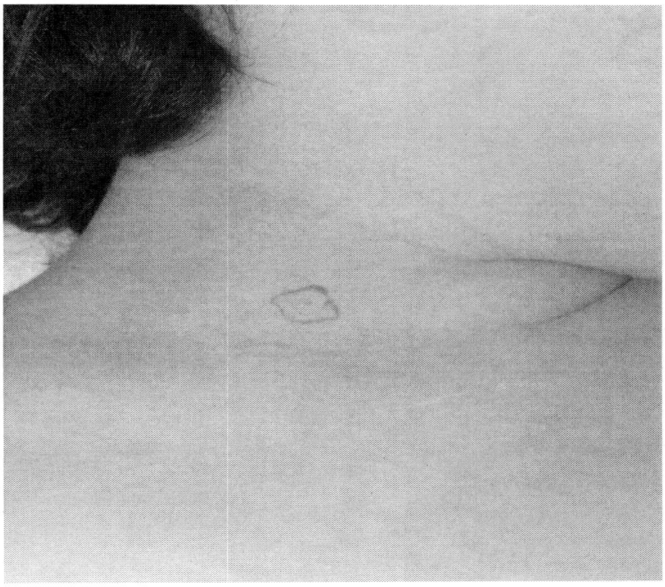

Figure 16. Bronchogenic cyst.

The cyst may enlarge and be a cause of stridor in the newborn. Neck abscess from secondary bacterial infection can also occur. The abnormal fistula may discharge mucoid fluid. Bronchogenic cysts should be differentiated from other congenital cystic and nodular lesions on the upper chest, neck and back areas. Ultrasonography is helpful in diagnosis.

Treatment of choice is surgical excision. Chest radiography, CT or MRI scan should be evaluated before surgery to ensure complete removal of the cyst track (22).

Supernumerary nipple/Polythelia

Supernumerary nipples are brown to pink umbilicated or elevated papules and patches along the embryogenic milk line. Chest and upper abdomen are the most common sites. Supernumerary nipple at back, thigh, vulva, sole and neck have also been reported.

There were several past reports of association between supernumerary nipple with urinary tract anomalies and testicular malignancy. Grotto et al. studied and reported no association between kidney, urinary tract malformation and supernumerary nipple. However Adams debates this conclusion because of inadequate sample size requiring larger studies to confirm this association (24). The vast majority of supernumerary nipples are isolated findings (see figure 17).

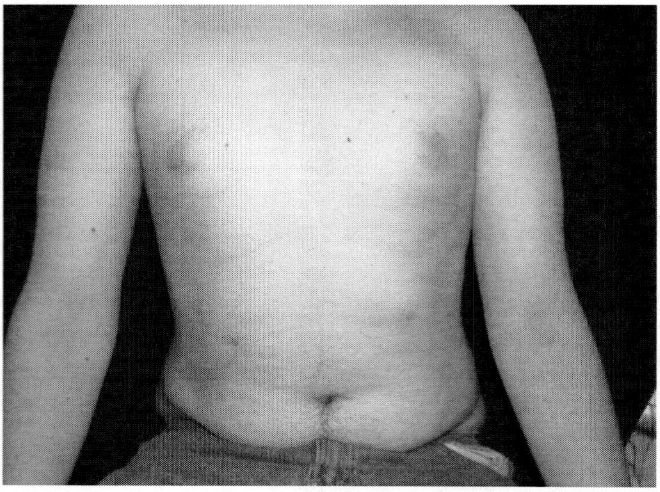

Figure 17. Supranumerary nipples.

Supernumerary nipples have also been rarely reported in association with several malformations e.g. spina bifida occulta, scoliosis, umbilical hernia, bilateral ovarian cysts and genetic syndrome such as Hailey-Hailey disease, spondylocostal dysostosis and Simpson-Globi-Behmel syndrome (24).

Dermoid cyst

Dermoid cyst is a congenital ectodermal growth that occurs at the site of embyonic fusion planes. The cyst wall is derived from an inward extension of an epithelial line that is a fusion plane of the ectodermal and neuroectodermal tissues. The cysts are usually asymptomatic, mobile, soft or rubbery, round and subcutaneous, size 1-4 cm. in diameter.

The most common locations are the upper lateral side of the forehead, eyebrow, overlying the anterior fontanelle, in the midline of the nose and submental region (see figure 18).

The majority of dermoid cysts are superficial and benign. However, nasal midline and glabellar lesions can have a dermal sinus extending into the intracranial compartment. This would present with recurrent infections. A midline small opening is the hallmark of nasal dermoid sinus cyst/tract. The sinus ostium may open along the midline of the nose between the glabella and the base of the columella, usually localized to the distal two-thirds of the dorsal nose. Another pathognomonic sign for dermoid sinus cysts is a tuft of hair emerging from the midline opening.

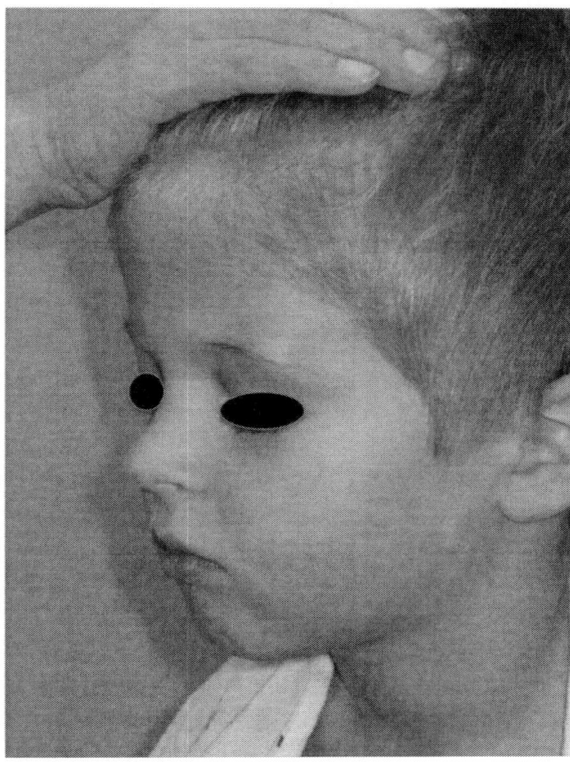

Figure 18. Dermoid cyst in a 6 year old WM. Note lump over left lateral eyebrow. It was present at birth and unchanged over time.

The differential diagnosis depends on the anatomical location, color, and surface characteristics. One should consider hemangioma, encephalocele, nasal glioma, epidermoid cyst when evaluating midline lesions of the face. Biopsy of midline nasal mass must be avoided until investigation of intracranial connection has been ruled out. MRI and CT scan have been used to evaluate the midline lesions of the face to rule in or out intracranial connection and structural abnormalities of bone.

Excision in early childhood around age 2 years is recommended. Surgical excision is performed to prevent the risk of local and penetrating infection. A multidisciplinary team of a pediatric dermatologist, pediatric otorhinolaryngologist, neurosurgeon and plastic surgeon should be assembled in cases of facial midline defects with intracerebral connection (25).

Congenital pedal papules of the newborn

Congenital pedal papules of the newborn are asymptomatic, bilateral, symmetrical skin-colored subcutaneous nodules, size 0.5-1 cm. in diameter on the medial aspect of the plantar surface of the heel (see figure 19). They go by various names in the literature such as congenital fibrolipomata, podalic papules in the newborn, bilateral congenital fatty heel pads, precalcaneal congenital fibrolipomatous hamartoma, congenital piezogenic-like pedal papules, bilateral congenital adipose plantar nodules and benign anteromedial plantar nodules of childhood.

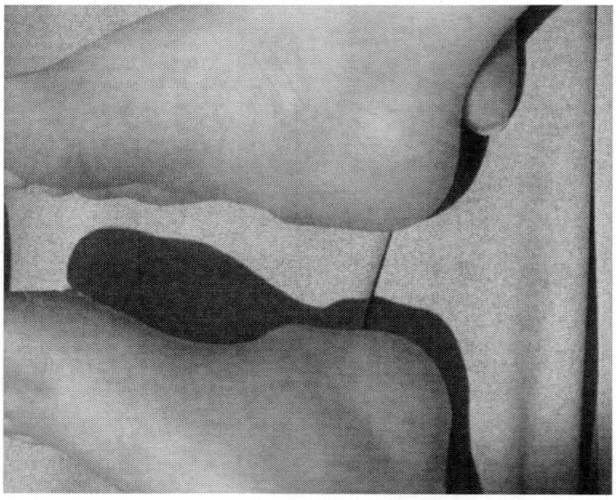

Figure 19. Pedal papules.

The incidence is probably underestimated. Greenberg et al. surveyed 263 newborns and 189 infants and the incidence of this condition was 5.9 % and 39.4 %, respectively. They were found by 1 to 3 months of age and tended to persist and /or enlarge proportionate with the child's growth.

The differential diagnoses are juvenile fibromatosis, plantar aponeurotic fibroma, childhood fibrous hamartoma and thickening of the heel pad associated with long-term dilantin therapy. Although, this condition is of unknown pathogenesis and tends to persist in the first few months to 1-3 years, treatment is not required because of its benign nature with frequent spontaneous regression (26).

Amniotic band syndrome

The amniotic band syndrome is a sporadic condition. The classic finding is constricting bands around the distal extremities. The incidence of this condition is 1:1,200-1:15,000 live births. This encircling band is said to be the cause of syndactyly, pseudodactyly, acrodactyly and amputation. The exact pathogenesis is unclear. One theory is that amniotic rupture initiates proliferation of mesodermal "strings" that cover, surround, encircle and then compress fetal structures. The severity is variable probably proportional to gestational age and the amount of amniotic leakage. Leakage of amniotic fluid in early gestational age causes more severe associated deformities including neural tube defect, facial, chest and abdominal wall defects. Late gestational age involvement causes more damage to the distal extremities (see figure 20).

There are reports of several familial cases of amniotic band sequence presenting with digital abnormalities. Inherited defects of the fetal membranes have been suggested for these familial cases. Possible risk factors are abdominal trauma including amniocentesis (27), connective tissue disorder, epidermolysis bullosa, uterine malformation, and first gestation in a mother younger than 25 years. Prenatal ultrasonography to diagnose amniotic bands has been described and three-dimensional ultrasound has also been reported to help secure the diagnosis. Surgical correction of the deformities is the treatment of choice. This may be performed pre-or postnatal.

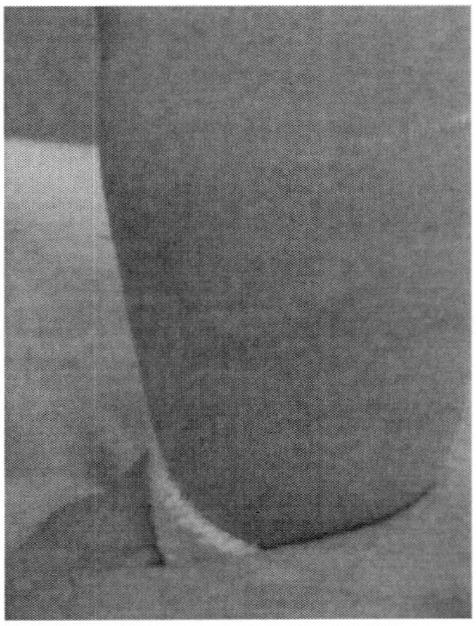

Figure 20. Amniotic band.

Aplasia cutis congenita (ACC)

ACC is defined as the localized or widespread areas of absence of all skin layers at birth. It is most frequently found as an isolated defect on the midline of the scalp. However other body locations can be affected (see figure 21).

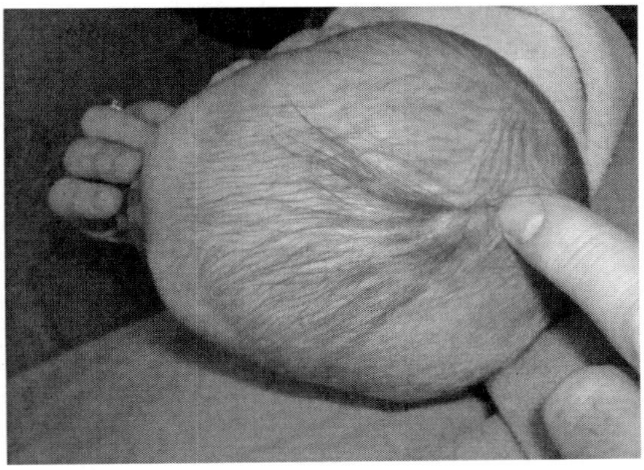

Figure 21. Aplasia cutis congenita, bullous type, with hair collar sign. There is a high risk of underlying brain abnormalities in this subtype, both because of the bulla and because of the hair collar sign.

This congenital skin disorder can occur as an isolated defect or as part of a genetic syndrome. The associated syndromes include Adams-Oliver syndrome, Opitz syndrome, chromosome 16-18 defect, trisomy 13-15 and oculocerebrocutaneous syndrome. In 1986, Frieden et al. classified this anomaly into nine groups based on the distribution of affected area, associated anomalies and the mode of transmission (28).

ACC coexisting with fetus papyraceus, group V in Friedan's classification has a typical distribution pattern over the trunk, buttocks and thighs bilaterally and symmetrically. Absence of skin is associated with fetal death during the late first to early second trimester.

The exact etiology of ACC remains unclear. The diagnosis of ACC could be confirmed by the clinical presentation. The differential diagnoses include iatrogenic injury (e.g. from scalp electrode, forceps delivery), focal dermal hypoplasia (Goltz syndrome) and epidermolysis bullosa. Ultrasonography may be performed to identify underlying skull defects.

The treatment of ACC depends on the condition of the infant, the body surface area, its location, and the experience of the local medical providers. The wounds of ACC gradually heal under conservative treatment in majority of cases. Secondary bacterial infection and trauma to this area of the scalp should be a concern especially with a skull defect. The skull defect can be related to internal brain involvement and an increase in risk of complications such as hemorrhage, thrombosis and infection.

Vesiculopustular and bullous disease of newborn

Acropustulosis of infancy is a pruritic, benign vesiculopustular condition in the neonatal and first few months of life. It can extend into infancy and early childhood. The exact etiology of this condition is unknown. It presents with 1-2 mm. papules, vesicles or pustules on the lateral aspects of fingers on palms and soles, as well as on the dorsal aspects of the hands, feet, wrists and ankles. Crops of lesions appear and recover as a cycle every 2-4 weeks (see figure 22).

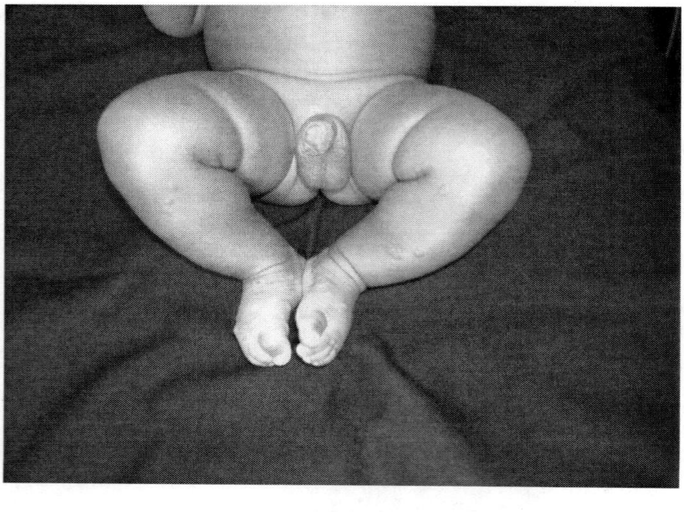

Figure 22. Acropustulosis. Note small pustules over distal legs (and arms.).

The differential diagnosis is neonatal scabies, eosinophilic pustular folliculitis of infancy, neonatal candidiasis, erythema toxicum neonatorum, transient neonatal pustular melanosis and dyshidrotic eczema.

Skin scraping for scabies, Gram stain, Wright stain and Potassium hydroxide (KOH) should be performed to rule out the other conditions. The lesion scraping reveals prominently neutrophils, occasionally eosinophils in Wright stain examination. Peripheral blood count may be reported with eosinophilia.

This condition spontaneously fades over 1-3 years. Supportive treatment with oral antihistamines and topical corticosteroids may be helpful to control pruritus. Oral dapsone is alternative treatment in severe cases and can be used as intermittent therapy to resolve the pustules rapidly (29).

Erythema toxicum neonatorum (ET)/Toxic erythema of the newborn

Erythema toxicum neonatorum is a benign, asymptomatic vesiculopustular neonatal condition. It is more commonly found in term infants. The incidence of this condition in preterm babies decreases parallel to their decrease in gestational age and birth weight. ET typically presents in the first 2 weeks of life with minute papules or pustules on an erythematous base or red macules or wheals on any part of the body. There is variability in both size and number of lesions (see figure 23).

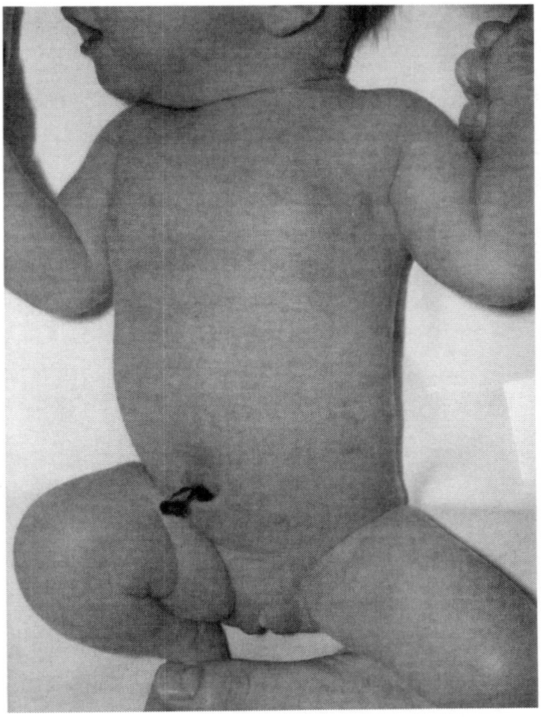

Figure 23. Erythema toxicum. Note discrete tiny pustules on a large red macules scattered mainly over the trunk.

The exact etiology is unknown. Postulated pathogenesis is inflammatory reaction to pilosebaceous orifice obstruction and mechanical or trauma stimulation. The recent proposal of this condition is a cutaneous response to commensal microbes penetrating into infant skin. Pustule contents reveal a prominence of eosinophils in Wright stain examination. Peripheral blood count also reveals eosinophilia. It may simply be another eosinophil migration disorder similar to EPF (see below) whose initial stimulus is unknown. Treatment is unnecessary, spontaneous resolution usually occurs within hours to days. Reassurance the parents should be provided (30).

Eosinophilic pustular folliculitis of infancy (EPF)/Eosinophilic pustulosis

Eosinophilic pustular folliculitis (EPF) of infancy typically presents with recurrent yellowish 1-3 mm pustules at birth or in the first few days of life. Boys are more frequently affected than girls. The common locations are scalp and face, but the trunk and extremities are also involved. The lesions generally turn to crust in 2-3 days. Recurrent crops of lesions usually appear and resolve over days to weeks. The total duration is about 3 months to 3-5 years (see figure 24).

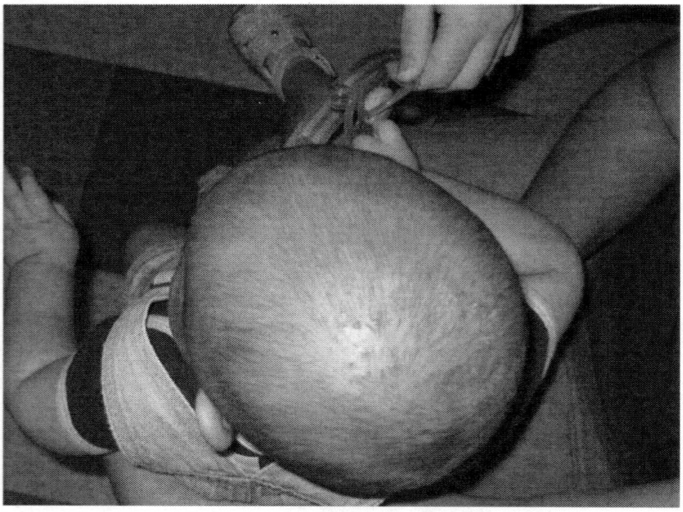

Figure 24. Eosinophilic pustular folliculitis. Note discrete yellow pustules on a red base on the scalp of this 33 week old Hispanic male. Tzanck stain showed sheets of eosinophils. The scalp is a common location. These are usually quite pruritic.

EPF is a variant of three eosinophilic proliferation disorders. This group consists of eosinophilic pustular folliculitis (EPF) (including classic EPF), immunosuppression-associated EPF (mostly-HIV related) and infancy associated EPF (EPF of infancy).

EPF of infancy is distinct from adult EPF or Ofuji's disease in distribution, configuration and histological features of the lesion. EPF of infancy is also distinct from EPF associated with underlying HIV infection in adult patients.

The exact etiology of this condition is unknown. EPF does not always have follicular involvement; therefore some investigators propose the term "eosinophilic pustulosis".

Pustular lesions reveal eosinophils with occasional neutrophils without organisms. Peripheral blood count can show eosinophilia in 70% of the cases.

Supportive treatment with antihistamines may be helpful to control pruritus. Antibiotics are usually ineffective. Topical corticosteroids may be helpful. There are a few reports of alleviation from alternative medication such as oral cimetidine and topical tacrolimus in older children. Spontaneous resolution of EPF may be responsible for case reports of success (31-32).

Transient neonatal pustular melanosis (TNPM)

TNPM is benign self-limited condition in term infants. It is more commonly found in African-American infants. The characteristic presentation is 1-5 mm. vesicles and/or pustules in single or clusters that progress to brownish crust. The vesicular rupture is followed by a fine white collarette of scale (see figure 25).

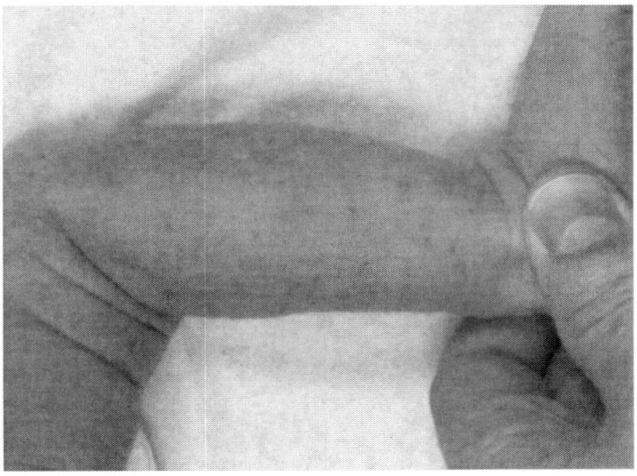

Figure 25. Transient neonatal pustular melanosis. Note small pustules that pop and leave behind dark macules in the exact location of the pustule.

The most common areas include forehead, neck, chin, upper chest, back, palms and soles. The lesions spontaneously resolve within a few days leaving hyperpigmented macules or patches. These pigmentations usually fade within weeks to months. Stain of the pustular contents reveals a variable number of neutrophils, occasionally eosinophils. Treatment is unnecessary (33).

Miliaria

Miliaria is the consequence of eccrine duct obstruction or sweat retention in the skin. This obstruction and/or retention are more common in premature infants because of incomplete differentiation of epidermis and appendages. This condition is most commonly found in the first few weeks of life. Multiple precipitating factors include immaturity of the eccrine duct, fevers, overheating and humidity. Bacteria have been suspected to be a risk factor in miliaria.

Miliaria is divided to four clinical groups according to the level of obstruction in the skin:

- Miliaria crystallina/Miliaria sudamina is the most common type of miliaria, frequently occurring in the first week of life. It characteristically presents with transient, asymptomatic, fragile, clear colored, minute flaccid vesicles without sign of inflammation, particularly on the forehead, upper trunk and intertrigenous area. This dew drop-like appearance results from superficial obstruction in stratum corneum of the skin layer (both intracorneal and/or subcorneal layer). Congenital miliaria crystallina has no particular association with prior maternal and infantile medical problems (see figure 26a).

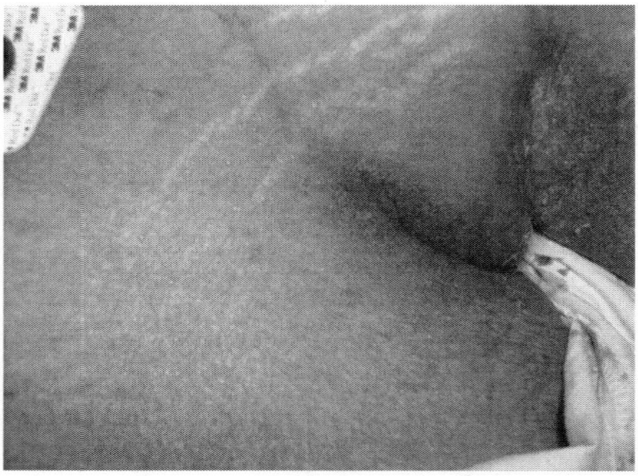

Figure 26a. Miliaria crystallina, seen in this photo just inferior to the striae distensae.

- Miliaria rubra / Prickly heat
- Miliaria pustulosa: Typical lesion reveals erythematous non-follicular papules, vesicles, pustules of face, neck and trunk. This condition results from intraepidermal obstruction of the sweat ducts with secondary local inflammation. They may be more erythematous in warm weather (see figure 26b). Miliaria pustulosa is a variant of miliaria rubra. These benign self-limited conditions spontaneously recover in days to weeks.

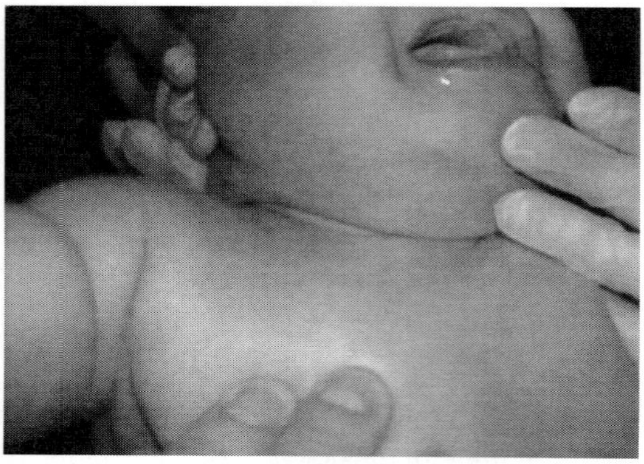

Figure 26b. Miliaria rubra in the folds of the neck and upper chest.

- Miliaria profunda: This lesion presents as a non-erythematous papulopustular eruption mainly on the trunk, extremities. It often localizes to hypohidrotic or anhidrotic areas. The obstruction occurs at dermoepidermal junction layer of the skin. This type can occur after repeated episodes of miliaria rubra extending to deeper tissues.

The clinical presentation of miliaria reveals asymptomatic, transient, skin-colored papules as well as goose flesh-like skin. They usually resolve within 1 hour after overheating has been corrected. The differential diagnoses of miliaria include neonatal herpes simplex infection, congenital candidiasis, incontinentia pigmenti, ET and TPM. Simple additional investigations, KOH preparation, Wright stain and Gram stain may be performed to rule out other diagnoses. Skin biopsy is also helpful for definitive diagnosis and level of involvement. Supportive treatment, avoidance of excessive heat, includes room temperature control, air-conditioning, appropriate clothing and bathing. The lesions spontaneously resolve without any scars or complications (34).

Neonatal acne/Acne neonatorum and infantile acne

Neonatal acne occurs in a first few weeks of life presenting with closed-head comedones (white-heads), opened-head comedones (black-heads) and inflammatory papules, and/or pustules on the forehead and cheeks. The presumptive pathogenesis of neonatal acne includes increased sebum excretion from sebaceous glands secondary to maternal and/or neonatal androgens. Neonatal acne usually presents during the first four weeks of life. It is more commonly found in boys than in girls (5:1) probably related to a distinct neonatal androgen. Neonatal androgens in boys originate from both adrenal glands and testes, whereas the girls have androgens only from the adrenal glands.

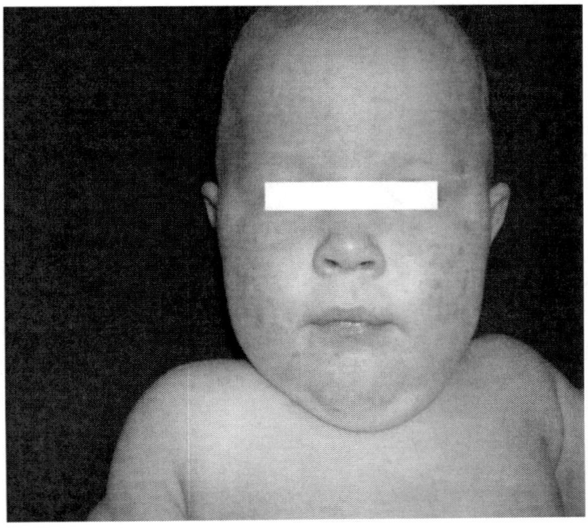

Figure 27. Infantile acne.

Infantile acne usually presents between 3 and 6 months (range 3-16 months), which is later than neonatal acne (the first 4 weeks of life). The course is variable, frequently resolving in 1 to 4 years. Infantile acne, unlike neonatal acne, can be severe and carries a higher risk of acne in the adolescent period (see figure 27). The differential diagnosis includes neonatal cephalic pustulosis, ET, TPM and folliculitis.

The natural history of neonatal acne is mild and transient. Most of these cases have spontaneous resolution without scarring in 4 weeks to 3 months. In cases of severe presentation, topical treatments are preferred over systemic treatments. Comedonal acne may be treated with 0.025-0.05% tretinoin cream. Topical erythromycin, clindamycin and/or benzoyl peroxide may be used in inflammatory acne (35).

Neonatal cephalic pustulosis (NCP)

Neonatal cephalic pustulosis (NCP) presents as minute papules, vesicles on an erythematous base on the forehead, and cheeks. These are no comedones and the lesions occur at 5 days to 3 weeks of life (see figure 28).

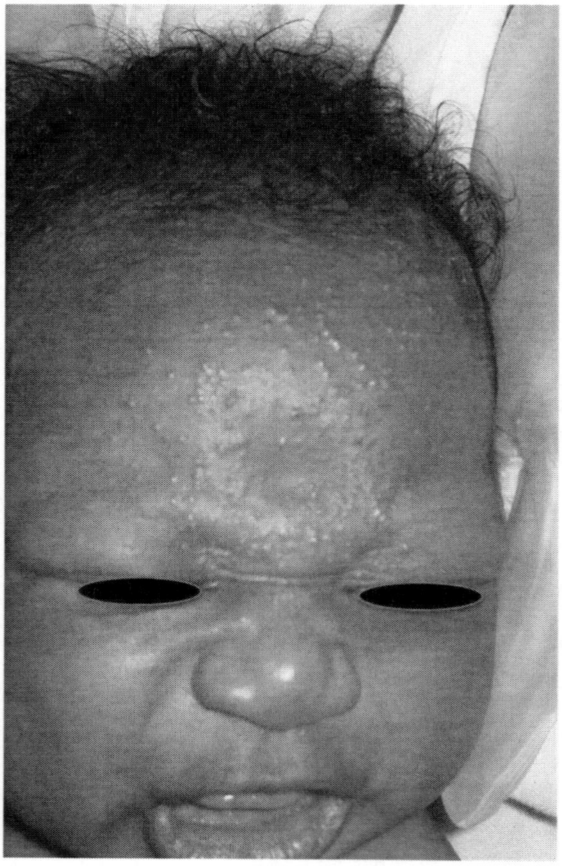

Figure 28. Neonatal cephalic pustulosis in a two week old black male.

Malassezia sympodialis had been proposed to be an etiology of NCP. This hypothesis is controversial. The isolation of this yeast may simply be colonization. Ayhan et al. supports the data that transient or persistent Malassezia spp. colonization may not correlate with the development of NCP. Skin colonization of patients with NCP (20.8 %) is not higher than in normal healthy newborns (37 %) (36). Moreover, there are marked differences from the previous studies both in decreasing number of colonies and in the species of Malassezia colonization in the first 3 days and few weeks of life. The authors report different species: M. furfur, M. dermatis and M. japonica. Other possible reasons for difference may be ethnicity, geography, culture media and collection methods of the study groups. KOH preparation may support the diagnosis.

Rapelanoro et al. in 1996 set forth diagnostic criteria including the presence of pustules on the face and neck, onset of lesion younger than 1 month of age, isolation of Malassezia by direct microscopy, ruling out other causes of neonatal pustular lesions and response to topical antifungal therapy.

This condition tends to resolve spontaneously. Topical antifungal (2% ketoconazole cream) twice daily for 1 week may shorten the course of the lesions.

Congenital Langerhans cell histiocytosis/congenital self-healing reticulohistiocytosis (CSHR)/self-healing reticulohistiocytosis of Hashimoto-Pritzker

Congenital Langerhans cell histiocytosis is a self-healing vesiculopustular and erosive condition from the clonal proliferation of activated Langerhans cell limited to the skin. It presents as asymptomatic small numbers of crusted brown to red to purple discrete papules and nodules on the body and trunk. The size and number of the lesions are variable. Systemic signs are usually absent (see figure 29).

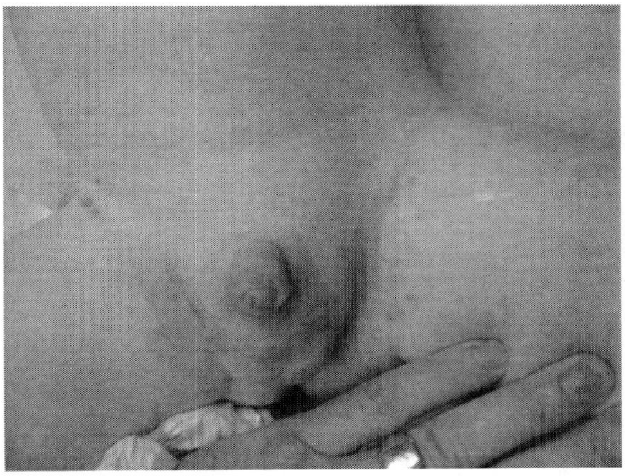

Figure 29. Langerhans cell histiocytosis.

Atypical presentation of CSHR had been reported such as vesiculobullous lesions, hemorrhagic bullae, blueberry muffin lesions, widespread irregular erythematous scaling, atrophic and erosive patches.

The definitive diagnosis is made by skin biopsy. Histopathological features are mononuclear and multinucleated histiocytes with multiple eosinophilic ground-glass cytoplasm in the dermis, with occasional epidermotrophism. Immunohistochemistry shows positive stains for CD1a, S100 or Langerin protein.

Systemic evaluation is recommended in all infants with this diagnosis. Currently, The Histiocyte Society recommends a protocol for all children with cutaneous Langerhans Cell Histiocytosis. Other organ involvement includes liver, bone, hematopoietic system, spleen, lymph node and lung. Children with multisystem involvement have a poorer prognosis than the skin-only group. Children should be monitored for months (some say years) for recurrence and systemic dissemination. The presenting symptoms of disseminated disease include the development of characteristic seborrheic-like lesions in the scalp and diaper area.

The treatment for cutaneous LCH is supportive. It tends to regress spontaneously by 1 to 4 months age. Topical corticosteroid may be effective (37).

Incontinentia pigmenti (IP)/Bloch-Sulzberger syndrome

Incontinentia pigmenti (IP) is caused by mutations in the NEMO gene (nuclear factor kappa B essential modulator) mapped to Xq 28. The NEMO modulator provides a protective function against tumor necrosis factor alpha from inducing cell apoptosis.

IP is rare X-linked dominant genodermatosis. Ninety seven percent of patients are female because it is lethal to male fetuses. The current literature does describe more than 42 surviving boys with IP. The International IP consortium proposed three possible pathogeneses for surviving males who have NEMO gene mutations. These mutations include hypomorphic alleles, somatic mosaicism and 47 XXY karyotype (Klinefelter syndrome). The chromosome defect maps to a different region in familial form versus non-familial forms (38). Ardelean et al. (39) reviewed the literature for male IP, and found the male phenotype had clinical and pathological features the same as the female phenotype.

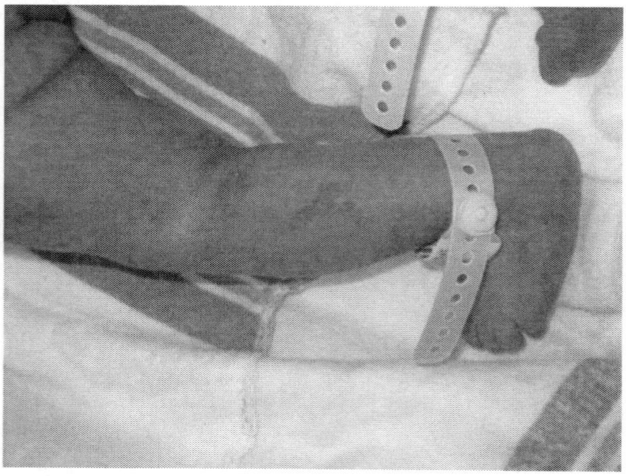

Figure 30a. Incontinentia pigmenti, vesiculo-.

There are four clinical stages of presentation including vesicular/vesiculopustular, verrucous, hyperpigmentation and hypopigmentation. Irregular sequence of these stages and overlapping presentation occurs commonly.The vesicular stage reveals inflammatory yellowish vesicles/vesiculobullous lesions in linear streaks following the lines of Blaschko. They are most commonly found on the trunk and extremities and usually present at birth or in the first few weeks of life (see figure 30a). The verrucous stage characteristically reveals lesions within 6 weeks following in the same areas as the pustules (see figure 30b). The hyperpigmented stage reveals linear and whorled hyperpigmentation slowly followed by a hypopigmented stage. Again the lesions follow Blaschko's lines in the same areas as the original pustules.

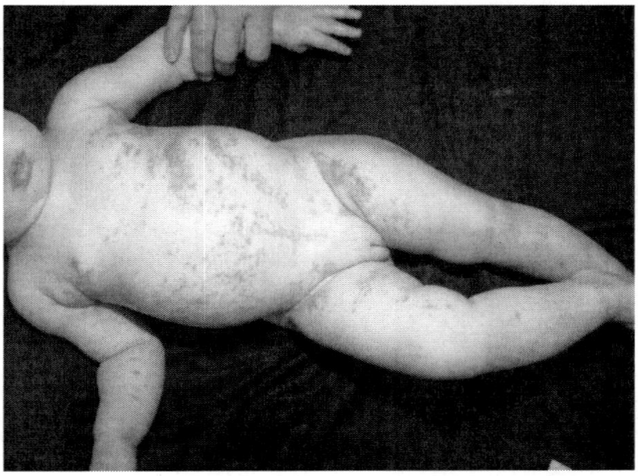

Figure 30 b. Incontinentia pigmenti showing a rare "recall reaction" where the former areas of vesicles and bullae long quiet, suddenly reactivate when the child gets a systemic inflammation such as the flu.

Extracutaneous manifestations are common including neurodevelopmental, dental, hair, eye and skeletal system problems and nail dystrophy. There are isolated cases of immune deficiency in I.P. Tooth abnormalities are the most common extracutaneous findings in male IP patients, followed by hair, eye and central nervous system anomalies. These should be evaluated and monitored. Skin biopsy usually helps make the diagnosis in suspected cases. The histopathological features of the first stage are spongiosis and intraepidermal vesicles with eosinophils commonly found in 74 % (18 to 89%). The second stage reveals acanthosis, hyperkeratosis and dyskeratotic cells. The treatment is supportive care. Educating the parents should be done regarding the genetic basis, the child's prognosis and the risk of affected future pregnancies (39).

See table 1 for clinical features of non-infectious vesiculopustular lesions in neonates.

Infectious group: Impetigo neonatorum

Neonatal skin is susceptible to Staphylococcal infection, especially Staphylococcus aureus phage group II type 55, 71. In addition there is decreased renal clearance of the bacterial toxin. This combined with immature skin barrier and immunity makes the neonate more susceptible to Staphylococcal infection and its toxins (40). The clinical spectrum from this pathogen includes impetigo neonatorum, Staphylococcal scalded skin syndrome (SSSS) and exfoliative dermatitis.

Table 1. Clinical features of non-infectious vesiculopustular lesions in neonates

	Onset	Presentation	Common site	Investigation: Wright/ KOH / CBC	Duration	Treatment	Remark
Acropustulosis of infancy (AI)	Birth - first few months	Papules, vesicles	Lateral aspect of fingers, palms, soles	Neutrophil > Eosinophil Eosinophilia	Months to years Complete recovery 1-3 years	Antihistamine ± topical steroid	Cycle every 2-4 weeks
Eosinophilic pustular folliculitis (EPF)	Birth - first few days	Yellowish pustules 1-3 mm.	Scalp, face > trunk, extremities	Eosinophil > Neutrophil Eosinophilia	Months (rarely in years)	±Antihistamine	Cycle days to weeks
Erythema toxicum neonatorum (ET)	Birth – first few weeks	Papules, pustules 1-2 mm. on erythematous base	Any part	Eosinophil > Neutrophil Eosinophilia	Hours to days	No	-
Transient neonatal pustular melanosis (TNPM)	Birth - first few days	Vesicles, pustules → crust→ fine collarette scale, hyperpigmentation	Forehead, neck, upper chest, back	Neutrophil > Eosinophil	Days	No	-Most in African-American -Leaving with hyperpigmentation
Neonatal acne	First few weeks	Comedones (opened, closed, inflammatory), pustules	Face, forehead, cheek	Neutrophil	Months	Optional - 2.5% benzoyl peroxide Cream	-
Neonatal cephalic pustulosis (NCP)	Days - weeks	Mutilple papules, pustules on erythematous base without comedones	Face, forehead, cheek	Yeast form	Weeks to months	Topical antifungal	Without comedones

Impetigo neonatorum typically presents with superficial vesicles or bullous lesions on an erythematous base at the neck, axillae, periumbilical and diaper areas. The bullae rapidly enlarge, spread and rupture easily leaving a raw surface with serum oozing. Impetigo neonatorum is usually found at 2 weeks of age but may be found as early as a few days of life.

The differential diagnosis includes herpes simplex virus infection, epidermolysis bullosa, Staphylococcal Scalded Skin Syndrome (SSSS), bullous mastocytosis and incontinentia pigmenti.

Complications of impetigo include osteomyelitis, pneumonia, septic arthritis and septicemia.Treatment is with systemic anti-Staphylococcal antibiotics. Supportive treatment is with drainage of bullae and vesicles to prevent local spreading, wet dressings to remove the crust and local wound care.

Neonatal scabies

Scabies, an infestation of the skin is caused by Sarcoptes scabiei, an obligate human parasite. The onset of presentation is as early as the first few weeks of life. The clinical presentation typically reveals generalized erythematous vesicles, papules, pustules and or burrows on the body, particularly in body creases, palms, soles, axillae, face and scalp. Nodular lesions are more common in infants than older children. They are usually found on the trunk, axillae and genitalia.

The presentation of scabies in infants is different from adults. The infants develop more inflammatory lesions of vesicles, pustules, and crusting. The lesions of palm, soles, face, neck and scalp are also more prominent in infants. The glans penis if often affected in boys presenting with burrows and nodules. Nodules of the scrotum are common. Nodular scabies in neonates frequently presents on the wrists and axillary vaults. They have been mistaken as solitary mastocytomas. The more typical cutaneous manifestations of scabies may present after the subsequent 2 months.

Typically scabies presents with itching. This can be difficult to assess in infants who lack the cerebral-digital coordination to scratch. More often they present with irritability, restlessness and poor feeding.

The diagnosis is confirmed by a skin scraping of fresh lesions. The identification of mite, eggs, larvae or fecal material is the gold standard for diagnosis. Classic cutaneous lesions in the parents or caregivers also support the diagnosis.

Skin biopsy is helpful in cases of unusual presentations and in skin scraping failures. Note, biopsy finding in scabies nodules is sometimes mistaken for histiocytosis X on H&E staining (41).

Most authors prefer 5 % permethrin cream for neonatal scabies which is effective and officially approved in infants over 2 months of age. There are many studies that show its efficacy and safety from zero to 2 months of age. The American Academy of Pediatrics recommends this medication as the treatment of choice for scabies infestation because of safety and efficacy profile. This cream should be applied all over the body including the scalp, head and face of the infants to eliminate scabies. It is then washed off after 8-14 hours. One treatment with this medication is usually effective in eradicating scabies but repeated application in 1 week later is recommended due to the possibility of misapplications during the first treatment. There are few reports in rats of neurotoxicity of permethrin 5 %, but there are no such reports in the human medical literature.

Treatment using 5 to 10 % precipitated sulfur in petrolatum is also effective. Sulfur treatment should probably be repeated in one week. Although, there are several reports of treatment failure, these authors state the safety profile of this medication makes it a reasonable choice.

Lindane 1 % lotion, (gamma benzene hexachloride) is usually not recommended in neonates because of systemic absorption and potential central nervous system toxicity due to high body surface area to mass ratio. However, Singal et al. reviewed and reported that the risk of Lindane neurotoxicity is minimal if used properly. Jin et al. supported the successful treatment scabies in a 2-month-old infant with Lindane because of unavailability the other medications of choice in their hospital.

Regardless of the scabies treatment in patients and caregivers, environmental decontamination must be done. Clothing and bed sheets should be laundered and dried at high heat. Items that cannot be laundered should be heated in a dryer for 20 minutes. Items that cannot be either laundered or put in a dryer can be placed in a plastic bag for one week. In this time any mites will have hatched, desiccated and died. In a dry environment the scabies mite dies quickly on the human skin. It is not necessary to clean carpets, curtains and other items that did not have prolonged skin-to-skin contact with the child (42).

Congenital candidiasis and neonatal candidiasis

Although several Candida species may cause of human infection, the most common cause is Candida albicans. Candidal infection in the newborn may be acquired from vertical transmission from mother or horizontally by nosocomial infection. They commonly manifest with several clinical presentations such as oral candidiasis, diaper dermatitis, systemic candidiasis, neonatal and congenital candidiasis (43). Table 2 reviews the comparison of definition, onset, presenting symptoms and risk factors between congenital and neonatal candidiasis

Table 2. Candidiasis in the newborn

	Congenital candidiasis	Neonatal candidiasis
Incidence	Very rare (< 100 cases in medical literature)	Common nosocomial systemic infection in NICU
Route of infection	In utero	**-Perinatal:** during pass through infected birth canal **-Postnatal:** externally acquired
Onset	At birth, first few days of life	After first few days to weeks of life
Pregnancy complication	Premature labor	Not applicable
Symptoms	**-Localized:** diffuse cutaneous eruption of erythematous macules, papulovesicles and pustules on erythematous base with/without systemic symptoms Nail dystrophy (diaper area and oral cavity are usually spared)	**-Localized:** oral thrush, diaper dermatitis **-Invasive fungal dermatitis:** primary skin infection; erosive, ulcerated, crusted plaques

	Congenital candidiasis	Neonatal candidiasis
	-Systemic: severe life threatening candidal systemic infection e.g. candidal septicemia, meningitis, urinary tract infection, disseminated diseases Systemic infection without cutaneous findings	**-Systemic:** extensive burn like dermatitis followed by desquamation Systemic infections, symptoms; apnea, bradycardia, hypotension, temperature instability, metabolic changes
Treatment	-Topical antifungal (only skin involvement) -±Systemic antifungal if systemic symptoms	-Topical antifungal -±Systemic antifungal
Risk	**-Risk of infection during pregnancy:** intrauterine device, cervical suture, foreign body, maternal candidal vulvovaginitis **-Risk of disseminated candidiasis:** prematurity/ ELBW, central catheter, antibiotic therapy, corticosteroid therapy, amniocentesis, maternal uterine device, cervical circlage	**-Risk of systemic infection**: primary immune deficiency, immunosuppression, prolonged antibiotics, hyperglycemia, invasive procedure with candidal contamination **-Risk of invasive fungal dermatitis:** VLBW infants, vaginal delivery, hyperglycemia, steroid administration **-Risk of invasive candidiasis:** ELBW infants, central catheter, broad spectrum antibiotics, intravenous lipid emulsion and/or endotracheal intubation
Remarks	**-ELBW** (birth weight < 1,000 g.): wide spread desquamating dermatitis, ecchymosis, necrosis **-Nail dystrophy** from candidiasis / Localized only nail plate candidiasis -Pustules on the palms and soles are a hallmark of congenital candidiasis	**Invasive candidiasis** is culture positive from blood and/or sterile body fluid

Congenital and neonatal Herpes simplex virus infection

Herpes simplex virus (HSV) infection is one of the most common human viral infections (see figure 31). The most important infection during pregnancy is the primary genital HSV infection, most often type II that causes the severest neonatal complications.

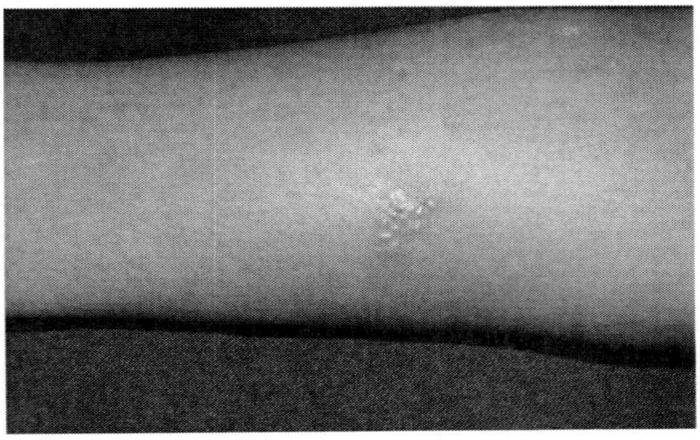

Figure 31. Cutaneous Herpes simplex in a six year old black female's lower leg. Note clear vesicles clustered together on a red base.

The outcome of this infection varies on the rate, time of infection and especially organ involvement (45). Table 3 reviews the comparison of definition, onset, presentation, risk factors and prognosis between congenital and neonatal herpes simplex virus infection.

Table 3. Aspects of neonatal Herpes infections

	Congenital HSV infection	**Neonatal HSV infection**
Incidence / rate of infection	5 % of all HSV infection in neonate	7/ 100,000 live births
Route of infection	In utero	-**Perinatal:** 85-90 % -**Postnatal:** 5-10 %
Source	Primary or recurrent genital HSV	Exposure infectious secretions or lesions in birth canal
Mode of transmission	Ascending intrauterine (with/without intact membrane)	Contact exposure
Type	90 % is HSV-2	70-80 % is HSV-2
Presentation onset	24-48 hours of life	First 28 days of life
Symptoms	**Triad** **-Skin:** diffuse erosive without vesicles, scar on scalp, face, trunk, extremities **-Eye:** chorioretinitis, microphthalmia, cataract **-CNS:** intracranial calcification, seizures, microcephaly	**-Localized (mucocutaneous):** (50 %) SEM *Skin-* group of vesicles on erythematous base at initial site of contact lesion (wide spread, zoster-like) *Eye-* conjunctivitis, keratitis *Mouth* **-Disseminated:** (17 %) visceral organ involvement; lung, liver, CNS **-CNS:** (33 %) infection, no visceral organ involvement with/without mucocutaneous involvement
Treatment	-Isolated (contact precaution) -IV Acyclovir 30 mg/kg/day 10 days -Ophthalmologic evaluation ± prophylactic treatment	-Isolated (contact precaution) -IV Acyclovir 30 mg/kg/day 10 days or 60 mg/kg/day 21 days in disseminated -Evaluate to rule out disseminated, CNS involvement -Ophthalmologic evaluation ± prophylactic treatment
Prognosis	-High mortality -Severe impairment and anomalies (mental retardation, seizures, blindness)	**-Mucocutaneous:** 90% good outcome if treated early **-Disseminated:** high morbidity, mortality (60%) **-CNS:** low mortality (5%), but increased risk of abnormal development
Remarks	Both primary and recurrent maternal infection can cause congenital infection	-Incidence of neonatal HSV is lower in cesarean section -Risk of acquired neonatal HSV related to maternal genital HSV infection -Primary infection carries more risk than reactivation -Recurrent of skin lesion up to 5 years of age in the same site or different area -Relapse CNS infection after 1 year of neonatal infection

Congenital and neonatal varicella

Varicella zoster virus (VZV) infection may be acquired from intrauterine or perinatal exposure. The incidence of varicella in pregnant women appears to be 2-3 per 1,000 pregnancies. Since Varicella vaccine had been prescribed routinely in medical practice, the incidence of congenital varicella infection has decreased. There is a question whether newborns from varicella vaccinated mothers still have the protective immunity that passes through the placenta during gestation.

Table 4. Varicella Infections

	Congenital/Fetal varicella syndrome	**Neonatal varicella syndrome**
Route	In utero	**Perinatal, postnatal**
Time of contact infection	Early in pregnancy (first 20 weeks of gestation age) : higher risk in 13-20 weeks of gestation age	21 days ante-partum 10 days post-partum (severe risk when expose 5 days ante-partum, 2 days post-partum)
Mode of transmission	-Transplacental (varicella viremia transmitted via transplacenta to fetus) -Ascending infection (possible from lesion in birth canal)	-Transplacental viremia -Ascending infection during delivery -Respiratory droplet/ direct contact with infectious lesion after birth
Onset	After birth	9-15 days after onset of maternal rash
Symptoms	**GA:** low birth weight **Skin:** cicatricial lesions correspond to a dermatome **CNS:** encephalitis, hydrocephalus, seizure, mental retardation, microcephaly **Eye:** chorioretinitis, microphthamia, cataracts **GI:** duodenal atresia, colon atresia **GU:** hydronephrosis, absence of kidney **Musculoskeletal:** hypotonia, abnormal ribs, mandible, limb contracture *most common is skin involvement afollowed by hypoplasia of an ipsilateral extremities	**Skin:** wide spread vesicles, hemorrhagic vesicles (severe) **CNS:** encephalitis **GI:** hepatitis **RS:** respiratory distress, pneumonia *lesion may involve lung, liver, brain, kidney, adrenal, myocardium
Treatment	-Supportive treatment (mild) -±Acyclovir 15 mg/kg/dose q 8 hours and Varicella zoster immunoglobulin (VZIG) in severe to systemic involvement (to stop progression of eye diseases and/or neurological diseases)	-VZIG 1 ml/kg -IV Acyclovir 30-60 mg/kg/day > 5 days • < 5 days ante-partum to 2 days post partum : immediately after birth • Premature < 28 weeks or birth weight < 1,000 g : within 96 hours after exposure • Preterm who had postnatal exposure : within 96 hours after exposure
Prognosis	-Mortality nearly 30% in first few months of life	-Mortality 5-30% -Varicella encephalitis increases neuropsychologic outcome
Risk	**-Highest risk**: 13-20 w gestational age (GA) -Risk of embryopathy: 1-2% (GA < 20 weeks), almost nonexistent (3rd trimester)	**-Highest risk:** < 5 days ante-partum, < 2 days post-partum exposure
Remark		**-VZIG recommendation:** *all infant GA< 28 weeks or weight < 1,000 g *prematurity with no evidence of maternal immunity **-Severity related to time of maternal infection:** *transplacental viremia; low *21 days ante-partum, 10 days post-partum; non-fatal course *5 days ante-partum, 2 days post-partum; death 20%, neonatal varicella

The incidence of congenital anomalies after maternal varicella infection in the first 20 weeks of pregnancy is approximately 1-2 %. There are several presentations following VZV infection based on infection time and mode of transmission. Varicella pneumonia is the serious complication with risk of life threatening ventilatory syndrome. The mortality is approximately 11 % (46). Table 4 reviews the comparison of definition, onset, presentation, risk factors and prognosis between congenital and neonatal Varicella infection.

Iatrogenic causes

Calcified heel nodule is the most common form of iatrogenic calcinosis cutis. This condition results from variety of local tissue injuries including repeated trauma from obtaining blood. They cause the formation of an epidermal inclusion cyst prior to its calcification. Although, most of the cases are derived from repeated trauma/multiple heel sticks, a calcified nodule resulting from only a single heel stick has been reported.

The onset of presentation is about 4-12 months after birth. They usually reveal minute whitish or yellowish papules localized at the heel, gradually progressing to form asymptomatic heel nodules. The lesions rarely exhibit transepidermal elimination of the cyst contents and recurrence after incision and drainage is common. Additional investigations that bolster the diagnosis are small radio-opaque nodules in plain X-rays of the heels and characteristic histopathological tissue.

Spontaneous resolution occurs by 2-3 years of life. Treatment is unnecessary, except in symptomatic lesions to reduce discomfort when standing or wearing shoes. Treatment with medical curettage followed by topical acids (trichloroacetic 25-35%) and cryosurgery can be helpful (47).

Chemical burn injury in the newborn

Neonatal skin is immature, thin, poorly keratinized and has an increased surface area to body ratio. Therefore the problems of discoloration, irritation, necrosis, burning and systemic absorption can easily occur.

Chlorhexidine is an effective broad-spectrum topical antiseptic agent. It is used as the first line of antiseptic choice in most neonatal units because of low adverse effects. Chlorhexidine alone has been proposed to be safe even to the concentration to 2% in pediatric patients. There is no report of burns from this medication used alone. However the formulations of chlorhexidine in alcohol base (alcoholic chlorhexidine 0.5% chlorhexidine in 70 % alcohol/methanol) are not safe in preterm babies under 28 weeks of gestational age. There are several reports of adverse effects of this formulation.

The stratum corneum of ELBW preterm infants is thinner with looser attachment to the dermis than in term infants. There is also increased percutaneous absorption of the medication. This can lead to serious complications such as excessive water loss, hypothermia, infection and septicemia. There is limited data for the optimal chlorhexidine preparation for the ELBW patients.

Other chemical agents found to cause skin burning include mercury (mercurochrome), topical povidine/iodine, and hexachlorophene-containing compounds. Thus, disinfecting agents in preterm and term infants should be chosen carefully (48).

Miscellaneous

Subcutaneous fat necrosis of the newborn (SCFN) is an idiopathic panniculitis in the neonatal period affecting apparently healthy full term newborns (see figure 32). The exact pathogenesis of this condition is unclear. Multiple risk factors include ante-partum obstetric complications, perinatal asphyxia (e.g. meconium aspiration) and postnatal events (e.g. hypothermia, hypoxemia). In theory these conditions induce physiologic blood shunting from the skin surface and cause adipocyte necrosis.

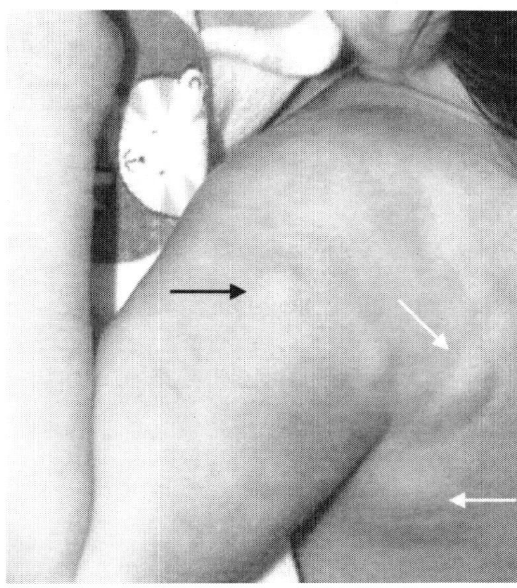

Figure 32. Subcutaneous fat necrosis.

The postulated cause of adipocyte necrosis relates to the saturated fat melting point. The neonatal adipocytes have relatively high concentration of saturated fatty acids which results in a higher melting point. Under stress these fatty acids solidify and crystallize leading to adipocyte death. However, because infants delivered with uncomplicated maternal and neonatal courses have also been reported to have SCFN.

The characteristic presentation is a well-circumscribed, indurated, erythematous to violaceous painful patch/plaque located on the buttocks, cheek, posterior trunk, arm, and leg. The anterior trunk is classically spared. The most common onset of presentation is in the first few weeks to months of life.

Histopathological features characteristically reveal lobular necrosis of the fat cell and a mixed inflammatory cell infiltrate (multinucleated giant cell, histiocytes, lymphocytes and eosinophils) and needle-shaped crystal clefts arranged in a radial pattern in adipocytes. The pattern of arranged clefts is not pathognomonic for SCFN. It is also seen in sclerema neonatorum and post-steroidal panniculitis.

Most babies with SCFN have normal laboratory evaluation. Hypercalcemia is the most serious complication. Hypercalcemia had been found in 26-56 % of SCFN babies, usually in the recovery phase. The mean age of hypercalcemic onset was 6.7 weeks of age. The pathogenic mechanism of this condition is still not understood. Multiple theories are proposed such as elevated prostaglandin E and elevated parathormone level and extra renal production of 1, 25 dihydroxyvitamin D by the different investigators.

Hypercalcemia in SCFN can be asymptomatic, particularly in mild cases. Hypercalcemic symptoms e.g. vomiting, irritability, dehydration, hypotonia, polyuria, polydipsia, constipation and seizures should be monitored. Successful treatment of hypercalcemia with hydration and furosemide and/or systemic corticosteroid has been reported.

Hypoglycemia and thrombocytopenia may be found and precede the clinical presentation. Hypoglycemia and thrombocytopenia may arise from perinatal complications. The natural history of SCFN is transient, self-healing and resolving within several weeks to months. Affected areas occasionally heal with atrophic changes. Observation and monitoring the clinical symptoms and serum calcium levels until 6 months of age is recommended (49).

Sclerema neonatorum

This condition usually presents in very sick and often preterm neonates. The presentation characteristically reveals a diffuse, rapidly spreading, symmetric, stiffness, and induration of the skin and subcutaneous tissue. The most common locations are on the buttocks, cheeks, thighs, lower legs and trunk. The induration continues to spread from the torso onto the legs, buttock and all areas except the palms, soles and genitalia. The skin becomes yellow, white, mottled, woody and waxy with a cadaver-like appearance.

The exact etiology and pathogenesis is unclear. Four theories currently proposed include neonatal fat (see above), abnormalities in fat metabolism, connective tissue edema and other underlying diseases. The serious underlying conditions that are associated with sclerema neonatorum include sepsis, congenital heart disease, respiratory distress, hypothermia and metabolic disturbances (hypoglycemia, hyperkalemia, metabolic acidosis and electrolyte imbalance).

The differential diagnosis includes subcutaneous fat necrosis of the newborn and other panniculitides. A newborn that had clinical and histological overlap with both SCFN and sclerema neonatorum has been reported.

There are multiple therapeutic interventions reported to treat this condition including systemic corticosteroids, systemic antibiotics, exchange transfusion and polymorphonuclear leukocyte transfusion. Systemic corticosteroids have been proven ineffective, whereas the repeated exchange transfusion seems to be helpful to reduce mortality. Control of all abnormalities and systemic support is recommended to limit spread. Even with maximum support, the mortality of newborns with sclerema neonatorum is still high. Skin of infants who survive is reported to be normal (50).

Conclusion

We have reviewed a range of neonatal dematologic findings including transient benign physiologic conditions, birthmarks, developmental anomalies, vesiculo-bullous disorders, iatrogenic and factitious issues and others. We included brief discussions and updates on these topics and provided illustrations for the more clinically significant conditions.

References

[1] Visscher MO, Narendran V, Pickens WL, LaRufffa AA, Meinzen-Derr J, Allen K, et al. Vernix caseosa in neonatal adaptation. J Perinatol 2005;25:440-6.

[2] Conlon JD, Drolet BA. Skin lesions in the neonate. Pediatr Clin North Am 2004;51:863-88, vii-viii.

[3] Amitai DB, Fichman S, Merlob P, Morad Y, Lapidoth M, Metzker A. Cutis marmorata telangiectatica congenita: clinical findings in 85 patients. Pediatr Dermatol 2000;17:100-4.

[4] Larralde M, Luna PC. Benign self-limiting cutaneous lesions. In: Schachner LA, Hansen RC, eds. Pediatric dermatology, 4th ed. Philadelphia, PA: Mosby Elsevier, 2011:311-3.

[5] Donley CL, Nelson LP. Comparison of palatal and alveolar cysts of the newborn in premature and full-term infants. Pediatr Dent 2000;22:321-4.

[6] Cunha RF, Boer FA, Torriani DD, Frossard WT. Natal and neonatal teeth: review of the literature. Pediatr Dent 2001;23:158-62.

[7] Berk DR, Bayliss SJ. Milia: a review and classification. J Am Acad Dermatol 2008; 59:1050-63.

[8] Lee HS, Chun YS, Hann SK. Nevus depigmentosus: clinical features and histopathologic characteristics in 67 patients. J Am Acad Dermatol 1999; 40: 21-6.

[9] Korf BR. Tuberous sclerosis complex and neurofibromatosis. In: Schachner LA, Hansen RC, eds. Pediatric dermatology, 4th ed. Philadelphia, PA: Mosby Elsevier, 2011:481-9.

[10] Reza AM, Farahnaz GZ, Hamideh S, Alinaghi SA, Saeed Z, Mostafa H. Incidence of Mongolian spots and its common sites at two university hospitals in Tehran, Iran. Pediatr Dermatol 2010;27:397-8.

[11] Paller AS, Mancini AJ. Disorders of hyperpigmentation. In: Paller AS, Mancini AJ, eds. Hurwitz clinical pediatric dermatology, 3rd ed. Philadelphia, PA: Elsevier Saunders, 2006:284-99.

[12] Krengel S, Hauschild A, Schafer T. Melanoma risk in congenital melanocytic naevi: a systematic review. Br J Dermatol 2006;155:1-8.

[13] Bett BJ. Large or multiple congenital melanocytic nevi: occurrence of neurocutaneous melanocytosis in 1008 persons. J Am Acad Dermatol 2006;54:767-77.

[14] Juern AM, Glick ZR, Drolet BA, Frieden IJ. Nevus simplex: a reconsideration of nomenclature, sites of involvement, and disease associations. J Am Acad Dermatol 2010;63:805-14.

[15] Cordoro KM, Speetzen LS, Koerper MA, Frieden IJ. Physiologic changes in vascular birthmarks during early infancy: Mechanisms and clinical implications. J Am Acad Dermatol 2009;60:669-75.

[16] Chapas AM, Eickhorst K, Geronemus RG. Efficacy of early treatment of facial port wine stains in newborns: a review of 49 cases. Lasers Surg Med 2007;39:563-8.

[17] Bruckner AL, Frieden IJ. Hemangiomas of infancy. J Am Acad Dermatol 2003;48:477-96.

[18] Paller AS, Mancini AJ. Vascular malformations and malformation syndromes. In: Paller AS, Mancini AJ, eds. Hurwitz clinical pediatric dermatology, 3rd ed. Philadelphia, PA: Elsevier Saunders, 2006:307-44.

[19] Rosen H, Schmidt B, Lam HP. Management of nevus sebaceous and the risk of basal cell carcinoma: an 18-year review. Pediatr Dermatol 2009;26:676-81.

[20] Kugelman A, Tubi A, Bader D, Chemo M, Dabbah H. Pre-auricular tags and pits in the newborn: the role of renal ultrasonography. J Pediatr 2002; 141:388-91.

[21] Geddes G, Butterly MM, Patel SM and Silvio M. Pediatric neck masses. Pediatr Rev 2013;34(3):115-24.

[22] Zvulunov A, Amichai B, Grunwald MH, Avinoach I, Halevy S.. Cutaneous bronchogenic cyst: delineation of a poorly recognized lesion. Pediatr Dermatol 1998;15:277-81.
[23] Brown J, Schwartz RA. Supernumerary nipples: an overview. Cutis 2003;71:344-6.
[24] Adams BB. Supernumerary nipples a risk factor? Pediatr Dermatol 2002;19:463-4.
[25] Morgan DW, Evans JN. Developmental nasal anomalies. J Laryngol Otol 1990;104:394-403.
[26] Greenberg S, Krafchik BR. Infantile pedal papules. J Am Acad Dermatol 2005;53:333-4.
[27] Ray M, Hendrick SJ, Raimer SS, Blackwell SJ. Amniotic band syndrome. Int J Dermatol 1988;27:312-4.
[28] Frieden IJ. Aplasia cutis congenita: a clinical review and proposal for classification. J Am Acad Dermatol 1986;14:646-60.
[29] Mancini AJ, Frieden IJ, Paller AS. Infantile acropustulosis revisited: history of scabies and response to topical corticosteroids. Pediatr Dermatol 1998;15:337-41.
[30] Leung AC, Wheeler BH, Robson WL, Kossakowska AE. Erythema toxicum present at birth. Pediatr Dermatol 1992;9:162-3.
[31] Nervi SJ, Schwartz RA, Dmochowski M. Eosinophilic pustular folliculitis: a 40 year retrospect. J Am Acad Dermatol 2006;55:285-9.
[32] Ellis E, Scheinfeld N. Eosinophilic pustular folliculitis: a comprehensive review of treatment options. Am J Clin Dermatol 2004;5:189-97.
[33] Weston WL, Lane AT, Morelli JG. Color textbook of pediatric dermatology, fourth ed. Philadelphia, PA: Mosby Elsevier, 2007:366-7.
[34] Gan VN, Hoang MP. Generalized vesicular eruption in a newborn. Pediatr Dermatol 2004;21:171-3.
[35] Lucky AW. A review of infantile and pediatric acne. Dermatology 1998; 196: 95-7.
[36] Ayhan M, Sancak B, Karaduman A, Arikan S, Sahin S. Colonization of neonate skin by Malassezia species: relationship with neonatal cephalic pustulosis. J Am Acad Dermatol 2007;57:1012-8.
[37] Minkov M, Prosch H, Steiner M, Grois N, Pötschger U, Kaatsch P, et al. Langerhans cell histiocytosis in neonates. Pediatr Blood Cancer 2005;45:802-7.
[38] Smahi A, Courtois G, Vabres P, Yamaoka S, Heuertz S, Munnich A, et al. Genomic rearrangement in NEMO impairs NF-kappaB activation and is a cause of incontinentia pigmenti. The International Incontinentia Pigmenti (IP) Consortium. Nature 2000;405:466-72.
[39] Ardelean D, Pope E. Incontinentia pigmenti in boys: a series and review of the literature. Pediatr Dermatol 2006;23:523-7.
[40] Sandhu K, Kanwar AJ. Generalized bullous impetigo in a neonate. Pediatr Dermatol 2004;21:667-9.
[41] Karthikeyan K. Scabies in children. Arch Dis Child Educ Pract Ed 2007;92:e65-9.
[42] Strong M, Johnstone P. Interventions for treating scabies. Cochrane Database Syst Rev 2007;3:CD000320.
[43] Darmstadt GL, Dinulos JG, Miller Z. Congenital cutaneous candidiasis: clinical presentation, pathogenesis, and management guidelines. Pediatrics 2000;105:438-44.
[44] Sauerbrei A, Wutzler P. Herpes simplex and varicella-zoster virus infections during pregnancy: current concepts of prevention, diagnosis and therapy. Part 1: herpes simplex virus infections. Med Microbiol Immunol 2007;196:89-94.
[45] Whitley R. Neonatal herpes simplex virus infection. Curr Opin Infect Dis 2004;17:243-6.
[46] Sauerbrei A, Wutzler P. Herpes simplex and varicella-zoster virus infections during pregnancy: current concepts of prevention, diagnosis and therapy. Part 2: Varicella-zoster virus infections. Med Microbiol Immunol 2007;196:95-102.
[47] Williamson D, Holt PJ. Calcified cutaneous nodules on the heels of children: Acomplication of heel sticks as a neonate. Pediatr Dermatol 2001;18:138-40.
[48] Upadhyayula S, Kambalapalli M, Harrison CJ. Safety of anti-infective agents for skin preparation in premature infants. Arch Dis Child 2007;92:646-7.
[49] Mahe E, Girszyn N, Hadj-Rabia S, Bodemer C, Hamel-Teillac D, De Prost Y. Subcutaneous fat necrosis of the newborn: a systematic evaluation of risk factors, clinical manifestations, complications and outcome of 16 children. Br J Dermatol 2007;156:709-15.
[50] Zeb A, Darmstadt Gl. Sclerema neonatorum: review of nomenclature, clinical presentation, historlotic features, differential diagnoses and management. J Perinatol 2008;28:453-6.

In: Pediatric and Adolescent Dermatology
Editors: D Greydanus, A Feinberg and J Merrick
ISBN: 978-1-63321-853-6

Chapter 3

Dermatology: Pediatric and adolescent medicine

Arthur N Feinberg, MD*[*]*, Tor A Shwayder, MD, Ruqiya Tereen, MD and Therdpong Tempark, MD
Department of Pediatric and Adolescent Medicine,
Western Michigan University Homer Stryker MD School of Medicine,
Kalamazoo, Michigan, United States of America

Dermatological conditions are a very important part of pediatric and adolescent medicine and can have considerable influence on an adolescent's medical as well as psychological health. This chapter presents a brief summary of etiologic and pathogenesis of these conditions followed by a standard case management including newer developments where pertinent. The paper reviews these areas: skin infections and infestations (bacterial, viral, fungal, and parasitic); dermatitis (non-allergic, allergic, and idiopathic); hypersensitivity reactions (urticaria, erythema multiforme, and drug eruptions); miscellaneous skin conditions (acne, nevi, papulosquamous disorders); dermatologic manifestations of systemic disorders (pruritis without rash, inflammatory bowel disease, collagen vascular disorders, and endocrine disorders); and disorders of the hair and nails.

Introduction

The goals of this chapter are to discuss the more common skin conditions encountered in children and adolescents in the day-to-day practice of a primary care physician. We present a brief summary of etiology and pathogenesis of the conditions followed by a discussion of standard case management including newer developments where pertinent. The chapter is divided into six main sections:

[*] Correspondence: Professor Arthur N Feinberg, MD, Department of Pediatric and Adolescent Medicine, Western Michigan University Homer Stryker MD School of Medicine, 1000 Oakland Drive, D48G, Kalamazoo, MI 49008-1284 United States. E-mail: arthur.feinberg@med.wmich.edu

- Skin infections and infestations (bacterial, viral, fungal, and parasitic)
- Dermatitis (non-allergic, allergic, and idiopathic)
- Hypersensitivity reactions (urticaria, erythema multiforme and drug eruptions)
- Miscellaneous skin conditions (acne, nevi, papulosquamous disorders)
- Dermatologic manifestations of systemic disorders (pruritis without rash, inflammatory bowel
- Collagen vascular disorders and endocrine disorders)
- Disorders of the hair and nails

Skin infections and infestations

Bacterial infections

Bacterial infections of the skin are summarized clinically in table 1 (1-6).

Table 1. Characteristics of common bacterial infections

Skin layers/ Structures	Disease	Common sites	Predominant organism	Secondary organism
Epidermis	Impetigo	Face	Staphylococcus Aureus	Streptococcus Pyogenes (GABHS)
	Superficial Folliculitis	Face, scalp,	Staphylococcus Aureus	
	Furunculosis	Face, scalp, axillae	Staphylococcus Aureus	
	Staphylococcal Scalded Skin Syndrome		Staphylococcus Aureus Phage group II	
	Scarlatina	Face and scalp can involve whole body	Streptococcus Pyogenes (GABHS)	
Epidermal/ Subepidermal	Toxic Shock Syndrome	whole body	Staphylococcus Aureus	
	Ecthyma	Legs, buttocks	Pseudomonas aeruginosa	Many gram negative and some gram positive organism
Dermis	Carbuncle Erysipelas	Back, thighs Face	Staphylococcus Aureus Streptococcus Pyogenes (GABHS)	

Skin layers/ Structures	Disease	Common sites	Predominant organism	Secondary organism
	Deep Folliculitis	Scalp	Staphylococcus Aureus	
	Folliculitis Deculvans	Scalp		
Dermis and upper part of subcutaneous tissues	Cellulitis	Legs	Staphylococcus aureus	Streptococcus pyogenes (GABHS)
Deeper Dermis, Subcutaneous Tissues & Fascia	Necrotizing Fasciitis Type I: Mixed aerobic & anaerobic infection	Legs Arms Less commonly; Trunk Perineum Buttocks Head & Neck	Facultative Strptococci, Stphylococci, Enterococci Gram-negative bacilli , such as Escherichia coli, Klebsiella, Pseudomonas, Enterobacter, and Proteus, and Anaerobes, such as Peptostreptococcus, Bacteroides, and Clostridium specie	
	Necrotizing Fasciitis Type II: Monomicrobial		Streptococcus pyogenes (GABHS)	Streptococcus Agalactiae & pneumoniae V vulnificus Clostridium Staphylococcus aureus aureus [28] and Aeromonas spp

Impetigo

A common skin infection, impetigo affects about 2.8% of children under 4 years and 1.6% of those 5 to 15 years of age. Certain conditions that compromise the immune system can lead to impetigo including, burns, diabetes mellitus, B-cell immunodeficiency states etc. Infection has a predilection for face especially around the mouth and nose area. Typical lesions can be bullous or non-bullous, as well as have a mixed presentation occurring within the same area. Previously beta-hemolytic Streptococcus (GABHS) was thought to be the main causative agent especially in the non-bullous form, but current literature suggests Staphylococcus aureus as the predominant etiology in both forms of impetigo.

Contact dermatitis presents with tiny vesicles on erythematous skin but they are very itchy and usually occur on exposed areas with a history of contact with a sensitizing agent. Small clear fluid filled vesicles of herpes simplex infection are more common on the lips and perioral area and can be quite painful. Varicella vesicles easily rupture and encrust like impetigo but involve the whole body and occur in crops with lesions of different stages present in same area. Ecthyma is usually a solitary ulcerative lesion surrounded by tiny vesicles which leaves a scar unlike impetigo which seldom does. Pemphigus foliaceus is a rare disease usually involving the face in a butterfly like fashion also presents with vesicles and occasional bullae on an erythematous base.

Bullous impetigo

Accounting for 70% of cases, this starts as innocuous reddish papules which coalesce and form small bullae which easily rupture forming erosions covered with the typical honey colored thick crust.

Non-Bullous impetigo

This less common form presents with expanding honey-colored crusts leaving a raw erosive area.

Secondary impetigo

Secondary infection of minor cuts, insect bites and excessive scratching of eczematous, scabies and other pruritic lesions especially in diabetic or immunocompromised children can result in impetigenous lesions, usually of the non-bullous type.

Management

Prevention of infection spread is important although topical disinfectants are not indicated. First line of treatment for small lesions confined to one or two area is a topical antibiotic like mupirocin, bacitracin or fusidic acid. Topical antibiotics are not only superior to placebo but mupirocin and bacitracin were found to be superior to oral erythromycin. Amoxicillin/clavulanate (125/30 mg per ml) three times daily, cephalexin 30 mg/kg/day in 2 divided doses, erythromycin 40 mg/kg/day in 2-4 divided doses and dicloxacillin 90 mg/kg in 2-4 divided doses per day, for 7-10 days resulted in satisfactory outcomes.

Cellulitis

A rapidly spreading infection of skin and subcutaneous tissues results from introduction of infecting organism through a minor cut, prick or any break in the skin. Any part of the body can be involved but it typically occurs on lower extremities, although in young children face involvement is common. The diffuse rapidly progressive lesion with no clear margins presents with typical signs of acute inflammation i.e. warm and tender to touch and shiny red in appearance because of swelling. Immunocompromised hosts are susceptible to cellulitis and its complications. Staphylococcus aureus, Streptococcus pyogenes and Enterococcus sp are common offenders. Rare infection with Hemophilus influenza especially in infants and with Clostridium difficile is possible. Cellulitis can present with signs of systemic infection like fever, malaise, pain, lymhangitis and lymphadenitis.

Periorbital (pre-septal) and orbital (post-septal) cellulitis

These are mostly unilateral and often are due to a spread of infection from the adjacent inflamed sinuses (7). Local skin infection may also be the initiating factor. Infections can be recurrent and often present in winter months in young children with average age of presentation being 6.8 years with a 2:1 male preponderance. Most common agents involved are Staphylococcus aureus, S. epidermidis, and Streptococcus pyogenes. Orbital cellulitis is an emergency as it can lead to serious complications like cavernous sinus thrombosis, meningitis, permanent loss of vision, and diplopia.

Management

Prompt recognition and initiation of antibiotics is required for quick resolution and prevention of complications. Penicillins, cephalosporins, amoxicillin-clavulanate and macrolides all are effective in uncomplicated cases. Adolescents with diabetes, immunocompromised status, may require hospitalization and intravenous administration of second or third generation cephalosporins with or without aminoglycosides. Attempts to isolate the organism are indicated if empiric treatment fails to show any signs of improvement. Orbital cellulitis should be treated as an emergency; intravenous antibiotics and hospitalization is necessary as well as a consultation with ophthalmology and otorhinolaryngology.

Erysipelas

This is a localized infection of skin and subcutaneous tissue caused by group A ß hemolytic streptococcus, usually affecting the face and extremities. Unlike cellulitis, lesions are sharply demarcated and may present with a prodrome of fever, chills, nausea, vomiting, and arthralgia. It responds well to oral antibiotics but at times intravenous antibiotics are indicated. Other well localized lesions with defined margins like a drug reaction or contact dermatitis may pose a diagnostic challenge but targeted questioning may delineate history of exposure.

Folliculitis

An infection of the hair follicle, it is divided in types based on the depth of hair follicle involved, infecting agent and area involved:

Superficial folliculitis

This is the most common form which can affect any area of the body with hair follicles, mostly in areas with poor hygiene and maceration. Staphylococcus is the usual causative organism. Small pustules with hair in the center generally resolve without treatment and with no scarring. Chronic recurring infection responds to topical antibiotics mupirocin 2%, clindamycin, or erythromycin.

Deep folliculitis

Less commonly, infection reaches to the base of follicle resulting in painful papules and pustules, healing with scarring. Treatment with oral antibiotics targeting Staphylococcus aureus is indicated.

Gram-negative folliculitis

This is common in adolescents with acne vulgaris who are being treated with a long term antibiotic regimen, which give rise an opportunity for gram negative bacteria like Klebsiella, Enterobacter, and Proteus to over populate and infect the hair follicles. Usually the folliculitis affects the areas where acne is predominant such as the face and chest.

Hot-tub folliculitis

Erythematous itchy papules or pustules overlying large areas of trunk, extremities and other areas usually present after few hours to up to 3 days after exposure to a hot-tub, whirlpool, or swimming pool which has not been chlorinated properly or if the water pH was suboptimal. Outbreaks have been reported with use of community pools, whirlpools and water slides. In cases of severe infection fever, malaise, sore throat and lymphadenopathy may occur. Lesions are self limiting over a few days. 1% acetic acid soaks can hasten drying.

Furunculosis

A perifollicular erythematous abscess due to Staphylococcus aureus, commonly affects intertrigenous areas but also can occur on scalp, and at other sites where hair follicles are abundant. Furuncles when they occur inside the auditory canal or nasal cavity can be very painful. Nasal carriage can be the primary source of infection. Hyperhidrosis can predispose to furunculosis and maintaining good hygiene of intertriginous areas may be the key to prevent autoinoculation and recurrence. Community acquired methicillin-resistant Staphylococcus aureus (CA-MRSA) is becoming a more frequent cause of furunculosis. Children with immunocompromised status like HIV or inherited immune deficiencies are susceptible to treatment-resistant and recurrent furunculosis.

Carbuncle

These are collections of multiple inflamed furuncles in a small area. Favored sites for carbuncles are where dermis is thick such as thighs, back of the neck and trunk. A carbuncle is a large erythematous, painful, indurated mass located within deep subcutaneous tissue. Multiple small furuncles which comprise a carbuncle connect to each other via subcutaneous tracts and ultimately drain pus to the surface.

Management

Solitary furuncles of less then 5 cm in diameters respond well to the excision and drainage only. Cases where multiple or larger lesions are present or where systemic signs of inflammation are evident an oral antibiotic like minocycline or doxycycline (children 8 years and older) 100 mg every 12 hours is indicated. Clindamycin can be used in cases of MRSA furunculosis at a dose of 2–8 mg/kg/dose every 6–8 hours. In patients with MRSA furunculosis leading to systemic infection hospitalization and a course of intravenous antibiotics such as vancomycin is necessary.

Incision and drainage is the treatment of choice for carbuncles. Surgical consultation may be indicated for large carbuncles to excise and drain the abscesses and to clean some of the tracts. Deep seated carbuncles are hard and fixed and feel like a malignant tumor on palpation. If they perforate they cause deep lesions which heal with scarring. Oral anti-staphylococcal antibiotics are only indicated in case of systemic involvement or when concomitant cellulitis is present.

Scarletina

Also known as scarlet fever it is a presentation of acute systemic Streptococcus pyogenes infection. It is given this name due to its distinctive reddish punctate sandpapery skin rash and mucous membrane involvement. A patient will have high fever, sore throat, vomiting and listlessness. The rash appears on second day and starts on the upper trunk and soon becomes generalized, sparing perioral area leaving a pale ring around the mouth. It soon concentrates in the axilla and groin. Mucous membranes also have a bright red hue with petechial lesions on the palate. The tongue becomes smooth and red strawberry tongue. Laboratory studies reveal leukocytosis and elevated anti-streptolysin O titer. A swab culture will confirm the hemolytic Streptococcus. Empiric treatment with penicillin should be started as soon as possible to avoid the non-suppurative complication rheumatic fever.

Staphylococcal scalded skin syndrome (SSSS) and toxic shock syndrome (TSS)

SSSS is predominantly a disease of younger children, 98% of cases are under 6 years and 62% are under 2 years of age. Inoculation of skin is usually via blood stream seeding from a distant infection from the pharynx, conjunctiva or middle ear. The pathogenesis of SSSS is Staphylococcus aureus producing an epidermolytic toxin (ET), mostly group phage II, causing lysis of epidermis at the level of granular layer. Cleavage of the epidermis results in positive Nikolsky sign with production of bullae with minor pressure which easily burst. Systemic signs of infection like high fever usually appear first followed in 24-48 hours by an orange-red macular rash resembling scarlatina with sandpaper like quality to touch. The skin becomes extremely tender and peels away easily leaving large denuded areas. The rash starts from the scalp and face, and descends downward with axillae and groins are commonly affected. It is important to consider other epidermolytic conditions in the differential diagnosis such as toxic epidermal necrolysis, erythroderma, and drug eruptions.

TSS

Staphylococcal TSS was first elucidated as a severe complication associated with usage of tampons during the menstrual period. Presently, about 50% of cases are menstrual-related and 50% are non-menstrual, specifically post-surgical or post-infectious. The pathogenesis is due to the TSST 1 toxin which accounts for 90% or more of menstrual cases. Staphylococcal enterotoxins are more prevalent in non-menstrual cases. It presents with a flu-like prodrome then progressing to high fever and hypotension. The dermatologic manifestations are diffuse erythema involving the palms and soles. In non-menstrual cases the erythema may be more concentrated at the site of surgery or infection. The patient may progress to shock adult respiratory distress syndrome (ARDS) and multi organ system failure (MOSF). The diagnosis is clinical as bacterial cultures are not reliably positive (only in 5% of cases).

Streptococcal TSS is due to increased virulence related to its M protein as well as presence of streptococcal pyrogenic exotoxins (SPEA). It occurs as a complication of delivery, surgery, viral infection such as varicella or use of NSAIDS. It presents with a prodromal flu-like picture and then proceeds to a diffuse erythema (10% of the time scarletinaform), but unlike staphylococcal infection is followed by ecchymosis and sloughing, appearing more like necrotizing fasciitis. Complications include sepsis, ARDS and MOSF.

Management

Blood culture may be negative in TSSS but one should attempt to obtain culture and sensitivity to ensure the targeted antibiotic treatment. Local treatment with potassium permagnate 1:9000 bath of the skin may provide some comfort although excessive use may cause dryness and further dehydration. The mainstay of treatment remains the Penicillinase-resistant systemic antibiotics like naficillin, flucoxacillin, and methicillin can be used in severe cases by intravenous route. Re-epithelization of the skin usually occurs quickly and without any scarring. Despite the severity of the rash the prognosis of uncomplicated SSSS is favorable with mortality rate of less than 5%.

Antibiotics of choice are for staphylococcal TSS are clindamycin 600 mg IV every 8 hours and vancomycin, 30 mg/kg/day in 2 divided doses. Intensive care support is critical in cases of shock. For streptococcal TSS, studies have shown that S. pyogenes does not respond well to penicillin, though susceptible, primarily because of the status of the host. Therefore, empiric antibiotics should include clindamycin 900 mg. IV every 8 hours and imipenem 500 gm IV every 6 hours for 14 days. Antibiotics may need to continue until no additional surgical debridement is needed or there are no systemic signs.

Necrotizing fascitis

A life threatening infection invading all layers of skin and going beyond subcutaneous tissues including fat and superficial layer of fascia, necrotizing fasciitis (NF) affects younger children and neonates especially if they have another infection like pharyngitis, chicken pox, respiratory tract or urinary tract infection (8). Children with lowered immunity and other debilitating conditions like diabetes, trauma or surgery are more susceptible. Two types of NF are known based on the organism involved. Type I NF is caused by multiple organisms both aerobic and anaerobic. Type II NF is caused mostly by a single agent, usually Streptococcus pyogenes but other organisms are also known to be responsible for it (Table 1). Infection is rapid and presents with severe systemic signs of infection. The skin becomes erythematous followed by development of severe edema and hemorrhagic bullae. The patient complains of severe unrelenting pain which later on can be replaced by numbness in the affected area once the nerve endings are damaged. Crepitus in subcutaneous tissue signifies infection with a gas producing organism like Clostridium or Enterobacteriaceae.

Management

Prompt recognition of NF and isolation of the organism is the key to recovery. A scoring system has been used to streamline the process for early diagnosis of NF known as Laboratory Risk Indicator for necrotizing fascitis (LRINEC) which includes the basic laboratory screens, total WBC, hemoglobin, sodium, glucose, serum creatinine, and C-reactive protein. A cut off score of 6 is used for a clinician to be alert to the possibility of NF. Tissue oxygen saturation of less then 70% has been used to identify NF in lower extremities in adults. In about 13% of cases of NF subcutaneous gas can be detected by radiography. Computed tomography is superior to plain radiographs as it can also detect early soft tissue changes like fat stranding, fascial thickening, and dissection along the fascial plains. Magnetic resonance imaging (MRI) has also been shown to be highly sensitive in diagnosing NF. Recently ultrasound has been used more frequently and has shown some efficacy.

A multidimensional approach to these patients is the key to resolution of NF, including surgical and infectious disease consultation, sterile precautions, hydration and nutritional status of patient. Emergency surgical exploration and debridement is the key component of treating NF, multiple debridements may be necessary. Hyperbaric oxygen and IV immunoglobulins with varying degrees of evidence for support have been used as adjunctive treatments to hasten the tissue healing process. Empiric treatment with broad spectrum antibiotics with coverage for MRSA as well as Streptococcus pyogenes should be started as soon as possible change it to a more specific regimen once results of culture and sensitivity are available. Refer to treatment of streptococcal TSS above for antibiotic selection.

Ecthyma gangrenosum

This is a relatively rare infection, resulting from occlusive vasculitis usually associated with pseudomonas septicemia. It mostly affects patients who are immunocompromised. Victims of burns have a high rate of pseudomonas septicemia. It usually affects the buttocks and anogenital area but can occur anywhere. It presents as a small innocuous macule, which becomes purulent and develops into a thick walled hemorrhagic bullous lesion, which ultimately becomes a gangrenous ulcer. The pathognomonic feature is a grayish-black eschar surrounded by an erythematous ring. A localized form at the site of infection is also reported, more common in immune deficient hosts especially children with hematologic cancers. Non pseudomonas ecthyma gangrenosum has also been reported. Differentiation between ecthyma gangrenosum and pyoderma gangrenosum can be difficult on clinical grounds. Histopathological features and absence of septicemia in pyoderma can distinguish between two almost similar gangrenous ulcers. In rare cases pyoderma can be complicated with superimposed ecthyma gangrenosum.

Management

Blood cultures and culture of aspirate from a lesion can confirm the Pseudomonas aeuroginosa. Biopsy and histopathology may be necessary at times. Localized smaller lesions can be treated with topical silver sulfadiazine. For larger lesions systemic antibiotics with pseudomonas the use of ß lactam penicillins including piperacillin-tazobactam, ceftazidime, cefepime, imipenem, or the aminoglycosides gentamicin, or tobramycin is efficacious.

Cat scratch disease (CSD)

CSD caused by the gram-negative bacillus Bartonella Henselae, a common infection acquired by playing with kittens and stray cats (9). It is more commonly seen in humid climates and especially during autumn and winter season. The initial scratch is followed by the development of a reddish papule within next 1-2 weeks, which later becomes larger and firmer with development of high grade fever in about 30% of patients. Regional adenopathy occurs most commonly in lymph nodes draining arms and legs especially in the axillae, groins and epitrochlear areas. The head and neck region is involved in up to 49% of cases. Lymphadenopathy may persist for weeks, and CSD is the most common cause of chronic lymphadenopathy in young children. The lesions heal completely within about two weeks with the symptomatic treatments warm soaks, analgesics and antipyretics. Skin lesions can be confused with pyogenic granuloma, Kaposi's sarcoma and epithelioid hemangoioma. Other disease with lymphadenopathy including tuberculous adenitis, infectious mononucleosis, tularemia and tumors can cause a diagnostic dilemma especially in about 10% patients where a typical CSD skin lesion was not present or noted.

Management

Immunofluorescent antibody (IFA) test or the enzyme immunoassay (EIA) test can be used to confirm diagnosis when in doubt. DNA polymerase chain reaction (PCR) assays are less commonly used but are highly sensitive. The atypical presentation Parinaud oculoglandular syndrome with high fever, regional lymphadenopathy and ocular involvement is seen in about 5% of patients. Encephalpathy and severe systemic disease occur in about 2.5 % of cases. Treatment is generally not necessary in typical CSD but in immunocompromised patients or patients with severe systemic infection treatment with antibiotics may be effective. Macrolide antibiotics are most commonly used such as azithromycin at doses of 10 mg/kg/day for 2-5 days and rifampin 20 mg/kg per day in divided doses for 2–3 weeks. Children over 12 years of age can be treated with cipro?oxacin 20 –30 mg/kg/day for 2-3 weeks or trimethoprim (8 mg/kg/day)- sulfamethoxazole (50 mg/kg day) for 7–10 days. In severely ill patients with systemic involvement gentamicin 5mg/kg/day IM or IV every 8 hours is efficacious.

Treponemal infections

Due to Treponema pallidum, syphilis has an incubation period of 9-90 days (average of 3 weeks). Supportive laboratory data are reviewed in chapter 17 (10). The spirochete gains access via mucosal abrasions during sexual activity with the induction of local immune response and secondary hematogenous spread. The dermatologic manifestation of primary syphilis is classic chancre, a well-defined painless erythematous ulcer with a firm (rubbery) base; there often is associated inguinal adenopathy, unilateral or bilateral, non-tender and non suppurative.

Secondry syphilis appears 6 weeks to 6 months after disappearance of the chancre and can present with a wide variety of findings in its role as “the great imitator” with fever, malaise, headache, arthralgia, generalized lymphadenopathy, hepatosplenomegaly, rhinitis, sore throat, alopecia (moth-eaten, patchy), polymorphic rash usually involving the palms and soles. The rash may be macular, popular, maculopapular, morbilliform and on occasion, pustular, papulosquamous, annular or nodular. Skin manifestations of secondary syphilis will resolve spontaneously over 2 or more weeks if not treated, but it would leave the patient at risk for further manifestations of syphilis.

Warts due to syphilis, known as condylomata lata are moist warty papules seen in moist areas of the body such as the perineum and intertrigenous areas. A mucous patch, usually a red papule is another manifestation of syphilis appearing in the mouth, tongue and genital areas.

Management

Primary, secondary and early latent stages of syphilis are treated with benzathine penicillin G (2.4 million units IM) in one dose; late latent and tertiary syphilis are treated with a similar dose for three weeks. Penicillin-allergic patients may be de-sensitized. Alternative antibiotic treatment includes tetracycline, 500 mg orally, four times daily, or doxycycline, 100 mg orally twice daily, for 14 days.

Lyme borreliosis (Lyme disease)

This is an infection transmitted by a deer tick Ixodes damini introducing the spirochete borrelia burgdorferi (11-13). Lyme disease is the most common vector-borne disease in United States with about 15,000 cases being reported annually. Initially confined to the wooded New England States it is now considered endemic in 15 States. The hallmark lesion is erythema migrans, which develops, in about 75-80% of patients at the site of tick bite in days to weeks. It can occur over any part of the body and typically leaves a central pale region which slowly expands. Low grade fever, malaise, arthralgia, myalgia regional adenopathy and headaches are common and in the absence of a definitive erythema migrans are difficult to distinguish from a common flu-like illness.

Atypical and chronic cutaneous manifestations can occur in a subset of patients including acrodermatitis chronica atrophicans usually affecting extensor surfaces of extremities and present as an indurated, hyperpigmented plaque. Systemic involvement can present in various forms, including about 15% of patients developing lymphocytic meningitis with signs of meningeal irritation, encephalitis and cranial nerve involvement. Facial nerve palsy in young children living in endemic areas is common up to 34 to 65% depending on different studies from different geographic locations. Other systemic manifestations include hepatosplenomegaly, chronic fatigue, migratory pain and cardiac and joint involvement.

Management

Prevention of tick bites should be emphasized to patients living in or travelling in endemic areas who should avoid heavily wooded areas, not sit on the ground, wear proper clothing, and apply n,n-diethyl- m-toluamide (DEET) sparingly, Permethrin can be sprayed on clothing. Prophylactic antibiotics to prevent Lyme disease after a tick bite are not recommended as up to 70-80% of deer ticks are not infective. Purified recombinant outer surface protein vaccine (OSP) has been approved for use in children 15 years of age and up, with 49% efficacy in the first year and ultimately 76% efficacy in preventing Lyme disease. Serologic testing is not useful in endemic areas as there is up to 30% chance of false results. Indirect florescent antibody and enzyme –linked immunosobent assay (ELISA) tests are available.

They may be negative in the early phase of infection, later becoming more sensitive and specific. Recommended treatment for early Lyme disease with children presenting with Bells palsy, mild carditis, and arthritis is based on age. In children less then 9 years of age penicillin or ampicillin 25-50 mg/kg/day in divided doses for a total dose of about 1-2 g/day is effective, while children older then 9 years can be treated with tetracycline 250 mg QID or doxycycline 100 mg BID. In complicated late Lyme disease where persistent arthritis, severe carditis, meningitis or encephalitis is present, ceftriaxone 75-100 mg/kg/day or penicillin G 300,000 U/kg/day is recommended.

Viral infections

Viral exanthems are summarized briefly in table 2 (14).

Table 2. Viral Exanthems of Childhood

Exanthems	Virus	Incubation	Hallmark
Measles	Paramyxovirus	10-12 days	Koplik's Spots
Rubella	Togaviridae/Rubivirus	14-21 days	Cephalo-caudal progression of rash

Table 2. (Continued)

Exanthems	Virus	Incubation	Hallmark
Erythema Infectiosum	Parvovirus B19	4-15 days	Slapped cheek, lacy reticular rash on extremities
Roseola Infantum	HHV-6 and -7	5-15 days	Rosy pink rash
Chicken pox	Varicella-zoster	10-21 days	Polymorphous lesions in crops
Hand-foot-mouth	Coxsackie A16, et al	3-7 days	Painful palmer, planter & buccal vesicles
Mollusum contagiosum	Molluscipox virus		Pearly umblicated dome shaped papules
Verucca Vulgaris (Warts)	Human Papilloma Virus		dome shaped/filiform/cauliflower/ flat lesions

Measles (rubeola)

This has been much a less common infection since the advent of a vaccination regimen in 1963, although in the late 1980s to early 90s, a resurgence of measles occurred in the USA mainly because of decline in levels of antibodies and in vaccination administration in certain populations. There have been other isolated outbreaks such as in San Diego CA in 2008, where a single case of a non-vaccinated child who returned from a trip abroad and exposed 839 people. Measles is highly contagious, is acquired by droplet infection and starts with high fever, sore throat, rhinorrhea, conjunctivitis, photophobia, cough and malaise. Simultaneous involvement of mucous membranes also occurs with the appearance of tiny grayish-white lesions on the buccal mucosa known as Koplik spots.

A maculopapular rash appears 3-4 days after the prodrome starting usually on the forehead and behind the ears and then spreading to involve the face, trunk and limbs. When rash is fully erupted fever subsides, and resolution of the rash is usually rapid without scarring. Complications that can occur during the acute phase of infection include superimposed bacterial infection leading to otitis media, gastroenteritis, and pneumonia and rarely encephalitis. A serious dematologic complication of is the appearance of purpura secondary to thrombocytopenia (black measles). Persistence of virus within central nervous system for months to years after initial infection and gives rise to a post infectious form of encephalitis known as subacute sclerosing panencephalitis (SSPE) which can occur in 1:100,000 patients.

Management

Supportive treatment includes rest, hydration, balanced nutrition, and protection from direct sunlight. Symptomatic treatment with antipyretics and cough suppression is helpful. In secondary bacterial infection, culture and sensitivity and targeted antibiotic therapy is indicated. Hospitalization is needed in patients with encephalitis and corticosteroid treatment is appropriate.

Varicella (chicken pox)

This is highly contagious and quickly spread by direct contact and droplet infection. After an incubation period of 1-2 weeks the disease starts with flu-like symptoms, fever, sore throat, and headaches. After 2-3 days of prodrome a rash first appears on trunk and spreads laterally. The mildly pruritic rash comes in crops starts as erythematous macules, which evolve in vesicles (dew-drop on a petal), and then into pustules. This eventually gives rise to a polymorphous rash with lesions in different stages of evolution and healing. Lesions rupture and become encrusted before completely healing. Usually there is no scarring or pigmentary change, though it may occur if pruritus is more severe than usual. Varicella usually runs a benign course but there may be rare secondary infections of the lesions with group A Streptococcus or Staphylococcus aureus. More serious complications such as necrotizing fasciitis, meningitis, encephalitis, transverse myelitis, or Guillain-Bare syndrome can occur.

Management

Supportive and symptomatic treatment is all that is needed in cases of an uncomplicated varicella infection. Aspirin should be avoided because of the possibility of inducing Reye syndrome. Antibiotic treatment will be indicated in secondary bacterial infections. Varicella vaccine became available in the USA in 1995 with the indication for routine vaccination for healthy children at 12-18 months of age or for older children who have not yet had a varicella infection. Varicella vaccine is considered effective in up to 85% of cases but it appears that protection against varicella declines one year post vaccination. Children vaccinated at younger than 14 months are more susceptible to breakthrough infection. Secondary infections are treated with appropriate antibiotics for group A streptococcus and staphylococcus as discussed above.

Rubella (German measles)

When acquired postnatally, it is a benign self-limiting disease which begins 2-3 weeks after exposure and presents with the prodromal phase comprising of mild fever, sore throat, eye pain, headache and lymphadenopathy of the head and neck. In next 1-5 days a maculopapular rash appears on the face, which then progresses to involve rest of the body. The rash begins to clear by day three without leaving any marks. Postpubertal girls are susceptible to persistent arthritis and arthralgia for several weeks. Encephalitis and thrombocytopenic purpura are rare complications.

Erythema infectiosum (fifth disease)

Due to Parvovirus B19 infection, this is usually seen in 4-10 years old children, but does occur in adolescents with outbreaks occurring in late spring and fall. Following a prodromal phase with low grade fever, sore throat, headache, myalgia and arthralgia a confluent erythematous maculopapular rash appears bilaterally on cheeks, in a butterfly fashion sparing the nasal bridge given the slapped cheeks appearance. Mucous membrane involvement is evident with reddish punctate lesions on the buccal mucosa. The rash then spreads to the trunk and on the extensor surface of the limbs, where it persists for about 5-9 days leaving behind a lacy or reticular pattern which fades over time. Exposure to an irritant like sunlight within next few weeks to months may cause recurrence of the rash. Transmission of acute infection from mother to fetus results in failure of erythropoiesis causing development of hydrops fetalis in 10%. Aplastic anemia is seen in patients who are susceptible due to underlying hemoglobinopaties or hemopoetic defects.

Hand-foot-and-mouth disease (HFMD)

This enterovirus (Coxsackie A and B sp) infection is highly contagious and spread by the oral fecal route with epidemics in the USA occurring about every three years. A brief prodromal phase of 12-36 hours presents with abdominal pain, anorexia, burning sensation in mouth, malaise, and low grade fever followed by development of painful erosive lesions on the hard palate and buccal mucosa. A painful vesicular rash on hands and feet appears, more pronounced on the hands especially on the palms and along the sides of the fingers. Symptomatic treatment including attention to nutrition is all that is needed, as painful oral lesions lead to avoidance of food.

Molluscum contagiosum

This common infection of school aged children, due mainly to Poxvirus 1, is highly contagious in close quarters, especially with community facilities such as shared bathtubs, swimming pools etc. Typical dome shaped skin-colored papules are 2-8 mm in size can occur as single or multiple lesions. They then become umblicated and turn pearly white. Common sites are face, hands, trunk and genitalia. Secondary bacterial infections can occur especially in the large papules which can reach up to multiple centimeters in size.

Management

Topical application of cantharidin as 0.7% cantharone is safe when applied sparingly and is effective especially in localized lesions. Other less common therapies include use of the immunomodulatory agent tarcolimus which although effective, may predispose to herpetic infection. Cryotherapy with liquid nitrogen application on each lesion for 6-10 seconds is effective and may need to be repeated in 3 weeks. Imiquimod has also shown some efficacy but evidence is limited. Excision and curettage and electrodessication can be employed when lesions are fewer and localized. Oral cimetidine may shown some efficacy especially when molluscum is associated with atopic dermatitis. As this condition is benign and self-limited, albeit over 6-12 months, watchful waiting is also appropriate in relatively mild cases.

Verruca vulgaris (viral warts)

This Human papilloma virus (HPV) infection is very common affecting up to 10% of children. The most common age group affected is between 12-16 years and it is transmitted by direct person-to-person contact and autoinoculation. Sun exposure can increase susceptibility to warts. Common warts are well circumscribed small papular lesions with a keratinized surface most commonly seen on hands, arms and legs especially on knees and elbows. Filiform warts have frond like projections usually found in the perioral area and on lips. Flat topped, smooth warts occur on sun exposed areas like face neck, and on the dorsum of hands. Planter and palmer warts are more commonly surrounded by an outer keratinized ring. Anogenital warts are cauliflower like soft lesions known as condylomata acuminata.

Management

Warts are self-limiting in 30% cases within 3 months and 78% involute in 2 years. Warts in children have higher spontaneous resolution rates. Topical therapy with keratolytic agents like salicylic acid 10-25% applied topically is effective in 67% of hand warts and 84% in planter warts within 12 weeks. Cryotherapy has a cure rate of 31 to 52% depending on the intensity of treatment. Pain and blister formation at the site of treatment has been reported. Only one study has reported use of topical immunotherapy with dinitrochlorobenzene in 40 children with an 80% cure rate. Imiquimod, an immune modifier has shown some efficacy in anogenital warts in adults but no data are available in children and adolescents. Intra-lesional bleomycin has also shown efficacy of up to 82-94% but the number of subjects studied was small. Mosaic warts are much more resistant to treatment.

HIV/AIDS

The acute exanthem of HIV infection is an erythematous morbilliform rash on trunk and extremities which manifests itself after 2-4 weeks incubation period with a prodrome of fever, lymphadenopathy, night sweats (15). The rash resolves within 5-7 days.

Non-infectious skin lesions

Sweet syndrome is a manifestation of underlying systemic disease characterized by painful violaceous indurated plaques with neutrophilic infiltration of the dermis has been reported in children with HIV/AIDS. Eosinophilic folliculitis is an altered immune response to the common skin antigens and is seen in advanced HIV infection especially when CD4 lymphocyte counts decrease to <200 cells/mm^3. Also, acute urticaria can become chronic urticaria with angioedema and gives rise to indurated lesions with a peau d'orange appearance. Many common skin diseases such as atopic and seborrheic dermatitis become more extensive and difficult to treat in patients with HIV/AIDS. Psoriasis, although not more common in this population, can be very problematic.

Trimethoprim-sulfamethoxazole is the most common drug-related cause of such reactions but other drugs can also caused eruptions including Stevens Johnson syndrome and toxic epidermal necrolysis.

Bacterial infections in HIV

Many bacterial skin infections such as impetigo, folliculitis, furuncles etc. have a very aggressive and extensive course in the HIV/AIDS population. Bacillary angiomatosis presents with pinpoint erythematous macular lesion which may form a larger lesion like pyoderma, is seen more commonly in HIV/AIDs patients and may be confused with Kaposi's sarcoma. Biopsy may be the only way to distinguish between them. It does respond very well to the macrolide antibiotics doxycycline or erythromycin. Incidence of Group B streptococcus (GBS) in infants exposed to HIV infection in utero, is late and more severe than in the non-exposed infants.

Viral infections in HIV

Herpes simplex (HSV) and Herpes zoster (HZV) infections are very common in HIV/AIDS patients. Both of these infections are much more serious, recurrent and recalcitrant to therapy. HZV infections can be debilitating and can involve multiple dermatomes at one time. Since lesions can be extensive, necrotic and atypical, laboratory testing with Tzanck preparation, biopsy of lesion or viral culture is necessary. Acyclovir is the treatment of choice. Incidence of HPV infection in HIV/AIDS patients has increased not only due to increased susceptibility to this infection due to due to immunosuppression but also due to decreased clearance of established infections and reactivation of latent infections. Condylomata Acuminatum (CA) is the most common presentation of HPV in HIV/AIDS patients. They tend to be much larger and numerous, and may spread to involve extensive areas of the body. Hypopigmented verruciform papules can spread easily in children. Common warts including veruccae vulgaris and veruucae plantaris are 16% to 17% more common in this population. Mulloscum Contagiosum occurs in 20% of HIV/AIDS patients which can become generalized affecting large area of body and reaching sizes up to 1 cm.

HPV is responsible for several carcinomas in situ or premalignant lesions including giant CA also known as Buschke-Loewenstein tumor (BLT) and intraepithelial neoplasia of anogenital region, which can progress to become anal, vulvar, or penile carcinoma. Acute cytomegalovirus (CMV) infections are seen in up to 90% of HIV/AIDS patients. Skin manifestations of CMV are varied ranging from vesicular, morbilliform rashes to indurated plaques to ulcerative lesions. These lesions respond well to foscarnet, ganciclovir, or cidofovir. Epstien-Barr virus can cause oral hairy leukoplakia and Burkitt's lymphoma or large cell lymphoma which can be treated with acyclovir at a dosage of 200 to 400 mg 5 times a day and highly active antiretroviral therapy (HAART).

Fungal infections in HIV

The most common fungal infection in HIV patient is candidiasis which could be the only presenting sign of HIV in early phase, with oral thrush. Other areas of involvement axillae, groin, vagina, and under other skin folds where maceration is likely. Systemic fungal infections are common in advance cases of HIV/AIDS like Cryptococcus neoformans presenting with pleomorphic rash. Histoplasma capsulatum may present with skin lesions in about 17% of cases. Spirotrichosis can cause ulcerative papules or nodules along with systemic involvement.

Yeast infections

Superficial candidal infection is most common, affecting skin and mucous membranes. Candida albicans is a budding yeast, which is a commensal organism of mucous membranes and is found around the skin adjacent to mucous membranes, gut and vaginal areas. Carriage in these areas is one other way of acquiring infection. Candidal mucocutaneous infections are common in very young and old and in debilitated populations. Any condition predisposing to defects in immunity especially of cellular immunity can predispose to candidal infections. Candida is known to have specific immunomodulatory effect which can also dampen the host's immune response. Diabetes mellitus is often complicated with mucocutaneous candidal infections. Other situations predisposing to candidiasis include use of antibiotics or corticosteroids, malnutrition, and HIV infection. Candida favors the moist occluded areas of skin most commonly intertriginous, perineal and perianal areas, perine especially in obese patients. Diagnosis can be confirmed by identification of pseudohyphae in a microscopic KOH preparation.

Management

Attempts should be made to keep the affected areas well aerated. Use of mild soap with water with gentle cleansing is recommended. Wet wipes without the strong additives like fragrances or preservatives are also effective. In recurring infection using barrier preparations like petroleum, Titanium oxide in paraffin, Zinc oxide cream can provide added protection against infection. Combination of corticosteroid plus antifungal preparations should be avoided. In any dermatitis where diagnoses is in doubt or which is present for more than 72 hours use of a topical antifungal agent twice daily with continuation for a week after disappearance of the rash is appropriate. Nystatin, ketoconazole, clotrimazole, econazole, miconazole, oxiconazole, and ciclopirox are effective anti-candidal agents.

Fungal infections

Fungal infections are summarized in table 3 (16,17).

Table 3. Clinical aspects of fungal infections

Clinical presentation	Fungi	Site of infection	Other presentations
Tinea Corporis	Microsporum equinum Microsporum fulvum Microsporum gypseum Trichophyton equinum Trichophyton gallinae Trichophyton rubrum Trichophyton tonsurans Epidermophyton floccosum	Anywhere on body Except groin, hair and nails	
Tinea Gladiatorum	Trichophyton verrucosum Trichophyton tonsurans	Highly contagious anywhere on body except groin, hair and nails	
Tinea Facie Tinea Barbae	Trichophyton mentagrophytes	Face and beard area	
Tinea Cruris	Trichophyton rubrum	Groin, perianal and perineal area	Tinea corporis, pedis, & manuum
	Epidermophyton floccosum		Tinea corporis & pedis
Tinea Pedis	Trichophyton interdigitale		Tinea pedis

Fungi are saprophytes, originally soil keratinophiles that have evolved to be able to infect animals and humans. They can be unicellular like Candida or multicellular like Dermatophytes. Candida sp can infect both skin and mucous membrane while dermatophytes can only infect keratinized areas like skin, hair and nails. Skin infections are localized to the stratum corneum, the superficial layer of skin, and never invade the deeper layers. Dermatophytes, also known as Tinea, and commonly called ringworm, have specific predilection for different sites of the body. Dermatophytes are divided in three main groups,

Trichophytons, epidermophyton and microsporum. They spread by direct contact with soil, infected surfaces, or contact with infected body area. The types of infections are classified based on the body area affected. Tinea capitis (head) and fungal nail infections, tinea unguum, as examples, are discussed below.

Tinea corporis

Dermatophyte infections of the body excluding groin area, feet, scalp, facial cheeks, and nails are known as tinea corporis. Trichophyton rubrum is the most prevalent organism. Most commonly infection is acquired via direct skin to skin contact. After invading the stratum corneum, the organism produces hyphae and grows outward producing the typical round or annular lesions with erythematous slightly raised margins surrounding a clear center .The expanding border is scaly and when scraped can provide sample to identify hyphae microscopically.

Tinea gladiatorum

A highly contagious variant of tinea corporis, this is common in populations where physical contact with bare skin occurs. Most cases are reported in wrestlers, but other physical contact sports have been sources of reports of outbreak of such lesions. The infection is more prevalent in seasons of active competitions and intense training. Skin lesions are unlike typical tinea corporis and may appear as scaly erythematous papules and plaques. Lesions have a predilection for the head, neck, and arms and are seldom seen on legs. Spread of infection to other athletes is frequent and covering of localized lesion during sports encounter should be practiced. In cases of extensive rash, there should be avoidance of contact sports. Resumption of such activities can occur after treatment for one week.

Tinea cruris

Commonly known as “jock itch”, this is a superficial fungal infection of inguinal folds, perineal and perianal areas, common in adolescent males, and post pubertal females. Moist, non-aerated areas of skin such as in between skin folds can give rise to maceration which is a perfect breeding ground for dermatophytes such as Trichophyton rubrum, Mentagrophytes sp or Epidermophyton floccosum. It is more common in summer months, and in children or adolescents who are obese or who wear tight fitting under garments, especially in young girls with nylon panty hose. In children participating in team sports the co-occurrence of tinea pedis and tinea cruris is common. At times it is difficult to differentiate between other rashes affecting this area like erythrasma, a chronic intertriginous infection due to Corynebacterium minutissimum which fluoresces orange under Woods lamp examination. Other fungal infection like Candida can be distinguished by presence of pinkish red smooth lesions without a definite border and satellite punctate lesions in adjacent areas. In younger children especially those wearing diapers contact dermatitis can present a diagnostic problem but usually a correlation to the offending agent will be clear. Psoriasis and seborrheic dermatitis are also included in the differential diagnosis.

Tinea pedis

This is a common condition in children and athletes commonly known as athlete’s foot. Sometimes the term “moccasin foot” is used to describe extensive infection where the whole foot is involved in the distribution of a shoe covering the foot. Infection is usually in between toes where moist skin nurtures dermatophytes, producing itchy, macerated lesions with fissuring and often a foul odor. Common risk factors are use of community shower stalls at schools, swimming pools, sports clubs, sharing slippers, socks and shoes, wearing shoes for long time, especially when not wearing absorbent socks and walking barefoot on sandy beach or other moist grounds which can harbor fomites. Most common organisms are the same as in tinea cruris (Table 4) Tinea rubrum affect relatively dry area of foot like heels, soles, and sides producing somewhat thickened pink lesions covered with fine silver scales. Differential diagnosis includes contact and atopic dermatitis, psoriasis, and candidal infection between the toes.

Pityriasis (tinea) versicolor

This superficial fungal infection it is caused by different genus Malassezia and especially by the species Malassezia fufur. It gives rise to typical fine scaly macular lesions mostly affecting the trunk, back and arms but can also involve other areas, especially in children where face involvement is common. It is more frequent in hot and humid climates and in those who use topical corticosteroid, and oil based skin products. It presents differently according to the color of skin of the individual affected hence the name versicolor. In light colored individuals typical leaf like macular lesions are hyperchromic or brownish while in dark colored skin the macules are hypochromic. Lesions have fine white scale on margins and occur in large numbers. A Christmas tree distribution is seen on the back and is pathognomonic of this condition. Lesions are completely asymptomatic and only reason patients seek help is for cosmetic concerns. Vitligo can be confused with tinea.versicolr especially in dark skinned individuals.

Management

Most infections are diagnosed purely on clinical judgment, although a potassium hydroxide (KOH) preparation can provide a cheap, quick and highly sensitive (88%) method of confirming the diagnosis within the office setting. Scrapings of the lesion border are placed on slide with a drop of 10-20 % of KOH and typical septate hyphae of dermatophytes are easy to detect. Wood's light Examination is not as useful in dermatophyte infections other than tinea capitis as Microsporum will fluoresce, whereas the more common Tricophyton will not.

Topical antifungals

These are highly effective in most cases of superficial infections except in tinea capitis and tinea unguium where systemic antifungal treatment is indicated. Commonly used topical preparations are Terbinafine, miconazole and clotrimazole, which can be applied twice daily for two weeks. Butenafine has advantage of once daily application for two weeks with same effectiveness but is more costly. The patient should apply topical medication to about 2 cm of surrounding area past the advancing edge of the infection and should be educated to avoid risk factors predisposing to reinfection.

Combination therapy

Combination preparations including antifungal and corticosteroids are widely used, mostly prescribed when diagnosis is not fully established. There is a growing concern that such treatment leads to partial resolution and quick relapse of infection resulting is prolonged treatment for months. One of the common such preparation available; Clotrimazole/ betamethasone has shown a 45% failure and a 36% relapse rate. Therefore they are not recommended.

Infestations

Head lice

Infestation with pediculosis humanus capitis is very common all over the world with prevalence rates ranging from 2% in United Kingdom to 13% in Australia and 100% in some remote communities of central and South America (18,19). Approximately 6-12 million people are infested with head lice each year in the USA. It usually affects children between ages of 3 to 12 years with a higher preponderance for girls and a lower predilection for African Americans. Head to head contact is the main source of transmission but sharing combs, hats, scarves, hair bands etc. or sleeping on the bedding of the infested person can also cause transmission. Outbreaks in preschools and elementary schools are common. In USA treatment cost associated with head lice infestation is estimated to be $1 billion annually. Head lice feed on the host's blood and can cause significant itching which leads to frequent scratching which in turn may give rise to secondary infections like impetigo. Diagnosis is best established by visualizing the live lice which at times could be very difficult as they tend to hide in areas where the hair is thickest as in the nape of the neck. Use of a louse comb can aid is diagnosis. Diagnosis cannot be established by finding occasional eggs especially >1/4 inch far from the skull as they are most likely dead nits from previous infestation, Finding many nits within ¼ inch of the scalp can be predictive of active infestation in about one third of cases.

Management

Prevention of spread is the most effective way of controlling the infection. Education not to share personal items like combs, hairbrush, hats etc. can be effective in limiting spread. Once the diagnosis is established application of 1% Permethrin, pyrethrins or 0.5% Malathion in children older than 24 months can be effective. 1% Permethrin is very effective in form of a crème rinse when left in the hair for 10 minutes and rinsed. The residue it leaves behind continues to kill the nymphs emerging from eggs. A second application is suggested in 7-10 days, preferably on the 9th day. Pyrethrin preparations are derivatives of chrysanthemums, and should be avoided in children with allergies to ragweed or chrysanthemums. Applied for 10 minutes and rinsed, with a second treatment on the 9th day is recommended. Alternatively, treatment on 0, 7, and between 13 to15 day has been proposed. Efficacy has decreased due to development of resistance. Malathion 0.5% is an organophosphate and is applied to dry hair and left for 8-12 hours with good ovicidal activity. Repeat application is not necessary unless live lice are detected, in which case reapplication on day 7-9 is recommended. Benzyl Alcohol 5% is approved for use in infants older than 6 months. Lindane 1% (gamma benzene hexachloride) shampoo is contraindicated in neonates and is not recommended for children less than 50 kg in weight because of seizure risk. A single oral dose of ivermectin 200 µg /kg has shown 74% effectiveness which increased to 95% when dose was repeated at 10 days. Prophylactic treatment of persons sharing the same bedding is recommended. All clothes, hairbrushes, combs and linens used 2 days prior to treatment should be washed in hot water (130° F). Floor and furniture can be vacuumed with minimal risk of transmission after 1-2 days.

Scabies

Scabies affects people of all social classes and ages, but it is more commonly seen in children and adolescents (20). It is estimated that about 300 million new cases occur worldwide each year. Caused by an arthropod Sarcoptes scabiei var hominis, this mite can not only transmit by skin-to-skin contact but also by contact with contaminated material like bedding or clothing where it can survive for up to 36 hours. Scabies is more common in crowded urban areas. Children are more at risk due to their propensity of being in close contact with each other. Teenage girls tend to be the highest group affected. After an incubation period of 3-6 weeks, the female mite burrows in the epidermis where it lays eggs. The larva emerges within 2-3 days and matures in an adult mite within 15 days increasing the population of mite thus the risk of transmission to others. The ensuing rash is highly pruritic due to a hypersensitivity reaction to the mite. Itching is worse during night when the skin is warmer. Scratching may cause excoriations and breaks in skin leading to secondary infections like impetigo. The initial lesion is a small erythematous papule, which can become a vesicle or pustule. Typical lesions are small linear brownish lesions called burrows, most commonly seen in between the finger webs, but also can be found along the sides of fingers, on the border of hand, flexor aspects of wrist. Other areas like, elbows, axilla, buttocks and genitalia can be affected.

Management

Diagnosis is confirmed by clinical examination and by finding typical burrow lesions in between finger webs. Attempt should be made to extract the mite, or eggs from these burrows by gently scraping and examination under light microscope. Failure to isolate mite or eggs does not rule out scabies and treatment can be started based on clinical judgment. Videodermatoscopy can provide high-resolution magnification of skin up to 600 times under incidental light and is a noninvasive and effective diagnostic tool to locate mites and eggs. Other techniques, epiluminescence microscopy and dermatoscopy have also shown diagnostic accuracy. Permethrin 5% cream is effective and safe when applied to the whole body including head and washed off after 8-12 hours, with reapplication recommended after 2 weeks. Transient burning and erythema can occur.

Malathion 0.5% an organophosphate applied to body and left for 24 hours is also effective. Lindane 1% has now become a second line treatment due to the concerns with neurotoxicity in cases of accidental ingestion, and wwith local irritation and continued itching. With randomized controlled trials, in comparison to topical crotamiton, lindane and oral ivermectin, permethrin has shown superior results. Permethrin was also found to be more effective in relieving itch in comparison to lindane and crotamiton. Oral ivermectin is shown to be effective treatment when topical treatment is not effective or disease is severe and widespread. Oral ivermectin is not indicated in children less then <15 kg in weight.

Cutaneous larva migrans (CLM)

Cutaneous larva migrans is a most common infestation acquired during travel. CLM is caused mostly by hookworm Ancylostoma brazilienseis, and less commonly by Ancylostoma caninum. Hookworms are most commonly found in tropical and subtropical countries in Southeast Asia, South and Central America and southern states of the USA. Ancylostoma brazilienseis and related hookworms are also common in Australia, Caribbean and in some parts of Europe. The adult hookworm lives in intestines of cats and dogs; ova are shed via feces in the soil where they larvae are hatched where they survive for several weeks. The most common risk factor for CLM infestation is walking bare foot on beach but any contact between uncovered skin and contaminated soil or sand can cause the transmission. Upon becoming attached to bare skin the larva secretes hyaluronidase to gain entry in the superficial layers of skin. After an incubation period of up to 6 days the typical erythematous serpiginous lesion develops known as creeping eruption or creeping dermatitis.

Vesicles and bullae also develop along the larva migration track along with local edema. Intense pruritus may also give rise to excoriation and secondary infection. Since humans are incidental hosts once the larvae cannot penetrate deep enough to gain entry in deeper tissue their journey comes to a natural end with death of the larvae. The lesion completely resolves within 8 weeks, but in rare cases it may persist for longer. On rare occasion systemic invasion can lead to development of Loffler's syndrome characterized by transient pulmonary infiltrate, eosinophilia, and hepatomegaly.

Management

Diagnosis can be established clinically with a temporal relationship with a visit to endemic areas, and finding the typical creeping eruption about 3mm wide which grows in length by few mm to few cm daily. No specific serological markers or specific diagnostic test are available for diagnosis of CLM. Eosinophilia can be present in about 20% of cases. Ivermectin is well tolerated and very effective when used as a single dose of 200 μg /kg with a cure rate of 94%. In cases of treatment failure the same dose can be repeated in 7 days to ensure complete eradication of infection. The rash and pruritus may take few days to resolve. Albendazole for children 6 years and older 15mg/kg//day in divided doses with maximum daily dose of 800 mg/day for 3 days is also effective. In younger children topical albendazole 10% ointment applied twice daily for 10 days can be effective.

Dermatitis

Irritant dermatitis

The most common irritant dermatitis occurs in infants in diapers secondary to contact with urine and feces. In children and adolescents caustics such as acids, alkali or hydrocarbons are the etiologic agents and usually cause an acute irritating reaction.

Management of irritant dermatitis consists mainly of identifying and ridding the patient of the offending agent.

Dry-skin dermatitis

This is generally due to excessive drying of the skin with agents such as soaps, alcohols, lotions or low humidity. It may occur in patterns, an example of which is "lip-smacking" dermatitis presenting as dry erythematous irritation around the lips. Another example of dry-skin dermatitis is Juvenile plantar dermatosis (JPD or "sweaty sock syndrome") presenting initially as erythema of the larger toes and subsequent peeling of the weight-bearing aspects of the plantar aspect of the feet. It is often mistaken for Tinea pedis (athlete's foot) which occurs initially at the smaller toes and more over the dorsum of the foot.

The goal of management of dry-skin dermatitis is to provide sufficient water to the skin plus a means of keeping it there, usually through liberal use of lubricants. The use of water-in-oil emulsions will also serve this purpose.

Seborrheic dermatitis

Seborrheic dermatitis is due to over-production of sebum from sebaceous glands and appears as a greasy accumulation of scales (21). The lesions are diffuse in infants, more over the face and scalp (cradle cap) as well as in the flexural areas. In adolescents, seborrhea is relegated mainly to the scalp (dandruff) the naso-labial folds, post-auricular area and the chest. It may be confused with fungal lesions, eczema, contact dermatitis or psoriasis. The etiology of this condition is unknown although association with the yeast Pityrosporum sp. has been demonstrated. It remains unclear whether this yeast is causal or acts as an agent in the inflammatory process. Treatment consists of low-potency topical steroids. Keratolytics (salicylic acid) inhibitors of epithelialization (selenium sulfide) and antifungal shampoos (ketoconazole) may be applied locally, but should be used judiciously around the face as they can be irritating to the eyes.

Allergic dermatitides

Atopic dermatitis

Atopic dermatitis is a hereditary condition associated with other allergic hypersensitivity such as asthma and/or allergic rhinitis (22,23). Often the respiratory problems are seasonal. When occurring in smaller children, the rash is more diffuse, but by early childhood and adolescence it appears primarily in the flexural creases and the dorsum of the hands. The skin is often dry.

The initial lesion may be erythematous papules, or in the case of darker-skinned individuals a follicular hyperkeratosis (chicken-skin) appearance. The skin is invariably pruritic, which then sets off the classic "itch-scratch-itch" cycle. The lesions then may start weeping, become excoriated, fissured and eventually lichenified. There also may be post inflammatory hypo- or hyperpigmentation in the affected areas.

There may be physical findings associated with allergy such as Dennie lines under the eyes or the "allergic salute" consisting of horizontal creases on the bridge of the nose. The may be peripheral eosinophilia or elevated serum IgE levels. Lesions may flare up due to overheating, over-drying, sweating or other contact allergens. Also, secondary bacterial infection or herpetic infection (eczema herpeticum, Kaposi's varicelliform eruption) may worsen the appearance considerably. The etiology of atopic dermatitis remains elusive.

Although there have been associations with other conditions causing dry skin, such as icthyosis, with food intake or presence of house dust mites, or with immunodeficiency, as in Wiskott-Aldrich syndrome, there are no studies that convincingly demonstrate a cause-effect link.

The management of atopic dermatitis is long term and is often fraught with relapses and much frustration on the part of both patients and physicians. If there is a family history of atopy, the patient may be more familiar with the necessary course of treatment, but it is nonetheless important for the clinician to stress the chronicity as well as the frequency of flare-ups.

Management of atopic dermatitis

There are four main goals to therapy:

- Dryness of skin: Emollients soften the surface of the skin, allowing for exposure of extra water-binding sites. Examples of this are a-hydroxy acids, lactic acid, salicylic acid and urea which remove excess scales form the skin. Lubricants will aid in retention of water either by attracting water to the skin or by containing vehicles that will prevent water from escaping the skin (occlusion). Petrolatum is a commonly used vehicle to aid in the retention of heat and moisture, but can feel greasy to the patient with subsequent low-compliance to therapy. Substances such as cetyl or stearyl alcohol when added to petrolatum will feel more comfortable to the patient as well as increase the ability of the petrolatum to take up water. Creams and lotions are oil-in-water emulsions and are effective in less-severe cases. They are more cosmetically pleasing to the patient and are more easily removable. Ointments contain more water-insoluble components which does have maximal occlusive properties. As they can be disagreeable to the patient, emulsifiers added to them may increase compliance, although they may diminish water-retention. Gels are primarily useful to facilitate penetration of other topical medications. Because they have an alcoholic base they can sting when applied.
- Pruritus: Management of prutitus consists of oral sedating antihistamines used primarily at night to prevent scratching and subsequent excoriation. Examples of such medications are hydroxyzine, 1 mg/kg/dose at bedtime or Cetirizine 2.5 mg under age 6 and 5 mg over age six at bedtime.
- Inflammation: The mainstay of anti-inflammatory management of atopic dermatitis is the use of topical steroids. The main issues for treatment revolve about the choice of the medication and the means by which it is applied. As the treatment of atopic dermatitis is multi-pronged, it is important to combine skin moisturization with the use of topical steroids, and flexibly, with the ultimate goal of diminishing the potency of the steroids and hopefully their use altogether, until the next relapse. The art of management of atopic dermatitis lies in the juxtaposition of different modes of treatment. The choice of a steroid should begin with one of low potency, such as Hydrocortisone 2.5% or Desonide 0.05%. If not effective, mid-potency steroids such as Fluocinolone acetonide 0.025%), or Triamcinolone 0.1% may be of help. Less frequently, high-potency steroids such as betamethasone dipopionate cream 0.05% may be necessary. It is important to recognize the consequences of overuse of topical

steroids, particularly in areas such as the face and genital area, such as skin atrophy and striae. Table 4 below lists topical steroid medications with their potencies.

Prior to resorting to high-potency steroid topical therapy, often moist occlusive dressings are effective, applying damp cotton gauze followed by dry cotton gauze over a moderate-potency steroid. This may be difficult in an adolescent who would be embarrassed to be seen in them during the day, so it may be employed while at home and during sleep. If is often necessary to encourage parents continuously to maintain this treatment. Patient and parental education is of foremost importance to maintain effectively the treatment plan, even in the face of many failures and frustrations along the way.

Treatment failure with the above may necessitate a dermatologist referral. Some primary care physicians may try coal tar applications to restore normal keratinization or immunosuppressive agents such as tacrolimus or pimecrolimus. Coal tar preparations stain and have an unpleasant odor, often a barrier to compliance. Immunosuppressive agents may be irritating to the skin when applied.

- Complications (secondary infection): Treating secondary bacterial infections is of paramount importance. The most common infecting agents are Staphylococcus aureus, Stpretococcus pyogenes and Herpes simplex. Appropriate antibiotic therapy, local or systemic, is necessary to treat these complications.

Contact dermatitis

Contact dermatitis occurs as the result of incomplete antigens, called haptens which penetrate the epidermis, are carried to lymph nodes where they are presented to T lymphocytes which then migrate back to the skin. Depending on the strength of the antigen (e. g. poison ivy or urushiol), it may take a week to process, or considerably longer for weaker allergens such as nickel.

Upon a second exposure to the antigen, the inflammatory reaction occurs with the T lymphocyte releasing inflammatory mediators resulting in acute erythematous, often vesicular, pruritic dermatitis. The hallmark of diagnosis is recognition of the distribution and pattern of the dermatitis.

Typically it occurs only at the area of contact. Often a streaky appearance is the clue to the patient having brushed against the allergen while in a wooded area. If the lesions due to contact with poison ivy or poison oak appear to be diffuse, it is due to the patient having spread the oil with his hands at the time of initial contact. Often the shape of the lesion is helpful. If it is close to perfectly round, it may be secondary to a metallic contact such as clothing snaps.

The location may also be helpful as in nickel in earrings causing lesions about the ear lobes. Allergens present in leather or rubber may cause sensitization of the feet and toes. Perfumes, soaps and make-up will cause dermatitis in the regions to which they are applied. Treatment consists of local applications of low potency corticosteroids and antihistamines to lessen the pruritic component. Generally symptoms last for 3-4 weeks with or without treatment.

Idiopathic dermatitides

Dyshidrotic eczema

This condition has been erroneously considered to be secondary to dysfunction of the eccrine, or sweat glands. However histopathology demonstrates normal sweat glands. As there is a clinical association with atopy and contact irritants, a single etiology remains elusive. It presents with highly pruritic vesicles starting at the lateral aspects of the digits which eventually progress to fissuring and cracking of the palms and soles. Treatment is similar to atopic eczema usually with low-potency corticosteroid ointments and, if necessary moisture applications followed by covered dry dressings.

Keratosis pilaris

This common condition presents as follicular plugs of stratum corneum and appear most often on the extensor aspects of the upper and lower extremities and buttocks. It may also appear on the facial cheeks in younger children, especially during colder and dryer months. The lesions feel rough and dry and may be either flesh-colored or erythematous. Associations with atopy and icthyosis have been reported, but this condition often occurs independently. This condition may be chronic and responds to moisturizers (Urea) and keratoltics (Lactic acid or Retinoic acid).

Nummular eczema

This condition may be associated with atopic eczema, but may also occur independently. It is characterized by coin-like lesions, can be intensely pruritic and is treated similarly as atopic eczema. The duration of treatment is considerably longer than that of atopic dermatitis.

Hypersensitivity

Acute urticaria

This condition is short-lived and more often a consequence of infection (24). Bacterial etiologies include streptococcus, viral include EB virus, hepatitis and others. Urticaria may be allergic in nature, with elevated IgE levels and histamine mediation of the skin reaction, although only 3-5% of cases have been reported with this etiology confirmed. Allergic agents include hymenoptera, scorpions and jellyfish stings, drug reactions, food allergies, particularly to peanuts, tree nuts, eggs, shellfish, berries and tomatoes. Scombroid fish with high amounts of histamine may cause this reaction. Urticaria may be a manifestation of systemic diseases which is discussed in the section below. The hallmark lesion of urticaria is the wheal and flare which is very pruritic. It is transitory in nature, but with several relapses and remissions over a few days.

The course is generally benign and self-limited; however, there may be associated angioedema with swelling particularly of the hands and feet. During more severe local reactions there may be blistering with weeping clear fluid, often mistaken for bacterial cellulitis. Over time, urticarial lesions may appear dusky and be mistaken for ecchymoses. One must always be mindful of a more severe generalized reaction with upper airway obstruction due to oropharyngeal swelling (anaphylaxis).

Several conditions may be confused with urticaria such as hereditary angiodedma (C'1 esterase deficiency), erythema multiforme (target lesions), vasculitis, urticaria pigmentosa (mastocytosis) and viral exanthems.

Chronic urticaria

This condition is defined by symptoms lasting for more than 4-6 weeks. About 15% of them are the physical urticarias which are secondary to heat, exercise, cold or pressure (25). Cold urticarias may be hereditary or of immunogenic origin. Cases of severe anaphylactic reactions have been reported in patients with this condition jumping into cold water. Pressure and some cold urticarias are histamine-mediated, but others may be mediated through cholinergic nerves.

Management of urticaria

Acute urticaria that is not severe is best treated with antihistamines. Sedating antihistamines such as Hydroxyzine 1-2 mg/kg/day and Diphenhydramine 5 mg/kg/day, are more effective than non-sedating antihistamines. In more severe cases, adrenergic medications may be necessary to manage angioedema. In severe cases of anaphylaxis, airway maintenance is the first priority. Epinephrine, subcutaneously 0.01ml/kg of a 1:1000 solution acts rapidly in this situation. Albuterol inhalers may be used, as well as oral pseudoephedrine, but these may cause significant adrenergic side-effects.

Patients should be counseled that the course may last up to 6 weeks. If longer, then further studies are necessary to identify the type of chronic urticaria. Simple placement of ice on a patient's skin for several minutes will produce the wheal and flare. Similarly, heat and exercise or pressure will reproduce urticaria. Cold-agglutinins and cryoglobulins may be identified. Further studies to look for an infectious or autoimmune etiology may be necessary.

Erythema multiforme

This condition presents as fixed erythematous lesions varying in size and shape without prodrome. They follow an outbreak of Herpes labialis in about 50% of cases. The lesions last several weeks and progress to the classical "target" or "iris" lesions, occurring most commonly over extensor surfaces in an acral distribution. They may turn dusky or become encrusted over time. Oral involvement occurs rarely and is not extensive. There are few systemic symptoms and the condition is self-limiting. Subsequent Herpes labialis infections will induce recurrences. Although formerly connected with Stevens-Johnson syndrome

(SJS,see below), it is now considered a separate entity. One should no longer use the terms "erythema multiforme minor "and "erythema multiforme major." Treatment is expectant and occasional use of antihistamines may relieve rare instances of pruritus.

Drug eruptions

The most common drug eruptions are morbiliform (measles-like), urticarial and fixed. Others include pustular, phototoxic, scarletiniform, bullous and lichenoid (26-28).

Morbilliform eruptions

These rashes are diffuse maculopapular which appear about 1-3 weeks after institution of the medication. They are the most common and account for up to 50% of drug eruptions. There may or may not be pruritus. The rash usually involves the trunk and extremities and may ultimately become confluent. The most common offending agents are antibiotics, anticonvulsants, antifungals and non-steroidal anti-inflammatory agents. It is paramount to elicit a drug history in all patients with rashes. It is also important to consider that the primary illness may be the cause of the rash (strep, EB virus). Amoxicillin may elicit a morbilliform rash in a patient with EB viral infection 50% of the time.

Urticarial drug eruptions

These IgE-mediated reactions are the second-most common drug eruptions accounting for about 25% of them. They present as a wheal-and flare from hours to days after exposure and may be associated with angioedema, although rarely anaphylaxis. The intravenous or intramuscular route is more likely to cause anaphylaxis than oral dosing. Drugs most commonly associated with this condition are non-steroidal anti-inflammatory medications, antibiotics (penicillins, cephalosporins and sulfonamides). Note that Cefaclor produces a reaction resembling serum-sickness.

Fixed drug eruptions

These present as erythematous lesions of varying size, appearing at first urticarial, but then becoming well-demarcated and eventually hyperpigmented. The main offending drugs are antibiotics (Trimethoprim, Sulfonamides, Tetracyclines, and Ciprofloxacin), anticonvulsants (Barbiturates, Carbamazepine) and oral contraceptives. They recover slowly over months and re-occur with re-introduction of the offending agent.

Less common drug eruptions

Less common drug eruptions include vasculitis, erythema nodosum, photosensitivity, lichenoid and bullous eruptions. Offending agents for vasculitis include anticonvulsants, NSAIDS, antibiotics (penicillins, sulfonamides and macrolides), gold, diuretics and cimetidine. Erythema nodosum is associated with oral contraceptives, NSAIDs, sulfonamides and opiates. Photosensitive reactions may be phototoxic, due to direct damage due to sunlight altering the drug. They occur in sun-exposed areas and are often quite painful, resembling severe sunburn. The more common offending agents are antibiotics, particularly Tetracycline, Sulfa drugs, griseofulvin, ANSAIDs, diuretics (furosemide, thiazides), psoralens and coal tar derivatives. The other photosensitive reaction is a true allergy presenting as severe urticaria in sun-exposed areas. Ultra-violet light acts directly on the drug, altering it to an allergenic form. The most common offending agents are perfumes, para-amino benzoic acid, phenothiazines and sulfonamides. Lichenoid reactions occur months after exposure to drugs such as diuretics, beta blockers and phenothiazines, and their violaceous plaques are often mistaken for rashes associated with collagen vascular disorders.

Life threatening eruptions

Stevens Johnson Syndrome (SJS) and Toxic Epidermal Necrolysis (TEN) were once considered part of the spectrum of "erythema multiforme" but are now separated from that condition (29). It is difficult to distinguish SJS from TEN clinically and pathologically (separation at the dermal-epidermal junction) and therefore, some consider the two conditions a continuum with TEN being a more severe form. Some experts have defined SJS as epidermal detachment of <10% of body surface area, TEN as >30%. They present with a 1-2 week prodrome consisting of fever, headache, malaise, vomiting and/or diarrhea. Skin involvement consists of blisters, progressing to bullae with epidermal necrosis. There is mucosal involvement, frequently occurring 1-2 days before the cutaneous lesions in at least two sites. Especially involved are the mouth and eyes with crusty hemorrhagic lesions, but involvement may extend to the lower gastrointestinal tract kidneys, liver, heart and genitourinary tract in more severe instances. Skin and mucosal lesions often result in severe scarring, contracture and dyschromia, and there may be permanent damage to the nails.

Triggers are most commonly antibiotics (sulfonamides, penicillins), anticonvulsants and NSAIDS. In rare instances Herpes simplex and Mycoplasma pneumonia have been implicated. There is evidence that there may be a genetic predisposition for these conditions. One study confirmed evidence of a gene, HLA-B1502 associated with SJS in Han Chinese population after intake of carbamazepine. Outcomes can be poor with a mortality rate of up to 30% reported

Management of drug eruptions

The hallmark of management of drug reactions is prompt discontinuation of the offending agent. If there is any concern about anaphylaxis, airway must be maintained and subcutaneous epinephrine 1:1000, 0.01 cc/kg up to 0.5cc should be administered immediately with intravenous fluids. Systemic steroids may also be of benefit. In the event of anaphylaxis, the patient should carry information of this allergy usually as a wrist-band. In addition, it is paramount to document all allergies on the patient's medical record.

Most other reactions (urticarial, fixed or lichenoid) are not life-threatening and may take several weeks to months to subside. Medication is generally not necessary, although antihistamines may be of benefit for pruritus in urticarial reactions.

Treatment of SJS and TEN is challenging. The conditions manifest themselves clinically as burns and appropriate fluid replacement is necessary. As with burns, the lesions must be kept clean and debrided with serial cultures and appropriate antibiotic therapy as warranted. The use of corticosteroids and intravenous immunoglobulin is controversial. It is important to obtain dermatologic and ophthalmologic consultation to prevent or treat keratitis, iritis and scarring. Oral and airway hygiene is important as is support with total parenteral nutrition.

Miscellaneous skin conditions

Acne vulgaris

Acne vulgaris is one of the most common skin problems in primary care and dermatology offices (30,31). It usually begins at the onset of puberty. Genetic susceptibility influences development of acne and relates to severity.

Pathogenesis of acne involves multiple factors including abnormal keratinization, hormone and sebum production (androgen stimulation), bacterial colonization (Propionibacterium acnes) and host immune response with inflammation.

The obstruction of a pilosebaceous unit on the face, a follicular plug, is a microcomedone caused by excessive amount of sebum from desquamated epithelial cells in the follicular wall. Adrenal and gonadal androgens during the adolescent period affect sebum production. Microcomedones subsequently change to comedones in black head (opened head) and white head (closed head) forms. Propionibacterium acnes a Gram-positive anaerobic bacteria, colonizes at pilosebaceous follicles. This bacterium hydrolyzes triglycerides to free fatty acids (FFA) and produces proinflammatory mediators and chemotactic factors that are the causes of inflammation. This results in papules, pustules and nodulocystic acne. The severity of acne correlates with stage of sexual maturity and rate of sebum production.

The proposed trigger factors of acne are stress (activation of androgen hormone), mechanical factors, topical products (obstruction pilosebaceous unit) and medications (anabolic steroid, progestin, isoniazid, phenytoin, vitamin B12).

The presentation of acne is variable and includes comedones, papules, pustules, cysts, nodules, scarring and dyspigmentation at the face, neck, chest, back area.

Management of acne

Topical therapy

- Benzoyl peroxide: The mechanisms of action are antimicrobial, comedolytic and anti-inflammatory. These actions are useful in mild inflammatory and/or comedonal acne. There are varieties of concentration (2.5-10%), preparation (gel, wash, foam, cream) and it also comes in combination with other medications (topical antibacterial, vitamin A). This agent is usually used as a thin coat (pea sized) to all acne prone areas once to twice daily. The common side effects are stinging, drying, redness, peeling of the skin and bleaching of colored clothes.

- Topical antibiotics: The mechanisms of action are reduction of bacteria on the skin surface, within follicles and anti-inflammatory effects. The most common topical medications are clindamycin and erythromycin. Less commonly used are metronidazole and sulfonamide (sulfacetamide). These medications are appropriately used in mild to moderate acne, mixed inflammatory and comedonal acne, usually once to twice daily. Data recently show topical antibacterial resistance of P. acnes to erythromycin or clindamycin. Multiple drugs resistance is also reported. Recommendations for topical antibiotics are short-term use and avoidance of concomitant oral and topical therapy with the same medication. The combination use of topical antibiotics with topical benzoyl peroxide or topical retinoid decreases the risk of resistance. Antibiotics used in the treatment of acne are summarized in Table 5.
- Retinoids: The mechanisms of action are normalization of keratinization, comedolytic and anti-inflammatory effects. There are varieties of concentration, 0.01 and 0.1%, preparations, gel, microgel, cream form, vitamin A, and.adapalene. One may combine retinoids with other products such as benzoyl peroxide or tazarotene. The combination of many products enhances therapeutic efficacy. This agents are usually used as a thin coat (pea sized) once nightly on the dry face because of the effects of skin irritation and sun sensitivity. Post-inflammatory hypo-hyperpigmentation may occur in darker-skinned individuals. To prevent these effects begin with a lower strength preparation. The evidence of teratogenicity from topical retinoid use is inconclusive (pregnancy category C classification, no controlled studies in women; risk to the fetus cannot be ruled out).
- Azelaic acid: This medication is produced from the yeast Pityrosporum ovale. The mechanisms of action are minimal both in antibacterial and anti-comedonal effect. It may be an alternative treatment for mild inflammatory and comedonal acne. The dominantly beneficial effect is ability to ameliorate hyperpigmented lesions. The available form is a 20% cream. The side effects are pruritus, burning and erythema.
- Dapsone: This medication has FDA approval for treatment of acne. The available form is 5% gel. The supportive evidence of efficacy is lesion reduction in number and improvement of acne severity.

Systemic therapy

- Oral antibiotics: Oral antibiotics are used in cases of moderate to severe inflammatory acne. The mechanisms of action are decrease P. acnes resulting in decreased inflammation from reduction of neutrophil chemotaxis and pro-inflammatory cytokines. They are generally used to control the acne for several months, with improvement in 4-8 weeks after initiation. The most commonly twice-daily antibiotics used are tetracycline, doxycycline, minocycline and erythromycin. Table 4 below summarizes antibiotic treatment of acne.

Table 4. Topical steroids in treatment of atopic dermatitis. Adapted from The Harriet Lane Handbook 18th edition Mosby/Elsevier 2009

Generic Name	Brand Name
Class I	
Clobetasol proprionate	Temovate 0.05%
Betamethasone dipropionate	Diprolene 0.05% cream or ointment.
Class II	
Betamethasone diproprionate	Diprosone 0.05% ointment
Mometasone furoate	Elocon 0.1% ointment
Halcinonide	Halog 0.1%
Flucinonide	Lidex 0.05%
Desoximetasone	Topicort 0.25% cream, 0.05% gel
Class III	
Triamcinolone acetonide	Aristocort A 0.1% ointment
Betamethasone dipropionate	Diprosone 0.05% cream
Betamethasone valerate	Valisone 0.1% ointment
Class IV	
Triamcinolone acetonide	Aristocort 0.1% ointment
Flurandrenolide	Cordran 0.05% ointment
Mometasone furorate	Elocon 0.1% cream, lotion
Triamcinolone acetonide	Kenalog 0.1% cream or ointment
Fluocinolone	Synalar 0.025% ointment
Desoximetasone	Topicort LP 0.05% cream
Class V	
Flurandrenolide	Cordran 0.05% cream
Triamcinolone acetonide	Kenalog 0.1% lotion, 0.025% ointment
Fluocinolone	Synalar 0.025% cream
Tridesilon	Desonide 0.05% ointment
Betamethasone	Valisone 0.1% cream or lotion
Hydrocortisone valerate	Westcort 0.2% cream or lotion
Class VI	
Triamcinolone acetonide	Aristocort 0.01% cream, Kenalog 0.25% cream or ointment
	Locorten 0.03% cream
Flumetasone pivalate	Desonide 0.05% cream
Tridesilon	
Class VII	
Hydrocortisone	Hytone 1% or 2.5% lotion cream or ointment

Table 5. Oral antibiotics for treatment of acne

Drug	Dose / Frequency	Age	Side effects	Remarks
Tetracycline Cap (250, 500 mg)	250-500 mg Twice daily	Age > 9 yrs.	-Dental staining -GI upset, esophageal irritation -Photosensitivity	-Empty stomach -Avoid taking with antacid, dairy products -Take with a large glass of water
Doxycycline Cap (50, 100 mg)	50-100 mg Twice daily	Age > 9 yrs.	-Dental staining (less) -GI upset -Photosensitivity / photo-onycholysis	-Avoid taking with dairy products
Minocycline Cap (50, 100 mg)	50-100 mg Twice daily	Age > 9 yrs.	-Dental staining (less) -GI upset, hepatitis -Blue-gray skin pigmentation -Drug induced lupus -Headache, vertigo (vestibular disturbance) -Serum sickness like reaction	-Empty stomach -Avoid taking with dairy products
Erythromycin Tab (250,500 mg)	250-500 mg Twice daily	Any age	-GI upset	-Empty stomach
Trimetroprim-sufamethoxazole Tab (80/400, 160/800 mg)	80/400, 160/800 mg Once / twice daily	Any age	-Drug hypersensitivity reaction -Bone marrow suppression -GI upset, hepatitis -Renal toxicity	-Avoid in G6PD -Use as second-line drug
Cephalexin Tab (250, 500 mg)	250-500 mg Twice daily	Any age	-GI upset	Use as second-line drug

- Isotretinoin: Isotretinoin is cis-retinoic acid, a derivative of vitamin A, usually used in recalcitrant acne with severe and nodulocystic lesions. The mechanism of action is to eradicate all types of acne pathogenesis. This medication is usually started on dose 0.5-1 mg/kg/day up dose to 2 mg/kg/day. A cumulative dose of 100-150 mg/kg associated with successful treatment. The dose and duration of therapy depends on individual response, and a repeated course maybe necessary. The potential side effects are dry skin and mucosa, alopecia, pseudotumor cerebri (esp. taken with oral antibiotics), abnormal lipid profiles and liver function tests, exacerbation of inflammatory bowel disease and teratogenic effects (pregnancy category X classification). Female patients must be tested to reassure that they are not pregnant before beginning isotretinoin and be supervised to have at least two methods of contraception during the course of treatment. Signature of a consent form with risks and benefits is required before initiation of treatment.

Hormonal therapy

Hormonal therapy is an optional treatment in female patients especially in hyperandrogenic acne (hirsutism, androgenetic alopecia, menstrual irregularity, polycystic ovarian syndrome). The mechanisms of action are reduction of active free testosterone and ovarian androgen production. Oral contraceptive pills, norgestimate and ethinyl estradiol are approved by FDA to treat acne vulgaris.

Spironolactone, anti-androgenic agonist, is also an optional treatment in females. The side effects are breast soreness, menstrual irregularities, hyperkalemia and fatigue.

Nevi

Melanocytic nevi

The melanocytic nevus is a common skin disorder and may be congenital or acquired (32). The acquired form may be due to internal factors (genetic, race, skin type, hormone, and pregnancy) or external factors (sun exposure, cutaneous surgery, systemic immunosuppression, medications). Melanocytic nevi result from benign proliferation of melanocytes leading to accumulation of nevus cells (nevocyte) in the layers of skin. This condition is divided into junctional nevi (nevocytes in dermo-epidermal junction), compound nevi (nevocytes in the junction and dermis) and intradermal nevi (nevocytes limited to the dermis).The risk of transformation from melanocytic nevus to malignant melanoma is extremely low.

Congenital melanocytic nevi (CMN)

These lesions usually present at birth or in the first year of life. CMN is most commonly classified based on the diameter into three groups:

- Small (<1.5 cm. in diameter)
- Medium (1.5-19.9 cm. in diameter)
- Large/ giant (>20 cm. in diameter)

Giant melanocytic nevi in the neonatal period are considered when the size is larger than the palm of baby (about 6 cm.). CMN usually are brown colored macules, papules or patches on any location of the body. Giant melanocytic nevi tend to have color, size and texture, variation and become hairy with increasing age. The posterior trunk is the most common location of giant melanocytic nevi.

CMN of all sizes carry an increased risk of malignant melanoma especially in giant melanocytic nevi. Higher malignancy risk of giant melanocytic nevus is associated with large diameter, increasing of satellite lesions and location of the back. Malignancy risk rates range between 2 and 4% for giant congenital nevi. The malignancy risk for small congenital nevi is unknown but is probably less than 1%.

Neurocutaneous melanosis (NCM) is due to proliferation of intracerebral melanocytes which may result in seizure, malignant melanoma of CNS, increased intracranial pressure and spinal cord compression. NCM is mostly found in giant melanocytic nevi with satellite lesions.

The treatment of giant melanocytic nevus is complicated and controversial. The vast majority are simply followed with biopsy or removal only when worrisome lesions arise. Factors in management include location, size, neurocutaneous melanosis, cosmetic result, risk of malignant melanoma and anesthetic issues. Multidisciplinary approach with the patients and families should be provided.

Spitz nevus

The presentation of a Spitz nevus is a well-circumscribed reddish-brown dome-shaped papules or nodule, mostly as a solitary lesion. Spitz nevi are predominant in the pediatric population and most commonly occur on the face, neck and lower extremities.

They are usually acquired proliferations of melanocytes with histopathological features which sometime overlap with melanoma.

The differential diagnosis consists of atypical melanocytic nevus, melanoma, pyogenic granuloma and early stage of juvenile xanthogranuloma.

Although the potential risk of malignant transformation is minimal, there is no definite consensus on the management of Spitz nevi. Surgical excision to confirm the diagnosis and risk of malignancy is the usual approach. Care should be taken to remove the entire lesion on the first biopsy as examination of the deep component is essential for a correct diagnosis.

Halo nevus (Sutton's nevus)

This presents as a halo or hypopigmented macule surrounding a pigmented nevus. The halo is usually symmetrical and with a regular in border differing from the irregular halo of melanoma. The most common location of halo nevi is on the back. Half of the patients have multiple lesions.

Pathogenesis of this disorder is unknown. It has been proposed to be an immune-mediated attack to the nevus cells in the lesion. Autoimmune conditions such as vitiligo and thyroiditis are rarely found together with halo nevi.

The treatment of halo nevi is observational. Excision is unnecessary when the central lesion appears benign.

Nevus spilus (Speckled lentiginous nevus)

The initial lesion may reveal a large brown patch in the first few years of life and gradually develops the secondary variable darker lesion of superimposed, small-pigmented macules and/or papules. It is typically solitary. The trunk and extremities are the most common locations. The lesion varies in size.

The characteristic presentation is multiple dark brown to black macules superimposed on the larger brown patch.

Nevus spilus should be monitored because of the potential risk of malignant transformation.

Becker's nevus

Becker's nevi are acquired. The clinical presentation is unilateral slightly thickened irregular border of brownish hyperpigmented plaque, usually found at the chest wall, upper trunk and shoulder of adolescent males. Hypertrichosis is a common concomitant finding.

Pathogenesis of this condition is unclear. Increased androgen receptors in the lesion are presumed to relate to hypertrichosis in these nevi. Becker's nevi are associated with smooth muscle hamartomas that affect arrector pili muscle contractions.

Hyperpigmented patch and hypertrichosis tend to persist for life. Laser therapy is not recommended in most cases because of the unpleasant results.

Epidermal nevus

The epidermal nevus is a hamartoma of the top layer of skin. It presents as localized flesh to brownish verrucous surface papules or plaques, single to linear in configuration, sometimes along Blaschko's lines. The differential diagnosis includes lichen striatus, linear lichen planus. Skin biopsy is helpful to distinguish these conditions.

Treatment of epidermal nevus includes surgical procedure (excision, liquid nitrogen, cryotherapy, dermabrasion, laser ablation) and topical treatment (tretinoin, podophyllin, keratolytic agents). Cutaneous findings of epidermal nevus are concomitant with an array of extracutaneous abnormalities/ systemic complications such as limb defect/deformity, seizures, developmental delay, macrocephaly, eye abnormalities, skeletal abnormalities (kyphosis, scoliosis). This is known as" Epidermal nevus syndrome (EPS)".

The inflammation of linear epidermal nevus is termed "Inflammatory linear verrucous epidermal nevus (ILVEN)". This condition is a chronic and inflammatory cause of epidermal nevus variants. The symptoms are characteristically extreme pruritus and recurrent inflammation. Treatment of ILVEN is very difficult. Choices include topical or intralesional corticosteroid, topical retinoid, topical calcineurin inhibitor, topical vitamin D derivatives, CO_2 laser and surgical excision. Responses are often poor.

Papulosquamous disorders

Primary forms of ichthyosis (non-syndrome ichthyosis)

We discuss congenital forms of icthyosis mainly because they persist into childhood and adolescence and will require treatment (33-36).

Ichthyosis vulgaris

Ichthyosis vulgaris is the most common form of ichthyosis, which is frequently associated with atopic dermatitis. The other minor criteria of atopic dermatitis include xerosis, hyperlinearity of palm-sole, keratosis pilaris. This condition transmitted as an autosomal dominant trait. The examination of parents' skin may be helpful in diagnosis.

The presentation reveals white to gray scales on the extensor surface of extremities particularly on the lower leg. The flexor surface and groin are always spared. Scale is characterized by small, white to gray, like a fish scale, worse in dry weather.

The diagnosis is clinical. Skin biopsy may be done only in cases of uncertainty. The treatments include hydration, then topical emollient and/or keratolytic agents such as urea and lactic acid.

Recessive X-linked ichthyosis

The mode of transmission of this condition is X-linked recessive. The affected patients are males. Females are mostly carriers. The pathogenesis is a defect of the gene encoding the enzyme steroid sulfatase. The onset of this condition usually begins in first few months of age. It presents as generalized large dark brownish scales accentuated on the lateral side of neck, pre-auricular area, abdomen, back, feet but sparing the palm, soles, central face and flexural areas.

Corneal opacity is usually found in affected adult males. Because of contiguous gene syndromes, hypogonadism and/or cryptochidism are sometimes present. The treatments include topical emollient and/or keratolytic agents such as urea and lactic acid.

Bullous congenital ichthyosisform erythroderma (BCIE)/Epidermolytic hyperkeratosis (EHK)/Bullous ichthyosis (BI)

The clinical presentation of BCIE is extremely variable. The classic presentation is superficial bullae and broad sheets of desquamation, generalized erythroderma in the first few days of life. The skin and bullous disease will change to hyperkeratosis in the next first few months.

The characteristic findings are thick, hyperpigmented verrucous scales on the flexural surfaces, intertriginous areas of the body and on dorsal surfaces of the hands and feet. Palms, soles and scalp are frequently involved. Unpleasant odor is very common due to fermented bacteria, yeast and fungi in the hyperkeratotic skin.

The pathogenesis is a mutation of the keratin gene leading to abnormal keratin protein. Thickening skin is believed to be a compensatory mechanism for skin protection.

Emollients are the proper management. Mechanical trauma and prolonged use of keratolytic agents should be avoided because of increased skin fragility. Mild antibacterial cleanser (e.g. chlorhexidine) or bleach bath is beneficial to decrease bacterial fermentation. Oral vitamin A derivatives (isotrentinoin, aciretin, etc.) help slough the scale.

Lamellar ichthyosis (LI)

This severe condition is transmitted as an autosomal recessive trait. The pathogenesis is the TGM1 gene mutation resulting in defect of transglutaminase-1 enzyme which is necessary to for desquamation of the top skin layer.

The diagnosis is based on clinical findings which are are large plate-like scales, ectropion, eclabium and scarring alopecia. Ectropion is eversion of the eyelid which exposes the palpebral conjunctiva and induces keratitis and madorosis. Eclabium is eversion of the lips. The patient usually presents at birth with a collodion membrane. There are generalized large quadrangular dark brown thick scales at the face, trunk and flexor surface of the extremities. The classic scales are centrally attached with raised borders. Palms and soles are frequently involved with a varying degree of keratoderma and fissuring. Scarring alopecia particularly at the hairline is a common finding. The thickened skin also causes the obstruction of sweat ducts resulting in heat intolerance.

Treatments include topical emollients and /or potent keratolytic agents. Oral retinoids (e.g. acitretin) may be helpful in severe cases. Ectropion should be corrected to prevent long term visual complications.

Congenital ichthyosiform erythroderma (CIE)/Non-bullous congenital ichthyosiform erythroderma (NBCIE)

CIE is transmitted as an autosomal recessive trait. The pathogenesis is mutation of TGM1 gene, the same as in lamellar ichthyosis.

The patient initially presents with collodion membrane at birth. After being shed, the skin turns red (erythroderma) and develops fine white powdery scales on the face, scalp and trunk. Hyperkeratosis of palm and soles with deep fissures are common. Ectropion and scarring alopecia may occur in variety of degrees.

The treatments include topical emollients and/or keratolytic agents such as urea, salicylic acid, alpha hydroxyl acid, propylene glycol or combination of them.

Harlequin ichthyosis

Harlequin ichthyosis is the most severe form of congenital ichthyosis with high morbidity and mortality. This condition is transmitted as an autosomal recessive trait. Most of them are usually born prematurely and suffer complications of prematurity (e.g. respiratory distress, sepsis, hypothermia). The clinical is characterized by hard, thickened armor-like skin with brownish fissures leading to polygonal, triangular plaques. Rigidity of skin results in facial deformity, ectropion, eclabium, everted O-shaped lip (fish mouth deformity). The limbs are limited in flexion of hands and feet. Constriction of the chest wall often results in respiratory and feeding problems.

The treatment of harlequin fetus is controversial. High mortality rate is due to severe infection, poor feeding, and electrolyte imbalance. The treatment for survivors is systemic retinoid (acitretin) which may improve, ectropion, eclabium and accelerate shedding skin. Risks and benefits of long term use of medication should be discussed before starting treatment. Supportive treatment with emollients may be adjunctive therapy.

Lichens

Lichen nitidus (LN)

This condition is most commonly seen in children of pre-school and school age. The exact pathogenesis is unknown. The characteristic findings are minute sharply demarcated flesh-colored flat-topped papules arrange in groups and may circumscribe the trunk, genitalia, abdomen and forearm. Koebner's phenomenon (lesions developing at site of trauma) can be found in many patients. The condition is seen on the glans penis.

The differential diagnoses include papular eczema, flat warts, keratosis pilaris, micropapular lichen planus and follicular psoriasis. The characteristic histopathological features are used to confirm diagnosis in uncertain cases.

The natural course of this condition varies from weeks to months and recovers spontaneously. Supportive treatment with oral antihistamines and topical corticosteroids may be helpful.

Lichen planus (LP)

Lichen planus is a common disorder, usually found in all age groups. The exact pathogensis is unknown.The characteristic findings are small flat-topped pruritic polyglonal purplish papules (the four P's). The distribution is usually seen in flexural surface of lower legs, ankles, wrist, genitalia, lower back, face and mucous membranes or along Blaschko's lines. Papules may develop at the site of trauma (Koebner's phenomenon).

The polymorphic variants of lichen planus in pediatric patients consist of bullous LP, actinic LP, annular LP, atrophic LP, hypertrophic LP, linear LP, ulcerative LP, LP pemphigoid, LP lupus erythematosus and lichen planopilaris. Linear LP is the most common variant in pediatric patients. Follicular LP on the scalp (Lichen planopilaris) can lead to scarring alopecia.

Mucous membranes of the mouth may demonstrate a characteristic reticulated delicate white line or annular-linear lacy reticulate pattern defined as "Wickham's striae". The buccal mucosa, lip and tongue are the most commonly affected areas.

Nail involvement is uncommon in pediatric patients with lichen planus, but may present with pitting, lusterless nail with thinning nail plate, longitudinal ridging and twenty-nail-dystrophy.

The differential diagnosis depends on the variants presenting and includes lichen striatus, Lichen nitidus, lichen simplex chronicus, lichenoid drug eruption and papular granuloma annulare.

The diagnosis of LP relies on the characteristic pattern of lesions. The typical histopathologic features from skin biopsy are helpful to confirm the diagnosis.

Treatment of choice of LP is moderate to potent topical corticosteroids and antihistamines. In cases of extensive or recalcitrant symptoms systemic corticosteroid injection (triamcinolone acetonide 5-10 mg/ml. dose or 1 mg/kg/dose) is effective. Other treatments include topical tacrolimus, oral dapsone, PUVA or UVB light therapy, oral retinoid, cyclosporine and thalidomide.

Pityriasis lichenoides

Pityriasis lichenoides is an inflammatory papulosquamous skin disorder with characteristic clinical and histopathologic features. This condition has been divided into two forms including the acute form: Pityriasis lichenoides et varioliformis acuta (PLEVA, Mucha-Habemann disease) and the chronic form: Pityriasis lichenoides chronica (PLC).

The exact pathogenesis of pityriasis lichenoides is unknown. Recent data reveal an abnormal response to an antigenic stimulus provided by unidentified infectious agents, possibly viral. Pityriasis lichenoides is primarily a cutaneous T-cell lymphoproliferative disorder. Nevertheless, the progression of pityriasis lichenoides to cutaneous T-cell lymphoma in children has been rarely reported.

PLEVA is a polymorphous papulosquamous eruption. It presents as asymptomatic or pruritic symmetrical erythematous macules and papules coalesce in crops and turn to vesicular, necrotic and purpuric lesions. Lesions are most common on the trunk, proximal thighs and upper arms. The natural course of disorder usually lasts -several weeks to months.

The differential diagnosis is chicken pox, insect bite reaction, leukocytoclastic vasculitis and vesicular pityriasis rosea.

PLC is a chronic form of pityriasis lichenoides. The course of PLC is variable form months to years. The skin lesions reveal scaling papules and plaques and usually resolve with post-inflammatory hypopigmentation, or less commonly with hyperpigmentation.

The differential diagnosis is pityriasis rosea, secondary syphilis, guttate psoriasis.

Histopathology from skin biopsy may helpful in cases of uncertain clinical diagnosis. Patients and families should be reassured of the self-limited natural course of this condition. There is no specific treatment. Optional treatments include oral erythromycin, topical corticosteroid and phototherapy. Topical corticosteroid or oral antihistamine may decrease the pruritus. Oral erythromycin, 30-50 mg/kg/day for 1-2 months is partially effective in some cases. Ultraviolet light therapy may be helpful in cases not responding to oral erythromycin. Spontaneous recovery usually occurs in several months to years.

Pityriasis rosea (PR)

Pityriasis rosea is an acute benign self-limited papulosquamous disorder. The exact etiology of this condition is unknown. There may be a viral like prodrome and/or history of preceding upper respiratory tract infection in some cases.

The clinical manifestation is initially a single isolated lesion defined as “herald patch”. The most common area of herald patch is on the trunk, upper arm, neck or thigh. The lesion is characterized by sharply demarcated oval shape with surrounding fine white scale “collar sign”, usually seen 1-2 weeks prior to appearance of other lesions. Only about 50% of cases begin with a herald patch.

The secondary lesions reveal generalized erythematous patches, papules with fine white scale bilaterally and symmetrically discrete to the line of skin cleavage, in a “Christmas tree pattern” on the upper arm, neck, back, trunk and upper thigh. The white scales reveal a “collarette of scale” surrounding the lesion, characteristic of pityriasis rosea. Each individual lesion is football-shaped with a raised red border, trailing scale and darker flat interior.

The duration of secondary lesions may be days to weeks. Spontaneous recovery usually occurs within 6-12 weeks but may be prolonged over a period of 6 months. There may be residual post-inflammatory hypo-hyperpigmentation. The diagnosis is based upon the history, distribution pattern and the characteristic of the lesions. Histopathology of pityriasis rosea is not diagnostic because of the similarity with subacute or chronic dermatitis.

Patients and families should be reassured of the self-limited natural course of this condition. The treatment is supportive with topical or systemic antipruritic medications. Optional treatments include oral erythromycin, topical corticosteroid and UVB light therapy. Mild to moderate corticosteroid may temporarily reduce pruritus in some patients. Oral erythromycin (dose 25-40 mg/kg/day over 2 weeks) may shorten the course of disorder. UVB light therapy over 5-10 days can significantly improve the eruption and reduce the degree of pruritus as well as hasten the resolution.

Psoriasis

Psoriasis is an immune-mediated papulosquamous disorder (34). Its pathophysiology is postulated to be a combination of genetic predisposition, environmental factors, and innate and acquired immune system problems resulting in hyperproliferation and abnormal differentiation of keratinocytes.

The characteristic lesions of psoriasis are erythematous plaques with well-defined borders and papules with grayish or silvery scales. The papules may coalesce to large plaque, usually seen in a symmetrical pattern on scalp, extensor surface of elbow, knee, lumbosacral and anogenital area.

The term "inverse psoriasis" may be used in a variant of flexural surface involvement of axillae, groin, perineum, central chest and umbilical region.

The "Auspitz sign" is a characteristic phenomenon that results from removal of the white scale leading to fine punctuate bleeding points. Koebner's phenomenon may develop at sites of trauma.

Facial psoriasis especially in the periorbital area is more common in children than in adults. These often present with small round psoriatic plaques in the upper inner eyelid area.

The scalp is one of the most common sites of psoriatic involvement. The presentation is a well-defined, white scale on an erythematous base resulting in variable degree of temporary hair loss. The distribution involves the scalp, eyebrows, pre-post-auricular area and beyond the hairline. The term "tinea amiantacia" or "pityriasis amiantacia" is used for the generalized white scale pattern.

The most common manifestation of nail change in psoriasis is pitting. The others are discoloration of nail (oil drops), onycholysis and subungual hyperkeratosis.

Extra-cutaneous involvement of psoriasis may include psoriatic arthritis and symmetrical anterior uveitis in adult patients, rarely in children.

There are variable patterns of presentation.

Guttate psoriasis

This is usually the first manifestation of psoriasis in children and young adult. The lesion is characterized by drop-like (guttate), round/oval shaped and white scale in a symmetrical distribution on the trunk and proximal aspects of the extremities. Group A Streptococcal infection is the most common trigger of this condition. The reason for this sequence of events is unknown.

Pustular psoriasis

This is the most severe variant of childhood psoriasis. The explosion of generalized sterile pustules on the erythematous skin with previous plaque psoriasis or on normal skin characterizes the lesion.

The overlying pustules may be discrete or rapidly coalesce to large plaque as "lake of pus" before drying over 3-4 days with desquamation. The repetitive explosions of pustules consequently develop over several weeks.

The trigger factors are withdrawal of systemic corticosteroids, potent topical corticosteroid and/or respiratory tract infection.

Pustular psoriasis palmaris et plantaris is a chronic eruption usually symmetrical on both palms and soles. The lesions are characterized by deep-seated sterile pustules with white scales on top of a bright erythematous base. They finally turn to dark yellow or brown scales in several days. The crop of pustular lesions is often recurrent, and sometimes is associated with secondary bacterial infection due to Staphylococcus aureus.

The diagnosis of psoriasis depends on the characteristic clinical findings. Histopathology from skin biopsy is used for confirmation.

The natural course of psoriasis is unpredictable but prolonged and chronic. The trigger factors may aggravate psoriasis are traumatization (Koebner's phenomenon), medications (lithium, antimalarials, beta-blockers, withdrawal of systemic corticosteroids) and infection (especially Streptococcal).

Management of psoriasis

Topical therapy

- Topical corticosteroids are the most commonly used in therapy children. The options depend on the site of lesion, body surface area and duration of treatment. Risks of side effects should be considered and minimized by monitoring the amount of usage, potency, proper site, and intermittent rotational or combination therapy. The combination of topical corticosteroids with other medications e.g. topical calcipotriene is beneficial in older children.
- Calcipotriene is an analogue of vitamin D3, usually combined with topical corticosteroid to facilitate the onset of action. This medication is one of the effective treatments for mild to moderate plaque type psoriasis in children and adult. The most common side effect is lesional or peri-lesional irritation especially on the face and in folds.
- Tars are anti-inflammatory and anti-proliferative. There are many forms of tar preparations such as 1-10% crude coal tar (CCT), 5-10% liquor carbonis detergent (LCD) and topical corticosteroid and salicylic acid combinations. The concentration of medications is appropriately selected to age and lesion sites. Tar shampoo is used as monotherapy for scalp psoriasis or in combination with other topical therapy.
- Tacrolimus ointment is a calcineurin inhibitor effective in the facial and neck area and in intertrigenous psoriasis (psoriasis inversus).
- Anthralin, 0.1-1% cream and ointment is primarily effective treatment for chronic plaque type psoriasis. Short contact therapy is initially applied for 5 min. and gradually increased over time as tolerated before being rinsed off. The most common side effects are irritant contact dermatitis and perilesional staining.

Phototherapy

Natural sunlight is beneficial in psoriatic patients. Phototherapy is the most frequently optional treatment in children with moderate to severe psoriasis who are recalcitrant to topical therapy.

Narrow band ultraviolet B (UVB-312 nm.) is the currently effective treatment of psoriasis. Administration 3 times per week is usually required until clearance occurs. The side effects of UVB therapy include skin darkening and burning.

Systemic therapy

- Antibiotics are used to eradicate Streptococcal spp. which is one of the trigger factors of guttate or plaque type psoriasis. This medication should be prescribed only in case of positive throat culture, although the culture may also be positive in the carrier stage.
- Methotrexate is started orally at 2.5 mg up to 15-20 mg/wk based on ideal body weight (dose 0.3-0.5 mg/kg/wk). The most common side effects are nausea, headache, and fatigue. The most common serious side effect is bone marrow suppression. Supplementary folic acid 1-5 mg/day diminishes the risk of mucosal ulceration and macrocytic anemia. Complete blood count and liver function tests should be monitored for patients on this medication.
- Retinoids (acitretin: dose 0.5-0.75 mg/kg/day) is often used in combination with topical treatment, UVB therapy. The most common side effect is dryness of skin and mucosa. Other complications are hypertriglyceridemia, teratogenic effects, premature epiphyseal closure and hyperostosis. Complete blood count, liver function test and lipid profiles should be monitored during administration of the medication.
- Cyclosporine is effective in pediatric plaque type psoriasis at a dose of 3-3.5 mg/kg/day. The supportive data in childhood psoriasis is limited to a small case series. The side effects are hypertension, immunosuppression and renal and hepatic toxicity.
- Biologic agents: Etanercept has been systematically studied in a small number of pediatric patients with plaque type psoriasis. Infliximab has only case reports of effective treatment in childhood psoriasis.

Dermatologic manifestations of systematic disorders

The goal of this section is to demonstrate dermatologic manifestations of other conditions. This will enable the clinician to ameliorate dermatologic conditions by approaching the primary cause, often in conjunction with specialty consultation. We select disorders not uncommon in adolescents.

Pruritus without rash

Pruritus can be a manifestation of several conditions. There may often be no physical findings until the areas become excoriated. While malignancies such as Hodgkin and non-Hodgkin lymphoma are associated with pruritus, relatively few patients with prutitis without skin findings actually have a malignancy. Other malignancies will be associated with abnormal dermatologic findings which may be prutitic. Examples of such are mycosis fungoides associated with leukemia, carcinoid, associated with histamine flush. Renal failure patients, especially at the time of dialysis will complain of pruritus. Cholestasis will frequently cause itching, especially in the palms and soles, primarily due to deposition of bile salts in the skin. Specific hepatic causes include primary biliary cirrhosis, sclerosing cholangitis, pregnancy and hepatitis. Endocrine causes include hyperthyroidism and diabetes mellitus. Other conditions common in adolescence associated with pruritus include Iron deficiency anemia and occasionally allergies. In patients with immunodeficiencies such as HIV, pruritus may be a complication of the primary condition (eosinophilic folliculitis in HIV), or due to a secondary infection or infestation such as scabies.

Inflammatory bowel disease (IBD)

Primary Skin manifestations of IBD consist of mouth ulcerations and perianal fissures and fistulae, more common in Crohn's disease (37; see chapter 23).

Erythema nodosum

This is the most common skin manifestation of IBD, slightly more common in Crohn's disease than in Ulcerative colitis. They are red tender red or violaceous subcutaneous nodules most commonly on the pretibial area. They often become more manifest during exacerbations.

Pyoderma gangrenosum

This occurs in about 5% of patients with ulcerative colitis and 2% of patients with Crohn's disease. They present initially as a red papule and progress to central necrosis with subsequent ulceration.

Less common skin manifestations

Other lesions associated with IBD include psoriasis, epidermolysis bullosa, Sweet syndrome (neutrophilic infiltrates, also seen in myelogenous leukemia) and primary granulomas (metastatic Crohn's disease).

Management

This consists of treating the primary condition and inducing remission. This should be done in conjunction with specialty consultation from a gastroenterologist for appropriate management of corticosteroid dosages, or, in more severe cases, immunomodulators (azathioprine or 6-mercaptopurine), calcineurn inhibitors (cyclosporine) and monoclonal antibodies (infliximab). Sometimes surgical intervention in IBD will allow for remission of skin manifestations.

Regarding the specific conditions mentioned above, Erythema nodosum usually responds well to corticosteroid therapy. Pyoderma gangrenosum may also respond to interlesional steroids, local Chromoglycate, oral Dapsone, hyperbaric oxygen and granulocytopheresis. Sweet syndrome is particularly sensitive to corticosteroids.

Collagen vascular disease

These conditions are not uncommon in adolescents and identification of dermatologic manifestations is paramount to proper diagnosis and management.

Lupus erythematosus (SLE)

Lesions may manifest as vesicles, bullae or ulcerations of the nasal or oral mucosa as well as the integument (38). Skin lesions may progress to atrophy or scarring. Typical lesions also consist of the malar "butterfly rash", generalized maculopapular rashes, dermatitis, frequently sun-sensitive, and vasculitis (periungual erythema, Livedo reticularis, Telangiectasia and Raynaud phenomenon). Dermatitis often results in post-inflammatory hypo- or hyperpigmentation (see chapters 31,33).

Discoid lesions may be present in 25% of patients with clinical SLE of may be its sole manifestation. They are erythematous plaques often on the face, neck and trunk. They often heal with scarring, atrophy, telangiectasias or hyper- and hypopigmentation. Lupus panniculitis, hypertrophic LE and Lupus tumidus (photosensitive pink plaques or nodules) may also be a sole manifestation.

SLE may have hair and nail manifestations including alopecia, scarring and non-scarring and pitting, ridging and onycholysis of the nails.

Dermatomyositis

Classic skin manifestations include the heliotrope rash (red-purple eyelids, telangiectasia of eyelid capillaries, periorbital edema and malar and facial erythema), Gottron's papules (red papulo-squamous lesions over knuckles and sometimes extensor surfaces), nail capillary dilatation and tortuosity and skin ulcers. Calcinosis may occur not only in the skin, but in muscle and fascial planes.

Juvenile idiopathic arthritis

The rash associated with JIA is salmon-pink in color, fleeting and becomes more prominent with heat, both external and with fever. Skin trauma may bring out the rash (Koebner phenomenon).

Management

The goal of management of skin and mucous membrane lesions in LE is to prevent scarring and atrophy. An important aspect of dermatologic management in LE is preventative. Patients with photosensitivity should avoid excessive sun-exposure, use sunscreens and select light bulbs for their homes that do not emit ultraviolet light. Patients should avoid triggers of Raynaud's phenomenon such as smoking, cold, vasoconstrictors and caffeine.

Skin lesions in LE that are isolated often respond to topical therapy. Topical steroids are often effective, starting with low-potency medications, although it may be necessary to advance to fluorinated corticosteroids for deeper lesions. However, it is important not to overuse these medications as atrophy, striae and telangectasia may be complications. Topical immunosuppressants such as Tacrolimus are presently under investigation and may be effective.

If systemic medications are necessary, antimalarial drugs such as Chloroquine and Quinacrine. It may take 6-12 months to see improvement. Ocular pathology is a serious side effect of these medications and the prescribing physician should always be mindful of this. Systemic corticosteroids and immunosuppressive agents may be helpful for bullous lesions, but generally are not necessary.

Endocrinologic disorders

Thyroid disorders

Patients with hypo- or hyperthyroidism will present with pruritus, sometimes idiopathic, sometimes due to dry skin (see chapter 21). In hyperthyoridism the skin is thin and diaphoretic; in hypothyroidism, it may be cool, pale and myxedmatous. There may be a yellowish hue due to carotenemia in hypothyroidism. Patients with thyroid disease have an increased incidence of vitiligo especially in patients with auto-immune conditions. Hair may be thickened in hypothyroidism and thinned in hyperthyroidism.

Diabetes mellitus

Pruritus in diabetics may be secondary to neuropathy, but also may be a consequence of fungal and yeast infections. Antifungals are the treatment of choice

Adrenal disorders

In patients with adrenal insufficiency, the skin is hyperpigmented especially in the palmar creases and areas exposed to trauma or sunlight. Pigmentation may be exaggerated in areas that are normally darker. Mucous membranes may display spots of pigmentation. Vitiligo may be present in patients with primary immune disorders.

Dermatologic manifestations of Cushings disease are primarily skin atrophy, bruisability and striae. Hyperpigmentation due to overproduction of ACTH may also occur.

Management

Treatment of skin manifestations of endocrinological conditions is contingent upon management of the primary disorder and should always be done with consultation from an endocrinologist.

Hair and nails

Alopecia areata

The sudden onset of localized alopecia is characterized by sharply demarcated round or oval patches of hair loss.

The pathogenesis of alopecia areata is proposed to be a combination of genetic susceptibility, relating to the inner root sheath and faint association with autoimmune diseases (39). The classic autoimmune disorders include thyroid diseases (Hashimoto's thyroiditis), vitiligo, lupus erythematosus, rheumatoid arthritis, pernicious anemia and myasthenia gravis. The association with these diseases is not clear and testing for them is directed by family history.

The skin is smooth almost totally devoid of hair with or without scale. The areas of hair loss may be single or numerous. The rim of alopecia reveals the pathognomonic sign of "exclamation hair". The inflammatory process of hair is located at the attenuated hair bulb resulting in easily loosening. The initial hair loss may reveal an irregular border, area of involvement, length of hair and duration of loss.

The typical pattern of hair loss along the bilateral parietotemporal to posterior occiput is called the "Ophiasis pattern", usually indicating a poor prognosis. The progressive terminal scalp hair loss including the eyelashes and eyebrows is "Alopecia totalis" and the total complete loss of body hair is "Alopecia universalis". This progression is more common in children than in adults.

One of the differential diagnoses is trichotillomania. Trichotillomania typically presents with irregular border of hair loss with bizarre shaped and variation in length of unplucked hair.

The diagnosis is clinical. Histopathology from skin biopsy may helpful in cases of uncertain history and atypical presentation. Nail changes may be found especially a fine pitting nail either in a horizontal or vertical pattern.

There is variability of the natural course of disease and treatment. Poor prognostic factors are autoimmune diseases, family history of alopecia areata, vitiligo, thyroid diseases, young age of onset, extensive hair loss, Ophiasis pattern, Down syndrome and nail dystrophy.

Management of alopecia areata

- Topical corticosteroid is the most common therapy for alopecia areata in children (40). Mid to high potency preparations are usually prescribed with monitoring of side effects. Re-growth of hair should be assessed 6-14 weeks after starting treatment. Intradermal corticosteroid injection is mostly used in older children and in cases of failure of topical treatment. The concentration of triamcinolone acetonide varying from 2.5 to 5 mg/ml is administrated as multiple intradermal injections of 0.1-0.3 ml/site, approximately 1 cm. apart and repeated every 4-6 weeks.
- Oral prednisolone dose 0.5-1 mg/kg/day for 4 weeks or until the hair loss stops is used in selected difficult cases, but high relapse rate often occurs after dosage reduction.
- Topical Minoxidil may stimulate follicular DNA synthesis with proliferation, differentiation of follicular keratinocyte and re-regulation of hair physiology. The concentrations of minoxidil are 2-5% and may be applied twice daily. Hair growth is usually seen after 2 months of treatment. The uncommon side effects are allergic contact dermatitis, hypertrichosis and local irritation.
- Topical immunotherapy (Contact sensitizer)has been used in chronic and extensive alopecia areata. These agents will sensitize contacted skin inducing erythema, scaling and pruritus. T suppressor cells are generated to contacted area that may result in a non-specific inhibitory effect on the autoimmune reaction in hair follicles and in re-growth of the hair.
- Diphenylcyclopropenone (DPCP) is the most commonly used topical sensitizer in children. The efficacy of DPCP in alopecia areata ranges from 48% to 85%. The side effects of DPCP include eczematous reaction, itching, edema of face, scalp and cervical, post-auricular lymphadenopathy.
- Anthralin (Dithranol), 0.25-1% Anthralin cream, is initially used as short contact therapy and with gradually increasing contact time as tolerated prior to rinsing. The side effects of this medication are scalp irritation, folliculitis and staining of the skin and clothes. It can be used in combination with twice daily topical corticosteroid therapy.
- PUVA (Psoralens with Ultraviolet A). The presumed mechanism of action is photoimmunologic effect by inhibition of local immunologic attack of hair follicle. The response rate and high relapse rates vary with the dose. There is a known incidence of induced skin cancers with oral PUVA treatment.

Telogen effluvium

The characteristic pattern is diffuse thinning of the scalp hair. There are several anecdotal trigger factors including emotional stress, high fever, systemic illness, severe infection, surgery, nutritional deficiency, thyroid abnormalities, and systemic lupus erythematosus. Medications (Albendazole, Amphetamine, Retinoids, Beta-blockers, Anticonvulsants, ACE inhibitors) also affect this condition. These factors may interrupt the normal cycle pattern of the anagen phase and result in early telogen phase. Telogen phase with >25% of hair count is significantly abnormal.

The diagnosis of telogen effluvium is supported by the prior history of illness or stress for 6 weeks to 4 months and the percentage of telogen hairs in the scalp biopsy of more than 12-15% of terminal follicles.

In cases of telogen effluvium without evidence of historical trigger factors, complete blood count, serum iron/ ferritin and thyroid function tests are useful screening tests.

The treatment of telogen effluvium is supportive. Spontaneous re-growth of the hair may appear in several months unless the trigger is repeated. Re-growth of the hair is usually complete within 6 months.

Androgenic alopecia

Androgenic alopecia (male-pattern baldness), with a genetic predisposition is the most common cause of hair loss in adults. Androgen hormones gradually transform large scalp hair follicles to smaller follicles and turn anagen phase to telogen phase in a faster than normal cycle.

Androgenic alopecia can occur in either gender but males are affected more severely than females. The male pattern reveals the symmetrical frontoparietal recession of the hairline and/or vertex thinning where as the female pattern is relatively unaffected at the hairline but seen the vertex and/or as diffuse thinning. Some cases begin during adolescence.

The diagnosis is based on the pattern of scalp hair loss. Hair plucking of frontal area reveals the increased ratio of telogen to anagen phase but it is usually unnecessary to do this to make the diagnosis.

Topical treatment with 2.5% Minoxidil solution is used to stimulate follicular proliferation, dermal papilla vascularization, increased anagen duration and enlargement of miniaturized follicles. This solution should be routinely applied to maintain hair growth. It works well on vertex and frontal scalp thinning. Topical Minoxidil may cause telogen effluvium to occur 2-8 weeks after initial treatment due to releasing of telogen hair as anagen promotion begins. Irritation, erythema and hypertrichosis are the common side effects of Minoxidil.

Oral fenasteride is a specific type II 5 alpha reductase inhibitor resulting in reduction of levels of dihydrotestosterone both in serum and scalp skin. Fenasteride 1 mg/day is effective treatment in men older than 18 years of age. Response time to this medication may occur as early as 3 months. Medication should be continued at least 24 months before reevaluation. The side effect is sexual dysfunction in 4.2% of men.

Spironolactone, an aldosterone antagonist, 50-200 mg/day is the optional treatment of androgenetic alopecia in women. Breast soreness and menstrual irregularities are side effects of this medication.

Trichotillomania

Trichotillomania is classified as an impulse-control disorder. The scalp is the most common area of involvement but the eyebrows and eyelashes may be involved as well.

This condition usually occurs in adolescents or older children predominantly in females. The characteristic hair pattern is bizarre configuration, irregular border, frequently distributing to the side of patient's handedness with varying length and/or broken hair from traction. The affected areas are commonly found at the frontal, frontotemporal and vertex areas of the scalp.

Direct evidence from observation hair plucking and indirect evidence of broken groups of hair in the patient's room are helpful to confirm diagnosis.

The management of trichotillomania is difficult. The patients should be reassured the cause of disease is stress and that stress reduction will improve the condition. Supportive treatment such as mild shampoo, mild topical scalp lotion (hydrocortisone) may be useful to relieve pruritus and irritation. The mainstay of treatment is psychiatric intervention and behavior therapy.

Traction alopecia

Traction alopecia is traumatic hair loss secondary to tensile force on the scalp hair. It presents as oval or linear areas of hair loss along the margin of the hairline depending on type of traction or trauma. This condition is common in females who pull braids, adolescents with ponytails, or who use barrettes and hair rollers.

Hair will re-grow in a few months after stopping traction. However, scarring and little re-growth may occur because of follicular destruction.

Hirsutism and hypertrichosis

Hirsutism is excessive hair growth in women and girls due to androgens. This may appear at the upper lip, neck, anterior chest wall, breast, abdomen, upper inner thigh and legs. Often it is genetic, with one or both parents being hirsuite.

Hypertrichosis is excessive hair growth in male and female of non-androgen etiology without evidence of masculinization or menstrual abnormality. The excessive hair growth may occur both in generalized and localized pattern.

The ideal treatment is correction of the cause of these conditions. The simplest methods to eradicate the excessive hair are cutting with razors, scissors or shaving. Side effects include pseudofolliculitis and irritation. Epilation includes plucking, threading and waxing. Plucking and wax epilation are usually painful and induce folliculitis, pseudofolliculitis and post inflammatory hyperpigmentation.

Chemical depilatory agents, 2-10% thioglycolates, mercaptans and sulfide may be effective but cause irritation, have an unpleasant odor and systemic absorption may occur in extensive areas of usage.

Electrolysis permanently damages hair follicles but difficult to use in younger children. The side effects include erythema, edema, pain and post inflammatory dyspigmentation.

Laser hair removal includes the ruby laser (694 nm.), the alexandrite laser (755 nm.), the diode laser (800-810 nm.) and Nd:YAG laser (1064 nm.).

Systemic medication to control hirsutism should be used under supervision of an endocrinologist or gynecologist.

Hair changes with systemic disease

Anagen effluvium

The effects of systemic treatment of radiation and chemotherapy may result in this condition. Hair loss may be prominent at the frontal, vertex, parietal area of the scalp or generalized. The severity of generalized hair loss depends on the toxicity of the causative agents.

Several manipulations may minimize hair loss such as applying ice packs or tourniquets to the scalp for 30 min. before drug administration.

The medical history, physical examination and microscopic examination of hair are useful to diagnose this condition.

The ideal treatment is cessation of the causative agents and to wait for hair re-growth.

Infection

Tinea capitis

Tinea capitis is the most common hair infection of childhood (41). The characteristic pattern is localized alopecia and broken hair with scaling. The most common age groups are prepubertal children because the effect of sex hormones in adolescence my change the sebum of scalp to free fatty acid with a protective effect.

There are varieties of dermatophytes that cause tinea capitis such as Trichophyton spp., Microsporum spp., Epidermophyton spp. The predominant species vary according to geographic location. The different pathogens may affect varieties of clinical presentation. Trichophyton tonsurans is the major cause of tinea capitis in the USA. Predisposing factors of tinea capitis are large family size, over-crowded living condition, low socioeconomic status, the postmenstrual period and an immunocompromised host.

Transmission of diseases usually occurs by contact with infected spores in shedding scale, hair or fomites from person-to-person or animal-to-person.

The classic manifestations vary as patchy alopecia, gray patch, scaling with or without hair loss, follicular pustules/papules, erythema, black dot, kerion, scarring and favus:

- Gray patch is a non-inflammatory type of tinea capitis. The clinical reveals the grayish patches of spores covering the hair shaft (Ectothrix) and usually present with scaling. Microsporum spp. is the common agent causing this form.
- Black dot presents with small black dots from broken hair shafts with alopecia. The cause of this form is dermatophyte invasion of the medulla hair (Endothrix). Trichophyton tonsurans is the most common etiologic agent.
- Kerion is an inflammatory type of tinea capitis. It presents as a boggy mass, an erythematous plaque with pustules and purulent discharge. Alopecia with loosening hair is also a significant presentation. Sinus drainage may occur, and it is frequently misdiagnosed as a bacterial abscess. This form often results in scarring alopecia from permanent damage to hair follicles.
- Favus is a severe chronic condition. The characteristic pattern is scaly erythematous patches with yellow-red perifollicular papules. Yellow cup-shaped fungal mycelia

called scutula are present. This lesion may result in scarring, atrophy and permanent alopecia.

The differential diagnosis of tinea capitis includes seborrheic dermatitis, psoriasis, alopecia areata, trichotillomania, follicultis, lupus erythematosus and lichen planopilaris.

A potassium hydroxide preparation of scaling and broken hair confirms the diagnosis. The microscopic examination reveals tiny arthrospores surrounding or within the hair shaft. However, the gold standard of diagnosis is fungal culture.

The treatment of tinea capitis is systemic therapy because of the requirement of penetration of medication to hair follicles. The drug of choice for tinea capits is griseofulvin because of its efficacy, safety profile and cost. The dose is 20 mg/kg of the ultra-microsize form administered once daily for a month. Problems with liver function are now not thought to be as significant as they once were and thus liver function tests should be obtained only if treatment is going to last > 1 month.

Topical therapy may be an additional treatment. Shampoo containing selenium sulfide, ketoconazole or zinc pyrithion twice-daily usage is adjunctive therapy to eliminate contagious spores of dermatophytes.

Contaminated individual hairbrushes, pillowcases and hats of infected patients should be cleaned and not shared with others. Symptomatic family members and contacts should be evaluated.

Herpetic whitlow

Herpetic whitlow is the localized form of HSV infection, usually seen in dentists and physicians who have contact with herpetic lesions. Autoinoculation to other sites also may occur. Clinical manifestations are a deep-seated painful group of vesicles with surrounding erythema. Ipsilateral regional lymphadenopathy may occur.

The differential diagnosis is blistering dactylytis, impetigo, burns and friction blisters. Viral culture or direct fluorescent antibody testing are helpful to confirm the diagnosis.

The proper treatment is supportive therapy. Spontaneous recovery usually occurs over 3 weeks. However, the oral antiviral therapy may relieve pain and speed recovery.

Bacterial

Paronychia

Paronychia is bacterial infection surrounding the nail. Acute paronychia, usually presents as painful, erythema, swelling of the proximal and lateral nail fold. The cuticle is sometimes obliterated. The most common pathogen is Staphylococcus aureus. The pathogen in ingrown toe nail is usually Pseudomonas spp. and Gram-negative organisms.

Chronic paronychia usually manifests as asymptomatic periungual erythema. The most common pathogen is Candida spp. particularly with repeated and chronic exposure to moisture at work or due to finger sucking.

Systemic candidiasis, acrodermatits enteropathica, multiple carboxylase deficiency, chronic mucocutaneous candidiasis and immunodeficiency should be considered in cases of multiple involvements of nails in both hands and feet.

The ideal treatment of paronychia is to eradicate infectious pathogens and keep the finger dry. Either alcohol-propylene glycol vehicle or thymol concentration 4% in chloroform is applied to dry the nail fold. Topical clindamycin solution may beneficial in secondary bacterial infection.

Ingrown nail

The distal-lateral edge of the nail curves inward and penetrates the underlying tissue. The causes of this disorder are improper cutting of the nail, tearing the nail plate and/or too tightly fitting footwear. There may be genetic predisposition.

It presents as painful erythema, swelling and may turn to granulation tissue over time. Complications of ingrown nail are paronychia and recurrent dactylitis.

Treatments are use of properly fitting footwear, special trimming, waiting for the nail to grow past the free edge and to control infection by compression dressings, topical and/or systemic antibiotics. Antiseptic soaks such as Hibiclens soap, Dakins solution or potassium permanganate may be helpful. Surgical procedure such as partial/total nail avulsion is necessary in painful cases or in frequent recurrence.

Fungal

Onychomycosis/Tinea ungium

The term "onychomycosis" refers to a fungal infection of the nail (42-44). However, "tinea ungium" is a specific term for dermatophyte infection of the nail.

Onychomycosis is more common in adults than children. Toe nail onychomycosis is usually associated with tinea pedis. This condition is classified in four patterns of infection site including distal subungual, proximal subungual, lateral subungual and superficial white onychomycosis.

Distal subungual onychomycosis is the most common form of fungal infection. The separation of nail plate and nail bed by fungal invasion leads to onycholysis and thickening of subungual nail. Proximal subungual onychomycosis is an uncommon presentation in a normal host and is usually seen in HIV or other immunocompromised conditions. The cuticle of proximal nail fold is initially disrupted. Proximal separation of the nail plate and nail bed results in onycholysis, scaling and discoloration.

Superficial white onychomycosis is the superficial infection of nail plate. The organisms directly invade to the dorsal nail plate. The infected nail plate is fragile and easily removed. Trichophyton spp. is the most common pathogen of the finger nails.

The common findings of onychomycosis are not usually symmetrical and only one to three nails of one hand or foot may be involved. If all of the nails are involved, other diagnoses should be suspected. Including psoriatic nail, chronic paronychia, drug induced onycholysis, trauma, lichen planus and pachyonychia congenita.

The treatment of onychomycosis is systemic therapy because of poor topical penetration to the nail plate. However, topical therapy (such as Amorolfine, Ciclopirox) is used as adjuctive therapy in some cases. Topical usage is appropriate in superficial white onychomycosis. Oral griseofulvin is the drug of choice for onychomycosis. Other oral antifungals such as terbinafine (Lamisil), itraconazole (Sporonox) and fluconazole (Diflucan) are increasing in usage with good supportive evidence. Table 6 below lists systemic antifungal agents for onychomycosis.

Table 6. Systemic antifungal agents for onychomycosis in children

Antifungal agents	Dose	Remark
Gresiofulvin (tablet)	*-Continuous therapy* : 15-20 mg/kg/day	*-Continuous* Toe nail 6-12 months Finger nail 3-6 months
Itraconazole (capsule, oral solution)	*-Pulse therapy* : 5 mg/kg/day *-Continuous therapy* : 5 mg/kg/day	*-Pulse* (1 week on, 3 weeks off) Toe nail 3 pulses, follow up Finger nail 2 pulses, follow up *-Continuous* Toe nail 12 weeks Finger nail 6 weeks
Fluconazole (tablet)	*-Intermittent therapy* : 3-6 mg/kg/day (one dose/week)	*-Intermittent* Toe nail 26 weeks Finger nail 12 weeks
Terbinafine (tablet)	*-Continuous therapy* : <20 kg - 62.5 mg/day 20-40 kg – 125 mg/day >40 kg - 250 mg/day	*-Continuous* Toe nail 12 weeks Finger nail 6 weeks

Onychodystrophy

Pitting nail

This is a common problem in children. The alteration of the proximal matrix results in pitting of the nail plate surface. The characteristic pattern is punctuate depression of the nail plate which may be small, shallow or large, deep involving few or all of nails. It frequently occurs in normal healthy adolescents. There are many disorders associated with this condition including atopic dermatitis, alopecia areata, psoriasis, trauma.

Beau's line/Onychomadesis

Beau's line is a transverse groove/furrow of the nail plate resulting from the interruption of nail formation. There are several causes of nail matrix interruption such as systemic illness, high fever or systemic maladies such as Kawasaki disease, severe bullous eruption, thyroid disease, radiation therapy, Stevens-Johnson syndrome and chemotherapy.

The duration time of systemic illness is associated with the distance between cuticle and the groove.

Onychomadesis is complete separation of the nail plate resulting from the arrest of nail matrix. The causes of Beau's line have also been reported to be the causes of onychomadesis. Trauma to nail matrix can lead to this deformity.

These conditions are transient phenomena and nails re-grow without nail plate scarring.

Trachyonychia (twenty nail dystrophy)

Trachyonychia is a deformity of nail with opaque discoloration, rough, sandpaper-like, ridging, grooves or striations. The number of nails involved may be used in lieu of the term "twenty nail dystrophy."

This condition may occur months preceding cutaneous signs of other diseases. Commonly associated disorders are lichen planus, atopic dermatitis, psoriasis and alopecia areata but it may occur commonly in a normal healthy adolescent.

The exact cause of this condition is unknown. The natural course varies from 6 months to 16 years. We do not see it in adults, so it is either self-limiting or progresses to another condition.

An optional treatment is watchful waiting especially if the primary causative condition recovers. Treatment with potent topical corticosteroid at the proximal nail fold may be helpful only in some cases, but reports are anecdotal. Some practitioners use intralesional corticosteroid, triamcinolone, 0.5-1 mg/kg/month for 3-6 months.

Nail changes with systemic and nutritional disorders

Spoon nail/Koilonychia

Koilonychia is a common disorder of the nail plate. Physiologic koilonychia may be found in the great toenail of newborns and young infants. The nail is characterized by a central concavity with turned up distal and lateral margins.

This condition may be a secondary feature of several dermatological disorders (lichen planus, trachyonychia), systemic diseases such as hypothyroidism, hemochromatosis and iron deficiency anemia.

Clubbing of finger/Acropachy

Clubbing of fingers is one of the presentations of multiple systemic disorders. The most common diseases in adolescent patients include congenital cyanotic heart disease, inflammatory bowel syndrome, chronic hypoxia of pulmonary disease and endocrinopathy.

Red lunula

This condition can be seen in several systemic diseases such as alopecia areata, lupus erythematosus, psoriasis, dermatomyositis, congestive heart failure and carbon monoxide poisoning.

Terry's nail

This discoloration is characterized by the pink distal portion and the proximal white portion of the nail. It can be seen in cirrhosis, chronic congestive heart failure and adult-onset diabetes.

Half-and-half nail/Lindsey's nail

This proximal nail bed is white and distal half is red, pink or brown usually seen in renal disease with azotemia.

Yellow nail syndrome

The triad of yellow nail syndrome consists of yellow nail, lymphedema and respiratory disease. The pathogenesis of this condition is unclear and it is persistent.

This syndrome is associated with severe long term lymphedema, respiratory distress (especially chronic bronchitis, bronchiectasis, interstitial pneumonitis, and pleural effusion), thyroid disease, lymphoreticular malignancy, rheumatoid arthritis, lupus erythematosus, Hodgkin's lymphoma and nephrotic syndrome. Treatment with vitamin E and/or zinc supplement may be helpful

Conclusion

We have discussed common conditions encountered in adolescents during routine practice with particular emphasis on management. Please consult the bibliography below for further details. The chapter contains six tables for quick reference.

Acknowledgments

This chapter is an adapted version of a chapter in the book "Adolescent medicine: Pharmacotherapeutics in medical disorders" edited by Donald E Greydanus, Dilip R Patel, Cynthia Feucht, Hatim A Omar, Joav Merrick and published with permission by Walter de Gruyter, Berlin and New York.

References

[1] Cole C, Gazewood J. Diagnosis and treatment of impetigo. Am Fam Physician 2007;75:859-64.
[2] Rhody C. Bacterial infections of the skin. Prim Care 2000;27(2):459-73.
[3] Stulberg DL, Penrod MA, Blatny RA. Common skin infections. Am Fam Physician 2002;66(1):119-24.
[4] King RW, Kulkarni R. Staphylococcal scalded skin syndrome in emergency medicine. Accessed 2011 Jun 15. URL: http://emedicine.medscape.com/article/788199-overview
[5] Hogan PA. Pseudomonas folliculitis. Australas J Dermatol 1997; 38(2):93-4.
[6] Eneli I, Davies HD. Epidemiology and outcome of necrotizing fasciitis in children: an active surveillance study of the Canadian Paediatric Surveillance Program. J Pediatr 2007;151(1):79-84.
[7] Hauser A, Fogarasi S. Periorbital and orbital cellulitis. Pediatr Rev 2010;31(6):242-9.
[8] Stoneback JW, Hak DJ. Diagnosis and management of necrotizing fasciitis. Orthopedics 2011;34(3):196.
[9] Florin TA, Zaoutis TE, Zaoutis LB. Beyond cat scratch disease: Widening spectrum of Bartonella henselae infection. Pediatrics 2008;121(5):e1413-25.
[10] Rawstron SA, Mehta S, Bromberg K. Evaluation of a Treponema pallidum-specific IgM enzyme immunoassay and Treponema pallidum western blot antibody detection in the diagnosis of maternal and congenital syphilis. Sex Transm Dis 2004;31(2):123-6.
[11] Steere AC. Lyme disease. N Engl J Med 2001;345(2):115-25.
[12] Murray T, Feder HM Jr. Management of tick bites and early Lyme disease: a survey of Connecticut physicians. Pediatrics 2001; 108(6):1367-70.

[13] Ilowite NT. Muscle, reticuloendothelial, and late skin manifestations of Lyme disease. Am J Med 1995;98(4A):63S-8.
[14] Scott LA, Stone MS. Viral exanthems. Dermatol Online J 2003;9(3):4.
[15] Aftergut K, Cockerell CJ. Update on the cutaneous manifestations of HIV infection. Dermatol Clin 1999;17(3):445-71.
[16] Andrews MD, Burns M. Common tinea infections in children. Am Fam Physician 2008;77(10):1415-20.
[17] Berg D, Erickson P. Fungal skin infections in children. New developments and treatments. Postgrad Med 2001;110(1):83-4,87-8, 93-4.
[18] Centers for Disease Control and Prevention. Accessed 2011 Jun 15. URL: http://www.cdc.gov /parasites/lice/head/diagnosis.html
[19] Burkhart CN, Burkhart CG. An assessment of topical and oral prescription and over-the-counter treatments for head lice. J Am Acad Dermatol 1998;38(6 Pt 1):979-82.
[20] Chosidow O. Scabies and pediculosis. Lancet 2000;355(9206):819-26.
[21] Naldi L, Rebora A. Clinial practice. Seborrheic dermatitis. N Engl J Med 2009;360(4):387.
[22] Williams HC. Clinical practice. Atopic dermatitis. N Engl J Med 2005;352(22):2314.
[23] Leung DY. Atopic dermatitis: new insights and opportunities for therapeutic intervention. J Allergy Clin Immunol 2000;105(5):860.
[24] Sackesen C, Sekerel BE, Orhan F, Kocabas CN, Tuncer A, Adalioglu G. The etiology of different forms of urticaria in childhood. Pediatr Dermatol 2004;21(2):102-8.
[25] Kaplan AP. Chronic urticaria and angioedema. N Engl J Med 2002; 346(3):175.
[26] Samel AD. Drug eruptions. Up to date. Accessed 2011 Jun 15. URL: http://www.uptodate.com /contents/drug-eruptions
[27] Weston WF, Lane AT, Morelli JG. Color textbook of pediatric dermatology, 4th ed. Philadelphia PA: Mosby, 2007.
[28] Cohen BA. Pediatric dermatology, 3rd ed. Philadelphia PA: Mosby, 2005.
[29] Koh MJA, Tay YK. An update on Stevens-Johnson syndrome and toxic epidermal necrolysis in children. Curr Opin Pediatr 2009; 21:505-10.
[30] Antoniou C, Dessinioti C, Stratigos AJ, Katsambas AD. Clinical and therapeutic approach to childhood acne: an update. Pediatr Dermatol 2009;26(4):373-80.
[31] Krowchuk DP, Gelmetti C, Lucky AW. Acne. In: Schachner LA, Hansen RC, eds. Pediatric dermatology, 4th ed. Philadelphia, PA: Mosby, 2011:827-50.
[32] Marcoux DA, Duran-McKinster C, Baselga E. Pigmentary abnormalities. In: Schachner LA, Hansen RC, eds. Pediatric dermatology, 4th ed. Philadelphia, PA: Mosby, 2011:700-46.
[33] Paller AS, Mancini AJ. Papulosquamous and related disorders. In: Paller AS, Mancini AJ. Hurwitz clinical pediatric dermatology: A textbook of skin disorders of childhood and adolescence, 3rd ed. Philadelphia, PA: Elsevier Saunders; 2005:85-106.
[34] Benoit S, Hamm H. Childhood psoriasis. Clin Dermatol 2007; 25(6):555-62.
[35] Shwayder T. Disorders of keratinization: Diagnosis and management. Am J Clin Dermatol 2004;5(1):17-29.
[36] Oji V, Traupe H. Ichthyosis: Clinical manifestations and practical treatment options. Am J Clin Dermatol 2009;10(6):351-64.
[37] Peppercorn, MJ. Skin and eye manifestations of inflammatory bowel disease. UpToDate. Accessed 2011 Jun 15. URL: http://www.uptodate.com/contents/skin-and-eye-manifestations-of-inflammatory-bowel-disease
[38] Schur PH and Moschella SL. Mucocutaneous manifestations of systemic lupus erythematosus. UpToDate. Accessed 2011 Jun 15. URL: http://www.uptodate.com/contents/mucocutaneous-manifestations-of-systemic-lupus-erythematosus
[39] Paller AS, Mancini AJ. Disease of hair and nails. In: Paller AS, Mancini AJ. Hurwitz clinical pediatric dermatology: A textbook of skin disorders of childhood and adolescence, 3rd ed. Philadelphia, PA: Elsevier Saunders; 2005:145-83.
[40] Alkhalifah A, Alsantali A, Wang E, McElwee KJ, Shapiro J. Alopecia areata update: part II, treatment. J Am Acad Dermatol 2010;62(2):191-202.

[41] Kakourou T, Uksal U. Guidelines for the management of tinea capitis in children. Pediatr Dermatol 2010;27(3):226-8.
[42] Gupta AK, Skinner AR. Onychomycosis in children: A brief overview with treatment strategies. Pediatr Dermatol 2004; 21(1):74-9.
[43] Berker D. Childhood nail diseases. Dermatol Clin 2006;24:355-63.
[44] Holzberg M. Common nail disorders. Dermatol Clin 2006;24:349-54.

In: Pediatric and Adolescent Dermatology
Editors: D Greydanus, A Feinberg and J Merrick
ISBN: 978-1-63321-853-6

Chapter 4

Psychocutaneous diseases in adolescents

Donald E Greydanus, MD, DrHC (Athens)*
Department of Pediatric and Adolescent Medicine,
Western Michigan University Homer Stryker MD School of Medicine,
Kalamazoo, Michigan, United States of America

The *sine qua non* of successful management of the adolescent patient with a dermatological condition and potential primary or secondary psychiatric conditions is to acquire a careful medical and psychological evaluation of this patient. Time is necessary for this evaluation and also to develop a clinical rapport with the adolescent to help develop management plans that may change to allow appropriate compliance in this patient. As professionals, physicians need to consider the needs of their patients and one of the best gifts health care clinicians can provide to their patients is their time. Principles of confidentiality and informed consent must be followed. The therapeutic alliance will be enhanced if both adolescent patient and clinician are engaged in clinical decision-making processes. Patients should be allowed choice of management options where appropriate while considerable care should be given to adverse effects of medications or other treatment plans. Recalcitrant cases should prompt both a reconsideration of the differential diagnosis but also attention for underlying psychological factors and potential reasons for limited compliance by the often challenging adolescent patient.

Introduction

A complete history and physical examination is important to be performed by the competent clinician when evaluating the pediatric patient with clinical concerns including psychocutaneous disorders. A focused history can be utilized as time permits but sometimes a

* *Correspondence:* Donald E Greydanus, MD, Dr. HC (ATHENS), Professor and Founding Chair, Department of Pediatric and Adolescent Medicine, Western Michigan University Homer Stryker MD School of Medicine, 1000 Oakland Drive, D48G, Kalamazoo, MI 49008-1284 United States. E-mail: Donald.greydanus @med.wmich.edu

more comprehensive evaluation is needed to find the correct diagnosis after a succinct differential diagnosis which leads to selective laboratory testing and the optimal management based on establishing the correct diagnosis.

History taking skills in adolescent patients

The interview process is a key component in evaluation of pediatric patients, particularly the adolescent who presents with dermatological disorders (1). The *medical interview* is typically separated into three core components: information gathering, relationship building, and patient education. The six basic aspects of successful clinician-patient communication is identified in Table 1 in which the opening discussion is the initial step followed by the ability to collect key information in addition to sharing information that the pediatric patient needs to understand for optimal management compliance (2-4).

Table 1. Elements of Physician-Patient Communication (2-4)

1. Opening Discussion (Kalamazoo Consensus Statement)
2. Process of gathering information
3. Understanding the patient's perspective
4. Sharing Information
5. Reaching agreement on problems and plans
6. Providing closure to the encounter

Understanding the patient's perspectives is an integral part of this overall process in order to reach a mutual agreement between clinician and patient in regards to identified dermatological problems as well as psychological issues and recommended management plans. This is especially important when dealing with older children and adolescents. The final step in this interaction is properly closing the medical interview to allow the patient (and family for children) to successfully leave the encounter feeling that their questions were answered and that they are willing to return after following the clinician's recommendations.

Table 2 lists various clinician-patient communication patterns (4). The least favorite pattern is the "*narrow biomedical interview*" model since it is very closely clinician-controlled as seen in this mini-scenario:

> ***Clinician**: What brings you (the patient) in today?*
> ***Patient**: I have pimples.*
> ***Physician**: Where are the pimples? When did it start? How long has it been bothering you? Are you taking any medications for it?*

In this example, the patient is quickly interrupted with a barrage of queries and the clinician fails to use the "continuer" technique to identify all the issues the patient (and/or family) may have. Also, it fails to appreciate nonverbal patient cues, such as: "You seem upset today—can you tell me about that?"

There is some dialogue on psychosocial and behavioral issues in the "*expanded biomedical model*"; however, it remains dominated by the interviewer. A much healthier model is the "*biopsychosocial"* one in which there is a better balance of control between the adolescent and clinician. Patients control the "*psychosocial model*" and this is more popular with adult patients. Finally, the model that is often not popular with clinicians is the "*consumerist model*" since it is fully controlled by the patient who seeks answers to miscellaneous questions.

Table 2. Patterns of Physician-Patient Communication (4)

1. Narrow Biomedical Interview
2. Expanded Biomedical Interview
3. Biopsychosocial Interview
4. Psychosocial Interview
5. Consumerist Interview

The American Academy on Physician and Patient (AAPP) has developed the *PEARLS* mnemonic to review core elements of the medical interview (Table 3) (2-4). The concept of the link between patient and physician is noted by the term *Partnership* that is between the patient and clinician. *Empathy* means that the clinician expresses an understanding of the patient (and family) for the newborn, child, or adolescent patient. *Apology* notes that the clinician should apologize for lateness in seeing the patient or lateness in getting laboratory tests. Clinicians should acknowledge the patient's suffering and difficulties as suggested in the term *Respect* while *Legitimization* means that the clinician acknowledges feelings of the patient or family (i.e., being upset, sad, anxious, others). Finally, *Support* suggests the critical idea that clinicians provide the patient (and family in younger patients) with the concept that s/he will not be abandoned by the clinician in the case of chronic or recalcitrant dermatological disorders (2).

Table 3. Clinical Skills of the Medical Interview (American Academy on Physician and Patient: AAPP): PEARLS (2-4)

1. **Partnership**
2. **Empathy**
3. **Apology**
4. **Respect**
5. **Legitimization**
6. **Support**

Interviewing the adolescent patient

It is important to note that the adolescent is in a process of emancipating from parents while becoming more invested in his/her peer group. The clinician's goal with each office visit should be to identify the concerns the patient has with regard to his dermatological condition, seek out other issues related to this concern, provide appropriate clinical recommendations, and deliver an educational experience for the youth as well his the family. It is vital to understand the thoughts and feelings of the adolescent patient, especially if there is a link between the dermatological condition and the mental health of this patient, as noted in the many chapters of this publication. It is difficult to develop a beneficial plan for a specific patient if the healthcare professional has little knowledge of this specific patient.

Key components to improve the office visit are listed in Table 4 in a mnemonic format of 6 "A's" (5). Certainly health care providers should be available to their patients in office hours that are convenient or assessable to them. Early morning hours may not be good for many adolescents who like to stay up late and get up late if possible. Evening or later afternoon hours may be more acceptable to many of these adolescents. The clinician and office staff should like this age group and this *approachability* should be evident to the youth and family upon entering the office.

The décor can be "teen-friendly" and the patient should not have to endure a hostile clinician or nurse who may not approve of adolescent dress or behavior. The patient is concerned enough with his/her dermatological condition (and/or other issues) to come to the office and needs a warm as well as accepting environment from the office setting. For example, the adolescent female taking contraception to prevent pregnancy should not have to encounter an office person who does not approve of "teenage' sexual behavior.

Acceptability suggests that the clinician understands and accepts the youth's developmental stage and need for increasing autonomy. One should provide *appropriate* healthcare that deals with the patient's needs and not those of the healthcare provider. Some time should be spent alone with the adolescent patient to let him/her know s/he is the central figure in this clinician-adolescent patient-family triad. Confidentiality is part of the care of all youth. Certainly, the patient and family need care that is affordable to them; otherwise recommendations may not be followed and follow-up appointments may be curtailed.

Though time is money, it is critical that enough time be spent with the adolescent patient to both identify the dermatological issue but also begin the process of developing rapport with the adolescent patient (5-7). One should be caring and honest with this potentially fragile patient---just being oneself is best while avoiding a false persona that the youth can spot quickly. Once turned off, this patient will not reveal salient (i.e., personal) information and may not follow treatment recommendations. This traveler through adolescence is on a journey, often a trek of turmoil and discovery; s/he needs a comforting health care guide and not a crusty critic! The fundamental clinician who judges the youth and conveys a non-accepting attitude toward the patient's lifestyle does not help this patient on their passage from childhood to adulthood.

Adolescents become very embarrassed when asked to take off clothes and get into a gown. One can spend time alone with the youth who is fully clothed and assess the cognitive and developmental stage of the youth. Is sh/e in a Piagetian concrete thinking stage where abstract thoughts and vague questions are not understood well? Failure to answer a question may mean the question was not understood and not a sign of negativity.

Non-adherence to a recommended treatment plan may indicate a failure to understand the plan or a conscious (subconscious) effort to sabotage the plan because of conflicts with authorities (i.e., parents) over issues of autonomy. As one gets to know the adolescent patient, it is easier to identify the reasons for such sabotage and ways to overcome it. Education of the youth is important but must be based on knowledge of the patient that simply takes time.

Certainly, time should be spent with the parent (s) or guardian(s) in fact finding and guidance as well.

Confidentiality

Adolescents are not large, still-dependent children nor are they small, autonomous adults. It is critical for the adolescent patient to understand what is confidential and what is not. Diseases related to sexual or other high-risk, personal behavior require the clinician to establish guidelines with what is and is not shared with parents without the adolescent's permission (8-10). This is based on local laws and should be understood by clinicians, adolescents, and parents. Some issues cannot be confidential such as thoughts of suicide or homicide. Others can be confidential. In such cases, the clinician can ask permission from the youth to share such data with parents. Not respecting the youth's confidentiality can result in the clinician sabotaging management plans!

Parental confidentiality

There are different models of care the clinician can utilize depending on specific circumstances. Parents may request a private meeting if sensitive issues are present. However, meetings without the adolescent present can led to resentment on the part of the youth and failure of this young patient to reveal sensitive data and/or fully cooperate with treatment plans. One model that can be used is to see parents with the adolescent together, and youth alone, and then, if needed, the parents alone. As the child matures into an adolescent, issues of patient and parental confidentiality must change as well. See chapter 12.

Health questionnaires

Questionnaires can be very useful to identify family history, past medical history, past surgical history, and other pertinent health information. Indeed, various healthcare questionnaires have been prepared that youth can complete in private while parents can complete their own questionnaires (11,12). Considerable clinician- and staff time can be saved and results may provide direction regarding what further details are needed in direct **tete`-a-tete´** interviews. If the answers are handled appropriately, confidentiality can be assured and questions can be in a safe, non-threatening tone that may ask for yes/no responses.

Interview techniques

A number of modus operandi can be utilized to aid in the interview process (Table 5) (5,6). One well-known one is represented by the *HEADS+ (HEEADSSS)* mnemonic (13). **H** represents *home* (how are things at home?), **E** represents *education* (school) and *eating patterns*, **A** is for *activities*, **D** is for *drugs*, and **S** represents the critical issues of *safety*, *suicidality*, and *sexuality* (5,3,14,15). In a general interview one usually starts with "safe" questions (i.e., general medical issues, school, others) before getting into personal topics as sexuality, drug use, others. The questions can be directed more specifically if the presenting concern is dermatological; however, sexual behavior or thoughts of suicide should not be missed if the differential diagnosis considers such factors (i.e., gonococcal dermatitis syndrome, dermatitis artefacta, others).

Youth with concrete thinking skills have problems with "time frame" questions such as "How long have you had your rash?" A better approach may be: "Did your rash start before or after….?" One can name an event that would be easily identified by the patient. Some adolescents have difficulty describing severity of symptoms and do better with "On a scale of 1-10 (10 is the worse), what number or range would you use for your pain?"

Sometimes a *mini-Likert* can be useful such as "How would you compare your school/home performance with your friends?" One could also ask: "Do you feel less troubled, more troubled, or the same about…than your friends?" Some health care professionals use the "*Three Wishes*" approach and ask the adolescent patient to make "three wishes" about their current situation. For example, "If you could change yourself, your friends, your family, and your life—what three things would you change and how." The answers may vary but it gives one a sense of the youth's thinking skills and what issues are important?

Another approach that can be useful to identify potentially anxiety-stimulating topics is the "empathic lead-in" as for example? "If I were you, I would feel….Is that true for you?" If the clinician is correct, the discussion from the patient may develop; if one is incorrect, it may prompt the patient to correct the clinician impression. When told that one is wrong, the clinician can say: "Well, OK, then, can you tell me how it is for you?"

The "advanced notice of understanding" approach may be useful in some situations in which the clinician tells the adolescent patient how s/he will respond to various subjects. For example, the clinician says:" Many adolescents today use drugs or having sex…where do you stand on this." This approach conveys a non-judgmental attitude on the health care professional's part and lets the patient know s/he will not be judged poorly if involved in various high risk behaviors. Also, the "indirection and projection" approach can be useful to reduce patient anxiety about certain subjects. For example, the clinician can say "What do teenagers your age think of sex, pot, (other subjects)…?" OR "What is going on at your school about….?" The adolescent patient can project his/her own range of experiences in the answers and the peer group often reflects the specific patient's actions.

Active listening skills

Active listening skills are important to utilize when interviewing patients in which one seeks to hear exactly what the individual is or is not saying in response to questions (5,6). Taking the wrong history by incorrect listening can encourage the wrong diagnosis and wrong management plans. Patients can sort out their issues much better if the clinician is actively listening and interacting with them. One technique is "clarifying" issues in which one repeats the stated problem back to the adolescent; this helps to avoid selective or imaginary listening by repeating what was heard. Repeating allows the adolescent to make corrections or clarifications. If the patient concludes you are not listening, s/he may change answers.

Paraphrasing can be helpful in which clinicians use short paraphrases or summaries about what was said or what one thinks was said. The clinician can say: "If I heard you correctly, you noted…Correct?" Or "do you mean you are telling me…" Certainly this is done in a gentle manner so the patient does not feel you are questioning the validity or truthfulness of his/her responses. The health care professional can also provide insights into issues; for example, one can note: "You are really worried about this rash" or "You seem very anxious about this condition, is that right?" Also, *silence* can be a very useful technique in some situations. There does not have to be constant chatter or conversation and if the adolescent stops talking, silence may provide time to gather thoughts or feelings. Silence on the part of the clinician for 10 or 15 seconds may lead to the youth to begin further dialogue.

Concepts of the physical examination

The extent of the physical examination is based on the presenting issues and history of previous examinations. Both the medical history and exam can be used to establish rapport with this patient and provide education in pertinent, important, aspects of their health as related to the reason for this health care visit (5,6,14,16,17). Clinicians and staff should seek to avoid unnecessary embarrassment as previously noted. Keep the youth fully clothed while doing the history.

Conduct the physical exam with full respect for the privacy of this patient and utilize proper draping at all times. Young adolescents may be more developed (i.e., higher sexually maturity rating) than one might think because of age. One breast can be examined while the other is covered. Genitalia and lower extremities can be covered while the abdomen is examined. There are many variations on how to do the specific exam but seek permission for examination of sensitive areas and seek to avoid embarrassing this young patient. The issue of chaperonage is done according to local custom as well as the wishes of the patient (5,6,16).

A *mental status examination* affords the opportunity to observe if mental health disorders are complicating the dermatological condition (s) that may be present (18-24). Is the patient fully oriented (i.e., time, place, person)? Is there a normal or flat affect? Is there good eye contact with the clinician? Is s/he cooperative with the examination? Is s/he dressed appropriately for age and local area? Does s/he appear depressed, angry, upset, and/or express thoughts of suicide? Is there an intact memory, judgment, and intellect? What is the cognitive state (i.e., Piagetian concrete vs formal operational)? Is there evidence of hallucinations or delusions? The rest of the physical exam depends on specific complaints of the patient and need for examination of specific areas of the skin.

Successful management of the adolescent patient

Informed consent

The rights of patients to consent to various treatments have been defined by the concept of informed consent. This has been a legal as well as medical term in Western medicine that was derived over many centuries out of the Hippocratic tradition. This practice was based on the concept that clinicians would always act in the best interests of their patients (25). Medicine in the United States gradually focused on rights of patients that included receiving education about their maladies and also included the concept that these patients may agree or not agree to receive recommended treatments. Patients have the right to received informed concept assuming they are capable of such consent. The atrocities of physicians as examined during the Nuremberg trials (including the Doctors' Trial) of 1945-1947 provided further impetus to rights of patients (25). The term, *informed consent*, was first used in a medical malpractice trial by Paul G. Gebhard in 1957 in the United States (26).

Those with mental retardation, comatose condition, Alzheimer's disease, childhood age, severe mental illness, and other states or situations provide direct challenges to this concept of informed consent. However, when the clinician is dealing with the adolescent patient, it is vital that this patient understand and agree to management options suggested by the clinician. Subservient to this concept is the principle that the clinician has conducted an appropriate evaluation, knows the patient, and can thus provide the best recommendations to this patient with rights of informed consent.

If the adolescent patient does not understand and agree to the management recommendations, s/he may sabotage the treatment, refuse to follow the suggested plan, and damage any potential therapeutic alliance between patient and clinician. Interwoven in this plan is that principles of confidentiality should be clearly established for this patient that takes into consideration rights of the adolescent patient and parents/guardians (8,9). Indeed, confidentiality is never absolute and the judgment of the knowledgeable clinician who understands the patient is always critical. Laws of the country must be followed, such as HIPAA (Health Insurance Portability and Accountability Act) rules in the United States (27).

Shared-decision Making

This is a critical concept if the professional clinician seeks successful treatment of the patient with dermatological, psychological, and/or other disorders (28,29). Shared-decision making can be complicated when dealing with adolescent patients but must be utilized when dealing with this age and with other patients (30). Youth who do not understand and agree to treatment options may sabotage the management efforts, as noted before. Even if an adolescent patient cannot legally provide consent in a specific situation, the clinician can still seek an *assent* from the youth that involves soliciting this minor's willingness and choices for management plans (31).

Improving compliance

The dedicated healthcare professional may find it challenging and even complex to improve management compliance with his/her patients. There is no evidence-based research that recommended plans improve medication compliance (or other treatment compliance) in all cases (32). Clinicians need to spend time to understand the patient and then provide some counseling regarding why the medication or other treatment option is being suggested and working on getting the acceptance from this patient. A rapid response to management failure by quickly changing a dose, changing drugs, or adding more medications without appreciating underlying issues will not improve the clinical outcome for this patient (33). This is particularly critical when complex interplays occur between the potentially thorny triad of developmental needs of adolescents, dermatological diseases, and psychiatric disorders.

Such counseling may change but sometimes must focus on behavioral strategies to improve compliance with proposed treatment options. Based on understanding the specific patient, one can discuss why the medication is important to use. Handouts of the condition (s) can be helpful for some patients (or parents) while others may be helped by additional healthcare personnel, such as the office nurse or this patient's primary care clinician (34). It does not help to seek any coercion in advocated plans, as this may lead to more refusal to follow the medical plan (35). The key is understanding the patient and underlying issues that may be complicating the patient-clinician alliance. Allowing the patient to choose options may help as well as discussing any side effects of current medications. Changing to medications with minimal side effects can be very beneficial to the patient and increase his/her acceptance of the dermatological and/or psychiatric medication (s). Communication with the teenager via e-mail is often a positive experience for the patient as well (36).

Table 4. The 6 "As" of Providing Clinical Care to Youth in the Outpatient Setting (5,6)

1. Availability
2. Accessibility
3. Approachability
4. Acceptability
5. Appropriateness
6. Affordability

Table 5. Useful Tools in the Medical Interview of Adolescents (see the text) (5,6)

1. HEEADSS
2. Time Frame Questions
3. Numerical Rating Scale
4. Mini-Likert Scale
5. Three Wishes Questions
6. Empathic Lead-in Approach
7. Advance Notice of Understanding Approach
8. Indirection and Projection Approach
9. Active Listener Approach
10. Clarifying and Paraphrasing Approach
11. Using Silence Approach

Conclusion

Patients with dermatological and primary or secondary psychiatric conditions can be challenging as well as time-consuming for clinicians. Indeed, for some clinicians, successful management of this patient may be like untying an intricately interwoven Gordian knot! The *sine qua non* of successful management of the adolescent patient with a dermatological condition is to acquire a careful medical and psychological evaluation of this patient.

Time is necessary for this evaluation and also to develop a clinical rapport with the adolescent. Principles of confidentiality and informed consent must be followed. The therapeutic alliance will be enhanced if adolescent patient and clinician are engaged in clinical decision making processes. Recalcitrant cases should prompt both a reconsideration of the differential diagnosis but also a look at underlying psychological factors and potential reasons for limited compliance by the potentially demanding and difficult adolescent patient.

Acknowledgments

This paper is a revised and adapted version of an earlier publication: Greydanus DE. A clinician's approach to psychocutaneous diseases in adolescents: Untying the Gordian knot. In: Tareen RS, Greydanus DE, Jafferany M, Patel DR, Merrick J, eds. Pediatric psychodermatology. A clinical manual of child and adolescent psychocutaneous disorders. Berlin: De Gruyter, 2013:83-94.

References

[1] Greydanus DE, Feinberg AN, Patel DR, Homnick DN, eds. The pediatric diagnostic examination. New York: McGraw-Hill Medial, 2008.

[2] Barrier PA, Li JTC, Jensen NM. Two words to improve physician-patient communication: What else? Mayo Clin Proc 2003;78:211-4.

[3] Makoul G. Communicative skills education in medical school and beyond. JAMA 2003;289:93-6.

[4] Roter DL, Stewart M, Putnam SM. Communication patterns of primary care physicians. JAMA 1997;277:350-6.

[5] Greydanus DE, Patel DR, Pratt HD, eds. Essential adolescent medicine. New York: McGraw Medical, 2006.

[6] Hofmann AD. Communicating with adolescents and their parents. In: Hofmann AD, Greydanus DE, eds. Adolescent medicine. 3rd ed. Stamford, CT: Appleton Lange, 1997:40.

[7] Mehta R. Approach to an adolescent client. In: Bhave S, ed. Bhave's textbook of adolescent medicine. New Delhi, India: Jaypee Brothers Medical Publishers, 2006:16-20.

[8] Lyren A, Silber TJ. Consent, confidentiality, and other related issues in the care of adolescents. In: Greydanus DE, Patel DR, Pratt HD, eds. Essential adolescent medicine. New York: McGraw-Hill Medical, 2006:29-42.

[9] Ford C, English A, Sigman G. Confidential health care for adolescents: Position paper for the Society for Adolescent Medicine. J Adolesc Health 2004;35:160-7.

[10] McDonnell WM. Adolescent health care. In: Donn SM, McAbee GN, eds. Medicolegal issues in pediatrics. Elk Grove Village, IL: American Academy of Pediatrics, 2012:131-9.

[11] Elster AB, Kuznets NJ. AMA Guidelines for Adolescent Preventive Service (GAPS): Recommendations and rationale. Baltimore, MD: Williams Wilkins, 1992.

[12] Chatterjee S, Chatterjee R. Adolescent screening questionnaires. In: Bhave S, ed. Bhave's textbook of adolescent medicine. New Delhi, India: Jaypee Brothers Medical Publishers, 2006:21-5.

[13] Goldenring JM, Rosen DS. Getting into adolescent heads: An essential update. Contempor Pediatr 2004;21:64.

[14] Kaul P, Kaplan DW. Caring for adolescents in their office. In: Greydanus DE, Patel DR, Pratt HD, eds. Essential adolescent medicine. New York: McGraw-Hill Medical, 2006:17-27.

[15] Coupey SM. Interviewing adolescents. Pediatr Clin North Am 1997;44:1349.

[16] Brown RT. Issues for the male clinician. In: Coupey SM, ed. Primary care of adolescent girls. Philadelphia, PA: Hanley Belfus, 2000:81.

[17] Greydanus DE, ed. Caring for your teenager. New York: Bantam Books and American Academy of Pediatrics, 2003.

[18] Harth W, Hillert A, Hermes B, Seikowski K. Niemeier V, Feudenmann RW. Suicidal behavior in dermatology. Hautartz 2008;59(4):289-96.

[19] Misery L. Consequences of psychological distress in adolescents with acne. J Invest Dermatol 2011;131(2):290-2.

[20] Chuh A, Wong W, Zawar V. The skin and the mind. Aust Fam Physician 2006;35(9):723-5.

[21] Sambhi R, Lepping P. Psychiatric treatments in dermatology: an update. Clin Exp Dermatol 2010;35(2):120-5.

[22] Barankin B, DeKoven J. Psychosocial effect of common skin diseases. Can Fam Physician 2002;48:712-6.

[23] Gupta MA, Gupta AK, Ellis CN, Koblenzer CS. Psychiatric evaluation of the dermatology patient. Dermatol Clin 2005;23(4):591-9.

[24] Kieć-Swierczyńska M, Dudek B, Krecisz B, Swierczyńska-Machura D, Dudek W, Garnczarek A, et al. The role of psychological factors and psychiatric disorders in skin diseases. *Med Pr* 2006;57: 551–5.

[25] Mallardi V. The origin of informed consent. Acta Otorhinolaryngol Ital 2005;25(5):312-27.

[26] Katz J. The silent world of doctor and patient. New York, NY: Free Press, 1984.

[27] English A, Ford CA. The HIPAA Privacy Rule and adolescents: legal questions and clinical challenges. Perspect Sex Reprod Health 2004;26(2):80-6.

[28] Légaré F, Ratté S, Stacey D, Kryworuchko J, Gravel K, Graham ID, Turcotte S. Interventions for improving the adoption of shared decision making by healthcare professionals. Cochrane Database Sys Rev 2010;5:CD006732.

[29] Perestelo-Perez L, Gonzalez-Lorenzo M, Perez-Ramos J, Rivero-Santana A, Serrano-Aquilar P. Patient involvement and shared-decision making in mental health care. Curr Clin Pharmacol 2011;6(2):83-90.

[30] Unguru Y. Making sense of adolescent decision-making: challenge and Reality. Adolesc Med State Art Rev 2011;22(2):195-206.

[31] Campbell AT, English A. Law, ethics, and clinical discretion: recurring and emerging issues in adolescent health care. Adolesc Med State Art Rev 2011;22(2):321-34.

[32] Haynes RB, Yao X, Degani A, Kripalani S, Garg A. McDonald HP. Interventions to enhance medication adherence. Cochrane Database Syst Rev 2005;4:CD000011.

[33] Lerman I. Adherence to treatment: the key for avoiding long-term complications of diabetes. Arch Med Res 2005;36(3):300-6.

[34] Eisenmann CM. Revising a medication education program on an inpatient child and adolescent psychiatric unit. J Psychosoc Nurs Ment Health Serv 2011;14:1-7.

[35] Molodynski A, Rugkåsa J, Burns T. Coercion and compulsion in community mental health care. Br Med Bull 2010;95:105-19.

[36] Menachemi N, Prickett CT, Brooks RG. The use of physician-patient e-mail: A follow-up examination of adoption and best practice adherence. J Med Internet Res 2011;13(1):e23.

In: Pediatric and Adolescent Dermatology
Editors: D Greydanus, A Feinberg and J Merrick
ISBN: 978-1-63321-853-6

Chapter 5

Acne

Donald E Greydanus**, *MD, DrHC (Athens)
Department of Pediatric and Adolescent Medicine, Western Michigan University Homer Stryker M.D. School of Medicine, Kalamazoo, Michigan, United States of America

Acne vulgaris is a chronic inflammatory disorder of sebaceous units and hair follicles (obstruction of pilosebaceous units) found in the majority of adolescents and many adults. Acne vulgaris involves abnormal keratinization, androgen-stimulated sebum production, *Propionibacterium acnes* colonization, and abnormal host immune response to inflammation. Management involves use of various topical and systemic medications. Topical medications include benzoyl peroxide, various retinoids (tretinoin, tazarotene, adapalene), azelaic acid, and topical antibiotics (erythromycin and clindamycin among others). Systemic agents include various antibiotics, oral contraceptives, and isotretinoin. Management of comorbid conditions that worsen acne should be carefully managed, such as causes of hyperandrogenemia. Drugs that worsen acne should be stopped and substituted for if at all possible. Psychological impact can be considerable and should be an important part of the overall management for this disorder. Development of scars is very upsetting to patients and management should be directed to scar prevention early in the course of acne management. Acne rosacea, acne excoriée, and other acne variants are also considered.

Introduction

Acne vulgaris is a chronic, multifactorial, inflammatory disorder of the sebaceous glands as well as ducts and the hair follicles with a strong genetic predisposition (1-5). It is found in areas of increased sebaceous density, i.e, the face, chest, upper arms, and back. Though acne

* Correspondence: Donald E Greydanus, MD, Dr. HC (ATHENS), Professor and Founding Chair, Department of Pediatric and Adolescent Medicine, Western Michigan University Homer Stryker M.D. School of Medicine, 1000 Oakland Drive, D48G, Kalamazoo, MI 49008-1284 United States. E-mail: Donald.greydanus@ med.wmich.edu.

can be seen at any age, it typically begins at puberty and its onset as well as severity is influenced by genetic factors as well as the host immune response to inflammation.

Epidemiology

Acne can be found in all ages of childhood (neonatal, infantile, childhood) and adulthood (6-8). Acne vulgaris is found in as many as 40% in those between 8 and 10 years of age, 90% of mid-adolescent males (i.e., ages 13 to 17) and 80% of similar aged females; severe acne is noted in 10% of adolescents and young adults. Severe acne may occur in young adults even if they only had mild acne as adolescents. Concern with acne accounts for 14% of visits to primary care clinicians and 27% of visits to dermatologists. Table 1 provides a classification of acne and its many variants. The direct cost of acne management is over $2.2 billion per year in the United States (9). Acne rosacea is reviewed in the next section (10).

Table 1. Classification of acne and variants*

Type	Comment
• Acne Vulgaris (Group I)	
Comedonal acne vulgaris	Disorder of sebaceous follicles with horny impactions. Graded according to percent of face involved: I=10%; II=10%-25%; III=25%-50%; IV=more than 50%.
Papulopustular acne	Rupture of the distended sebaceous gland (inflammatory acne)with varying degrees of inflammation. Graded V-VIII.
Acne conglobata	Severe nodulocystic acne vulgaris. Described in 3% of white adolescent males, with severe scarring. Extremities and buttocks often involved, as well as groin, scalp and axilla. Persistence into adulthood can occur.
	SAPHO: syndrome of acne, pustulosis, hyperostosis, and osteitis; this is classified as a seronegative spondyloarthritis.
Tropical acne	Severe inflammatory acne vulgaris seen in those exposed to tropical conditions.
Acne fulminans (acute febrile	Rare variant described in males ulcerative conglobate acne) characterized by large nodules with scarring on trunk and sometimes face; also fever, ulcers, polyarthritis or arthralgia and leukocytosis. Sacroiliitis often noted. Osteolysis and periosteal reaction can occur.
• **Acne Vulgaris Variants (Group ii)**	
Infantile acne (acne neonatorum)	Comedonal acne on malar region of males during first few weeks to 1 year of life. Occasionally noted in either sex from 1-2 years of age. Acne neonatorum refers to acne limited to the first month of life.
Premenstrual acne	Cyclical microcomedonal acne developing before the menstrual period.
Gram-negative folliculitis	Associated with long-term broad-spectrum antibiotic use. Variable patterns of facial nodules due to *Proteus*, *Pseudomonas*,

Type	Comment
	Klebsiella, or *Enterobacter* organisms. Treat with isotretinoin or high-dose ampicillin. amoxicillin, or others.
Excessive androgen acne	Severe acne related to high androgen levels (eg, polycystic ovary syndrome). Treatment with antiandrogens such as cyproterone acetate and ethinyl estradiol reported to be therapeutic; close medical supervision is necessary due to adverse drug effects.
Folliculitis keloidalis	Chronic, recurrent low-grade pustular dermatitis of the occipital and posterior neck regions. May result in scarring, keloid formation, and alopecia. Most commonly noted in black males with closely shaved areas and ingrown hairs. Avoid certain shaved hairstyles and occlusive hair oils; topical or systemic antibiotics may be necessary. Intralesional corticosteroids or surgical excision of scar or keloids may be necessary.
Acne mechanica	Exacerbation of acne vulgaris by excessive rubbing to cause friction, as with overzealous face washing or even tight helmets or clothing (leotards); use of absorbent material under the occlusion can help, such as a cotton T-shirt under a leotard.
Chemical acne	Exacerbation of acne vulgaris by cosmetics, detergents, hair creams or oils, chlorinated hydrocarbons, tars, emollient skin or bath oils. Pomade acne refers to hair oil or grease inducing comedonal acne at the hair line and forehead. High-potency steroid cream should *never* be used on the face!
Acne due to physical agents Exacerbation of acne vulgaris by sunlight,	ionizing radiation; Mallorca acne (acne aestivalis) is a sunlight-induced, winter variant with papular folliculitis of arms, shoulders, and trunk; no comedones, nodules or scarring.
Drug-induced acneform rashes	Iodides, bromides, barbiturates, rifampin, phenytoin, lithium; others may be associated. Steroid acne can occur secondary to steroid (systemic, oral) use and responds poorly to antibiotics. Fluorinated steroids are particularly implicated, but fluorinated creams should *never* be used on the face! Patients with acne should be screened for medications and foods that might contain high levels of "acnegenic" substances. Athletes should be advised to avoid anabolic steroid use, which has many side effects, including a drug-induced acneform disorder.
• **Nonacne Acneform Rashes (Differential Diagnosis)**	
Pyoderma faciale	Progressive facial inflammatory lesions (nodules, hypertrophic scars, and absence of comedones) occurring in adult females 20-40 years of age.
Acne rosacea	Facial papules and pustules associated with dilated blood vessels in the nasolabial areas in adults age 30-50. See text.
Folliculitis-associated immunological defects	*Example*: Chronic granulomatous disease.
Perifolliculitis capitis abscedens	Diffuse, explosive scalp cellulitis associated with severe acne and hidradenitis suppurativa. Treat with antibiotics and retinoic acid.

Table 1. (Continued)

Type	Comment
Hidradenitis suppurativa	Keratin obstruction of aprocrine ducts with secondary infection of apocrine glands in axillae, areolae, labia, scrotum, or perineum. Fluctuant nodules with purulent drainage and sinus tract formation. Associated with obesity, severe acne vulgaris, tropical climates, poor hygiene. Unusual cases can be associated with fever, anemia, and arthralgia. Treatment is as for abscesses in general; intralesional steroid injection, exteriorization of sinus tracts, or excision of involved tissue may be required. Acne surgery is the ultimate choice for most, though oral isotretinoin (40 mg, bid) is helpful to some. Oral antibiotics (tetracyclin 1-2 g/day) can also help some. Avoid tight clothes over affected areas. Antibacterial soaps may help. Hygiene and aluminum chloride (6.25% in anhydrous alcohol) may help to reduce perspiration. Benzoyl peroxide and topical antibiotics may be helpful for a few patients, but not the majority. Response to all treatment measures is variable.
Pseudofolliculitis barbae	Chronic folliculitis in beard area (especially black males) aggravated by shaving. Treat by growing a beard, avoiding a close shave, clipping hairs, and systemic antibiotics if pronounced. Electric razor use is essential for most, though some may find frequent straight-edge razor changes acceptable. Multiple small keloids may form in persons predisposed to keloid formation.
Trichostasis spinulosa	Facial eruption resembling blackheads but made up of follicular papules containing vellus hairs, keratin, as well as melanin and distributed over the nose and malar regions. Treat with isotretinoin.
Adenoma sebaceum	Pinkish yellow sebaceous papules on face; commonly clustered in groups around the nose. Part of the classic stigmata of tuberous sclerosis.
Keratosis pilaris	Hereditary, self-limiting, hair follicle keratinization disorder which peaks in adolescence. Can be associated with atopic dermatitis or ichthyosis vulgaris. Flesh-colored 1-2 mm papules are noted on lateral upper arms, anterior thighs, or the face. The lesions can be red or white. Moisturizers (with lactic acid), topical keratolytics (with propylene glycol) and tretinoin may be helpful.
Neurotic excoriations	Superficial excoriation or deeper ulcer in acne areas and other generalized areas. Found in individuals with severe mental illness. Some distributed individuals use cigarettes, knives, acids, or alkalis to produce facial injury often called factitial dermatitis. Treatment is attention to the injured skin with psychiatric treatment.
Also see molluscum contagiosum and verrucae	

[*] Used with permission from: Greydanus DE: Disorders of the skin. In: AD Hofmann, DE Greydanus (eds). Adolescent Medicine, 3rd Edition. Stanform, CT: Appleton & Lange, 1997; ch. 18:377.

Pathogenesis

The pathogenesis of acne vulgaris involves three main components: sebum, keratin plug, and the microbial skin flora (11). Sebum is made by the sebaceous glands and is composed of approximately two thirds triglycerides and one-third wax esters along with steroid esters and squalene. The protein secreted by keratinocytes is called keratin while sebum is secreted into hair follicles through the sebaceous duct. Sebum production is influenced in adolescence by the adrenal and gonadal androgens. Acne is an inflammatory condition and starts with follicular keratinocytes becoming so sticky that a keratin plug forms which then occludes the follicle with trapping of sebum. Trapped sebum leads to perifollicular inflammation and secondary impaction. Seborrhea may be mild to severe and is not specifically linked to acne vulgaris.

Local bacteria contribute to the acne process and this flora includes *Propionibacterium acnes* (formerly known as *Corynebacterium acnes)* that has been implicated in acne pathogenesis since 1896. This bacterium is an anaerobic Gram-positive diphtheroid that increases during adolescence and colonizes at pilosebaceous follicles. This important microbe converts triglycerides to free fatty acids and produces mediators as well as chemotactic factors that lead to the inflammatory nature of acne (*vide infra*). Other flora implicated in acne include coagulase-negative *Staphylococcus epidermidis* and the yeast *Pityrosporum ovale*.

An important etiologic component in adolescent acne development is the increasing level of plasma testosterone in which testosterone is converted in the skin to dihydrotestosterone by 5-α-reductase. This conversion leads to direct stimulation of sebaceous gland enlargement via a cyclic cAMP (adenosine monophosphate) mechanism. Estrogen can inhibit gland stimulation and acne exacerbations in females may occur during periods of reduced estrogen stimulation, such as before menstruation. Youth can have normal hormonal levels but still have severe acne, partially due to increased free testosterone levels and dihydroepiandrosterone sulfate (D-HEAS) along with lowered levels of SHBG (sex hormone-binding globulin).

Acne vulgaris typically initiates with the development of microcomedones, the primary, noninflammed acne lesions which are due to occluded hair follicles. The microcomedone is due to excessive sebum from desquamated epithelial cells in the follicular wall, as noted above; microcomedones become overt comedones. Closed comedones are called whiteheads while open comedones or blackheads have pigmented epithelial cells and are due to retained melanin. The open or closed comedone obstructs the follicle duct and sebum outflow leading to follicle distention and potential rupture.

Inflammatory pathogenesis

Ongoing distention results in local tissue injury that is worsened by conversion of sebum triglycerides to irritant free fatty acids. The follicle ruptures which allows bacterial infection or invasion of the follicle and surrounding tissues that is complicated by *Propionibacterium acnes* which stimulates chemotactic substances that enhance polymorphonuclear neutrophils (PMNs). *P. acnes* interacts with Toll-like receptors (TLRs) in this process (9,12). TLRs are a class of proteins playing a significant role in the immune system and recognize molecules from microbes.

The pathogenesis of acne vulgaris involves inflammation with genetic overlay. Proinflammatory lipids, chemokines, and cytokines assume the role of mediators in this process that develop acne lesions with the stimulation of bacterial antigens (13). Current research invokes the influence of neuropeptides and peroxisome proliferator-activated receptor (PPAR) ligands. Those with acne have peripheral blood mononuclear cells (PBMCs) with increased interferon-gamma, and interleukins (IL-12p40 and IL-8). Antimicrobial and proinflammatory cathelicidins are involved in acne pathogenesis and these are a family of polypeptides found in lysosomes of macrophages and polymorphonuclear leukocytes; they are important parts of the immune system protecting against bacterial invasion (14).

The result of this complex inflammatory process--that is initiated by rising androgens of adolescence and influenced by environmental and genetic factors--is varying degrees of erythematous papules, pustules, nodules, cysts, scarring, and depigmentation that characterize inflammatory acne vulgaris. The severity is influenced by genetic factors, sexually maturity rating of the individual, and sebum production rate. Both dermatological and emotional scaring may also result. Scars can hypertropic (keloid) or atrophic (i.e., rolling, boxcar, or ice pick-types) (15).

Classification

Noninflammatory acne (Grade I) involves acne with both closed and open comedones. Further grades of inflammatory acne can result from the closed comedone (whitehead). Grade II (early inflammatory acne) reflects comedones and papules; papules are raised, red lesions which are obstructed follicles. Moderate, localized, inflammatory acne with pustules defines Grade III while Grade IV refers to severe, generalized acne vulgaris with cysts that are typically painful and warm. A wide variety of scoring systems have been used by clinicians over the years, such as the Investigator's Static Global Assessment Scale (16).

Management

The course of a patient's acne vulgaris and its management runs a highly individualized pathway. Clinicians should be sure of the diagnosis and of the differential diagnosis of acne vulgaris that includes drug-induced acneiform eruptions, acne rosacea, bacterial folliculitis, perioral dermatitis, angiofibromas, trichostasis spinulosa, adenoma sebaceum, keratosis pilaris, and various acne variants (17) (see table 1). One clue to acne vulgaris is to find the presence of both open and closed comedones. Some individuals have a mild course with comedonal lesions lasting only one or two years. Those at the other end of this spectrum have extensive, persistent disease with pustules and cysts lasting many years as well as emotional scars lasting a lifetime. Acne vulgaris may continue or even begin in adulthood.

Management seeks to control and not cure the acne in which primary goals involve improvement in appearance as soon as possible as well as prevention of scarring (18). Various recommendations are given that include gentile face washing and use of topical agents (bacteriostatic and/or peeling). Careful attention to skin color is important as skin of color is at risk for hyperpigmentation due to acne lesions and irritating topicals (19).

Improvement of simple Grade I acne vulgaris may be seen with gentile washing of the face or other involved areas two to three times a day with mild soap. Instruct the patient to avoid excessive or harsh washing as this may irritate the skin and lead to *acne mechanica* (Table 1). Also, the patient should avoid irritating the skin by use of rubbing alcohol, mechanical abrasives, or astringents. Teach the teenager to avoid squeezing or otherwise injuring the comedones since this increases damage to skin tissue and introduces more infection; a comedonal extractor can be helpful to safely remove unsightly comedones. Teach the patient that acne is not due to poor hygiene or dirty skin. Teach that acne is not a disease of shame but, in fact, a complex inflammatory disorder of the skin that affects billions of humans.

Diet per se is not usually causative in acne though some patients anecdotally noted that certain foods do exacerbate their acne, such as soft drinks, chocolate, French fries, nuts, or others (17). Research is evaluating such issues as the role of lipid-soluble antioxidants (vitamin A and E), omega-3 fatty acids, low fat/low glycemic foods, and other potential dietary factors (17). Cosmetics should be cautiously used and only apply oil-free or water-based types; avoid oily creams and any topical that consistently irritates the skin. For example, pomade acne (Table 1) can be improved by instructing the patient to use a less oily gel or lotion on hair ends. Also, less grease or oil exposure in restaurants or automobile shops can be beneficial to some persons with acne.

Table 2. Outline of Acne Vulgaris Management

1. Grade I or mild comedonal Acne
   a. Benzoyl peroxide (5% - 10%) once or twice a day OR
   b. Tretinoin: once or twice a day
   c. Caution using benzoyl peroxide and tretinoin together as this will increase skin irritation and erythema
   d. Azelaic acid as monotherapy
2. Grade II
   a. Benzoyl peroxide (5% -10%) with topical antibiotics (twice a day)
   b. Tretinoin with topical antibiotics twice a day; antibiotics are used for the inflammatory component of acne; increase tretinoin strength if necessary and tretinoin can be helpful for inflammatory component as well
   c. Can use product that combines benzoyl peroxide and topical antibiotic
   d. Azelaic acid with topical antibiotics
3. Grade III
   a. Antibiotics (oral) with 10% Benzoyl peroxide (twice a day)
   b. OR oral antibiotics with tretinoin (once or twice a day); increase tretinoin strength as needed.
4. Grade IV
   a. Use Grade III scheme.
   b. Use isotretinoin (Accutane)
   c. Dermatology consultation

A wide variety of regimens are utilized by different clinicians in the care of patients with acne vulgaris. Management of inflammatory acne typically involves topical and systemic antibiotics along with retinoic acid and/or benzoyl peroxide. Retinoic acid is the acid form of vitamin A and is also called all-trans retinoic acid (ATRA) (20,21). There are a variety of over-the-counter topics that can be used such as combinations of resorcinol and sulfur. Application of topicals is usually with a pea sized amount on a finger split into four parts of the face and a thin application gently applied over the face. Some patients (such as some males) are reluctant to consistently apply topical medication to their face because this is equated with a feminine task. They can be taught that this is simply applying medication and has nothing to do with masculine or feminine tasks. Clinicians should never underestimate the fact that acne scars (or scars from any cause) are very upsetting to patients and aggressive management is necessary to reduce scar prevention early and throughout the treatment course (22).

Table 2 outlines basic acne vulgaris medical management. Combination products include clindamycin or erythromycin with benzoyl peroxide. These antibiotics are generally not used alone for a long time since this may increase risk for antibiotic resistance. Typical dose of tetracycline or erythromycin is 250 to 500 mg daily (vida infra). The combination of benzoyl peroxide and oral antibiotics may reduce the risk for emergence of antibiotic resistant *P acne*. Various anti-acne vulgaris medications are now reviewed.

Benzoyl peroxide

Benzoyl peroxide is a commonly-used organic compound of the peroxide family consisting of two benzoyl groups connected via a peroxide link. It is listed in the World Health Organization Model List of Essential Medicines. Benzoyl peroxide is useful for comedonal acne because it leads to keratin dehiscence with resultant desquamation; benzoyl peroxide is also bacteriostatic (antimicrobial), anti-inflammatory, and leads to local reduction of free acid levels in the skin (23,24). Its work as a peeling agent leads to heightened skin turnover, pore clearing, and reduction in amounts of local bacteria.

Benzoyl peroxide is available in different formulations (cream, gel, foam, and wash) and topical concentrations: 2.5%, 5% or 10%. Water-based gels are less irritating than acetone or alcohol-based gels. It is also found as soap or a 5% and 10% wash that is very useful for back acne or application to other large areas. It is also available in different combinations with other chemicals, such as sulfur, salicylic acid, adapalene, vitamin A, and antibiotics (erythromycin or clindamycin) (23).

Side effects of this chemical include dryness and erythema particularly in atopic, black, and/or fair-skinned individuals. Liquid and cream forms are less irritating than gel forms, though gel forms seem to be more efficacious. Other side effects include excessive peeling, pigmentary changes, transient acne worsening by stimulation of existing comedones, and increased photosensitivity. Benzoyl peroxide can lead to bleaching of colored articles (i.e., towels, clothes, bed coverings).

One regimen is to advise the patient to start with a thin layer of 5% benzoyl peroxide and use it for a few hours a day or every other day; then, use a gradual build-up plan as tolerated to an overnight application and eventually to a twice a day regimen that allows comfortable dryness and peeling but avoids excessive redness, chapping, cracking, or discomfort.

Eventually the patient should seek to use a 10% gel formulation. Combination products as noted may be helpful in recalcitrant situations.

Tretinoin

Tretinoin is also called all-trans retinoic acid (ATRA) and is the acid form of vitamin A. It is very commonly used in the treatment of acne as a cream or gel and is also used for other dermatological conditions such as alopecia, stretch marks, and wrinkling associated with aging. It is also used in capsule form to treat acute promyelocytic leukemia. A number of brands are available in its topical form. Tretinoin is available in increasing potency: cream (0.025%, 0.05%, 0.1%), gel (0.01%, 0.025%), micro-gel (0.04%, 0.1%) and liquid (0.05%).

Tretinoin targets the main factors of pathogenesis for acne: it heightens the rate of cell turnover in the follicular epithelium, reduces the cohesiveness of the epithelial cell, thins the skin horny layer, heightens antibiotic activity, and leads to less formation of comedones. Many clinicians use tretinoin or other topical retinoids as the first line of management for acne since topical retinoids target the microcomedo which is the precursor to other acne lesions; other advantages to topical retinoids include anti-inflammatory and comedolytic effects. Topical retinoids are combined with oral antibiotics for moderate to severe acne with discontinuation of the antibiotic within 8 to 12 weeks; the retinoid can then be continued as maintenance management (18).

Tretinoin topical application may lead to skin erythema, itching, scaling, burning, and even a severe sunburn. Thus, a gradual increase in its use (as noted with benzoyl peroxide) is recommended and appropriate sunscreen needed with sun exposure. Avoid para-aminobenzoic acid (PABA) sunscreens due to increased hypersensitivity risks. A post-inflammatory increase or decrease in pigmentation may be seen in darker-skinned patients. Side effects may be reduced with lower strength formulations. Evidence of teratogenicity is unclear at this time and it is listed with a category C classification.

Patients using tretinoin should avoid hair removal waxing since removal of the wax leads to removal of the epithelium leading to more erythema and pain. Cautiously use tretinoin with benzoyl peroxide, as for example one topical (i.e., benzoyl peroxide) is used in the morning and then tretinoin at night; however, use of both products increases the risk of severe skin sensitivity.

Use a mild soap and also use a 30 to 45 minute delay between face washing and tretinoin application to reduce skin irritation risks. Liquid or solution forms are most irritating to the skin. Start with a less concentrated from with gradual build-up from once every second or third day to every day as tolerated. Educate the patient that initial use can lead to transient irritation of formed comedones with a temporary pustular rash within two to three weeks of use. This can occur in half of those using tretinoin and may lead to discontinuation because of complaints that the medication made their acne worse. The skin should be dry before coming into contact with bed sheets or clothes due to potential bleaching action of tretinoin.

Adapalene

Adapalene is a third-generation topical, anti-inflammatory retinoid used to treat mild to moderate acne vulgaris because of its ability to reduce microcomedone development. It is available as a 0.1% cream, 0.1% gel, and 0.3% gel. In contrast to tretinoin, adapalene can remain effective even when applied at the same time as benzoyl peroxide. It can heighten the effectiveness of topical clinidamycin though increased side effects may result. It can be used with antibiotics (topical or oral) for mild to moderate acne and combined with oral antibiotics for moderate to severe acne (25). Adapalene was FDA-approved for acne in 1996 and is also used to treat keratosis pilaris.

Tazarotene

Tazarotene is another topical, anti-inflammatory retinoid used to treat mild to moderate acne vulgaris; it is also FDA-approved to treat psoriasis and skin damaged from sun exposure. It is available as a gel or cream and has side effects similar to other topical retinoids; for example, severe skin dryness and cracking may be seen. It is available in two concentrations: 0.05% and 0.1% and it is usually taken once at night after using a mild face cleanser. As with other retinoids and benzoyl peroxide, it may take some weeks for clear evidence of improvement to be seen often leading to patients becoming discouraged and prematurely stopping this medication. Education by the clinician about this possibility may reduce such compliance issues.

Azelaic acid

Azelaic acid is part of the dicarboxylic acid group and is used for mild to moderate acne vulgaris. It is developed from the yeast *Pityrosporum ovale* (*Malassezia furfur*) that lives on normal skin and is industrially made by oleic acid ozonolysis. It is also found in barley, rye, and wheat. Azelaic acid prevents skin pore occlusion (i.e., anti-comedonal effect) and reduces local bacterial growth (i.e., anti-bacterial effect). It is available in a 20% cream or 15% gel form and can be used twice a day as tolerated. Its use may cause tingling, burning, stinging, or itching of the skin which is usually temporary. Hypopigmentation is also reported especially in those with dark skin. However, it also used to treat skin pigmentation disorders since it is a tyrosinase inhibitor that decreases melanin production. Thus, a major benefit of this product is to improve hyperpigmented lesions.

Antibiotics: Overview

Antibiotics are not utilized for mild comedonal acne but are indicated in mild to moderate acne with inflammatory and/or cystic lesions often with other medications (i.e., benzoyl peroxide or retinoids) (Table 2) (26,27). Oral formulations are used for moderate to severe acne and may take 1 to 2 months to see improvement and can be used for many months.

Improvement occurs because of *P acnes* suppression, bacterial lipase inhibition, and interference with neutrophil migration by local chemotaxis improvement. Topical formulations should be used for short-term use (as under 3 months) and not combined with the same antibiotic in oral form to reduce the risk of antibiotic resistance which is especially noted with topical erythromycin and clindamycin. Such resistance may also be lowered with the combination of antibiotics with topical benzoyl peroxide or topical retinoid. The development of such resistance leads to poor response to anti-acne treatments.

Topical forms of erythromycin (1.5%-3.0%), or clindamycin (1%) are used as well as oral forms of tetracycline, erythromycin, doxycycline, and minocycline. Irritation and dryness may occur with topical formulations. Pseudomembranous enterocolitis is an unusual side effect to use of topical clindamycin. A gel form may be more efficacious for those with oily skin. Combination with benzoyl peroxide is available as seen with erythromycin or clindamycin.

Oral tetracycline

Tetracycline hydrochloride has been a commonly used oral antibiotic for acne vulgaris with a dose usually between 250 mg to 1,000 mg per day. Dosages over 1 gram per day are seldom used. One regimen is use 250 mg four times a day (500 mg twice a day) with gradual reduction to 250 mg once a day as efficacy is seen. Occasional patients require 2 to 3 grams per day for significant improvement. Inhibition of MMP (matrix metalloproteinase) enzymes are part of the effectiveness of tetracycline in acne treatment (28).

Optimal absorption is seen when taken on an empty stomach (i.e., 2 hours after a meal or 1 hour before a meal). It may take two to four weeks for improvement to be appreciated. Failure of efficacy may arise because of issues with compliance, antibiotic resistance, absorption problems, and/or persistence of deep nodular lesion.

Tetracycline has proved to be a safe antibiotic that can be used for many years. Periodic screening should be done that includes a complete blood count (CBC), blood urea nitrogen, creatinine, and liver enzymes. Side effects tend to be dose-related, particularly if daily doses are over 500 mg (Table 3). Clinicians should carefully monitor for gastrointestinal (esophageal) irritation, photosensitivity, and with chronic use, renal complications as well as microbial resistance. It should be taken on an empty stomach with a large glass of water; avoid taking it with an antacid or with dairy products. Gram-negative folliculitis (especially around the nose) may occur in some with severe acne taking tetracycline chronically. Using with ibuprofen may heighten the efficacy of tetracycline.

Monilial vaginitis responds to anti-fungal treatment and tetracycline discontinuation is usually not necessary. Tetracycline is not used in those under age 9 years since it may cause enamel defects in unerupted teeth and can be deposited in teeth as well as bones of a fetus of a pregnant individual. Tetracycline is contraindicated in pregnancy. Anecdotal cases of pregnancy are reported in females on both oral contraception and tetracycline; however, there is no clear evidence-based research that antibiotics, such as tetracycline, actually reduce efficacy of oral contraceptives.

Table 3. Potential side effects of tetracycline

Allergic reactions
Bacterial resistance
Esophagitis
Gastrointestinal irritation
Gram-negative folliculitis
Headache
Hemolytic anemia
Inhibition of leukocytosis during acute infections
Monilial vaginitis
Photoonycholysis – separation of the nail from its plate after sun exposure (rare)
Photosensitivity
Pseudotumor cerebri.
Teeth discoloration (do *not* use in those younger than 12!)
Transient blood urea nitrogen elevation
Transient leucopenia
Transient liver enzyme elevation

Other oral antibiotics

Erythromycin is also widely used for acne vulgaris and is used in doses of 500 mg to 2,000 mg per day. Erythromycin may also lead to gastric irritation including when taken on empty stomach. Side effects also include nausea and diarrhea which can be reduced by taking enteric-coated erythromycin. It can be given at any age.

Doxycycline (50 mg twice daily), trimethoprim-sulfamethoxazole, and minocycline (50-300 mg per day) have also been used. *Doxycycline* has similar side effects to tetracycline, though with less dental staining. Gastrointestinal upset, photosensitivity, and photo-onycholysis are well known adverse effects of this antibiotic. Do not give to those under 9 years of age. Oral *clindamycin* (150-600 mg per day) is not used for acne since it can lead to colitis. Bacterial resistance is a growing phenomenon and it is recommended to avoid using oral or systemic antibiotics over 3 months in attempts to control this problem.

Minocycline can lead to dizziness, headaches, photosensitivity, vertigo (vestibular disturbance), tooth discoloration, and, with chronic use, increased skin pigmentation as well as localized facial marks that are dark bluish; also, rarely seen are autoimmune syndromes with hepatitis, serum sickness-like reaction, lupus-like syndrome, and a hypersensitivity syndrome. It should be given on an empty stomach and avoid taking it with dairy products. It should not be given to those under 9 years of age. Dosage is 50 to 100 mg twice a day. Its high price and significant potential adverse effects both suggest it is a second-line oral antibiotic for acne vulgaris treatment (29).

Trimethoprim-sulfamethoxazole can be given at any age but should only be used as a second-line drug for acne vulgaris. It can lead to drug hypersensitivity reaction, bone marrow suppression, gastrointestinal upset, hepatitis, and renal toxicity. It should be avoided in glucose-6-phosphate dehydrogenase deficiency (G6PD) and used only as a second-line antibiotic. Dosage is once or twice daily of the 80/400 or 160/800 mg formulations. Some clinicians prescribe *cephalexin* at 250-500 mg twice a day; it can be used any age but can lead to gastrointestinal upset and it is considered as a second –line drug.

Dapsone

Dapsone (diamino-diphenyl sulfone) is a white to creamy-white, odorless crystalline powder used to treat a number of disorders, including mild to moderate acne vulgaris as a 5% gel. Oral dapsone is also used for acne fulminans and acne conglobata if other treatments do not work and is used for its anti-inflammatory and immunomodulatory effects.

Miscellaneous acne treatments

Oral zinc sulfate has been used with mixed results by clinicians and has been limited by gastrointestinal side effects (17). The role of topical sulfur, salicylic acid, and resorcinol remains unclear though they have been used for many years (17). Patients with severe cystic acne and thick walls can be improved with intralesional steroid injection (triamcinolone acetonide) or incision and drainage. Use of antiandrogens may be helpful in some, such as spironolactone (50-200 mg per day) or cyproterone that can reduce sebum production (*vida infra*).

Oral contraceptives can improve acne vulgaris by lowering gonadotropin secretion with reduced ovarian-induced androgens and also by increasing SHBG (sex hormone binding globulin) levels that lower free testosterone levels. Oral contraceptives can serve as an adjuvant treatment for acne, particular in a female who is sexually active. Pills with low androgenic progestin are recommended, such as norgestimate which is FDA-approved for the treatment of acne vulgaris or others (3, 30-32). Sexually active females with acne may notice worsening of this condition if placed on long-acting progestin implants or depo-medroxy-progesterone acetate.

Ultraviolet light therapy does not significantly improve acne vulgaris and may lead to skin aging and possibly melanoma. Research is focusing on newer research treatments such as use of low-dose isotretinoin plans, chemical peels, photodynamic therapy (PDT), light and laser treatments, anti-inflammatory agents as lipooxygenase inhibitors, insulin-sensitizing drugs, 5-alpha-reductase type I inhibitors, oral probiotics, and others (33-35). PDT uses a photosensitizer, light source, and molecular oxygen to kill specific cells in the pilosebaceous units and is being used by dermatologists to treat inflammatory acne vulgaris (36). Scars can be treated with a chemical peel, dermabrasion, collagen injection, or intralesional steroids or keloids.

Isotretinoin (13-cis-retinoic acid)

Isotretinoin is a powerful anti-acne medication identified since the 1980s to be effective in many cases of severe, recalcitrant, nodulocystic acne, milder acne resistant to other more traditional treatments, and various forms of acne with scarring and psychological distress (37-39). It is a derivative of vitamin A and is used in other conditions including hidradenitis suppurativa, acne rosacea, acne fulminans, acne conglobata, some forms of ichthyosis, and others. Its precise mechanism of action is unclear but may be related to its effect on NGAL (neutrophil-gelatinase-associated lipocalin) in skin which lowers sebum production and exerts an antimicrobial effect on *P. acne*. It decreases sebum production and shrinks sebaceous glands in addition to having anti-inflammatory effects; it also improves abnormal keratinization. Though its effect on sebum production is temporary, the remission on acne can be permanent.

Dosage includes 0.05 to 1.0 mg (up to 2.0 mg) per kg per day over a twice a day course for 15 to 24 weeks (up to 9 months); improvement is typically seen with an accumulative dose of 100 to 150 mg per kilogram. A second course is occasionally needed after 2 months or more off the medication. Most patients receive significant improvement, including 40% or more with complete acne resolution. Lower doses (i.e., half the usual dose) may be effective in some with lower side effects but a higher relapse rate. Prior to isotretinoin prescription the clinician should order a complete blood count (CBC), chemistry profile (including liver function tests), and fasting lipids (triglycerides and cholesterol). The CBC and chemistry profile are typically obtained again at 4 to 6 weeks into treatment with isotretinoin.

A large number of side effects are possible with isotretinoin (Table 4). Triglycerides are particularly increased in those with diabetes mellitus, alcohol abuse, obesity, and/or positive family history for hyperlipidemia. Patients with a history of intestinal disorders may develop severe diarrhea or rectal bleeding; some research notes a possible link to inflammatory bowel disease in some patients that includes both ulcerative colitis and Crohn's disease. Diffuse skeletal hyperostosis may develop with prolonged use of isotretinoin. There is an association between pseudotumor cerebri with tetracyclines and isotretinoin; vitamin A supplements may increase this toxic risk as well. Final closure of epiphyses may not occur in youth until the late teens or even early 20s and thus, use of isotretoinoin in this age group may result in decreased potential growth by reducing long bone growth. High doses of isotretinoin can result in toxicity that looks like vitamin A toxicity. It is not used with a history of allergy to paraben because paraben is used as a preservative in the isotretinoin gelatin capsule.

Frequent (even hourly) application of white petrolatum to the lips is helpful in dealing with the often present cheilitis due to isotretinoin; steroid ointment may be helpful such as 1% hydrocortisone or stronger formulations. Xerosis may improve with application of lipid-free moisturizers or lotions without worsening the acne. Ocular dryness may improve or stabilize with artificial tears. The risk of photosensitivity is lowered with use of sunscreens in an oil-free, non-acnegenic base. A lower dose of the isotretinoin may be necessary to deal with such irritating adverse effects. Use of isotretinoin can lead to the appearance of lesions that look like pyogenic granulomas and may require discontinuing the isotretinoin if steroids do not ameliorate this development. Apply antibiotic ointment (i.e., mupirocin) to the nose two times a day to reduce *Staphylococcus aureus* infections, which if this develops, requires appropriate antibiotics. The clinician should be vigilant in observing and managing these potentially serious infections.

Table 4. Potential side effects of isotretinoin

Teratogenicity (see text; Table 5)
Cheilitis (90%)*
Severe dry skin and pruritus (80%)*
Dry nose and mouth along with epistaxis (80%)
Conjunctivitis (40%)
Dry eyes*
Decreased night vision*
Difficulty with contact lenses (40%)
Increased cholesterol and triglycerides (25%)*
Musculoskeletal aches (16%)
Alopecia and hair thinning (10%)*
Photosensitivity
Arthralgia*
Corneal opacities (5%)
Headache (5%)
Fatigue (5%)
Depression (<5%)*
? Suicide risk?
Elevated liver enzyme and blood sugar levels
Severe rectal bleeding and diarrhea
Acne rosacea* (with high doses of isotretinoin)
Inflammatory bowel disease* (including exacerbation of previous disease)
Low back pain
Keloids*
Degenerative disc disease*
Increased susceptibility to sunburn
Osteopenia*
Peeling of palms and soles
Pseudotumor cerebri (especially when combined with oral antibiotics)
Premature epiphyseal closure
Cervical spine hyperostosis
Erectile dysfunction*
Others
*May be permanent side effects

Teratogenicity and isotretinoin

Isotretinoin is a *major* teratogenic agent and Table 5 outlines some of these defects; it is contraindicated in pregnancy and is classified as an FDA Pregnancy Category X and ADEC Category X. The use of this drug during pregnancy leads to a 25-fold increase in teratogencity that includes mental subnormality in 50% even without external evidence of other defects. Isotretinoin does affect the fetal dividing cells but not the spermatozoa or ova.

Table 5. Teratogenic effects of isotretinoin*

Affected Area of the Body	Teratogenic Effects
Head	Microcephaly, abnormal cranium, anencephaly, seizures, psychomotor retardation.
Eyes	Microphthalmia, blindness, down-slant of palpebral fissures.
Ears	Atretic ears, hypoplastic auditory meatus, absent eighth nerve, deafness, rudimentary, or malformed pinnae.
Mouth	Cleft palate, cleft lip, micrognathia.
Heart	Patent ductus arteriosus, atrial septal defects, ventricular septal defects, truncus arteriosus, others.

Used with permission from: Greydanus DE: Disorders of the skin. In: AD Hofmann, DE Greydanus (eds). Adolescent Medicine, 3rd Edition. Stanford, CT: Appleton & Lange, 1997; ch. 18:380.

The FDA announced the *iPLEDGE* program in 2005 to emphasize the need for pregnancy females to avoid taking isotretinoin. Since 2006 only clinicians officially listed in this program can prescribe this drug and only patients who are officially registered can received this drug. This also includes males though there is no evidence that their sperm is affected. Females taking isotretinoin should have negative pregnancy test (s) at least 2 weeks prior to its initiation and should take two types of contraception at the same time for at least 30 days prior to starting it and for at least 30 days following use of this drug. If one if taking isotretinoin, s/he is not allowed to donate blood during the time on this drug and also for at least 30 days after stopping it. The program for isotretinoin management recommended by the manufacturer is called *S.M.A.R.T.* (System to Manage Accutane Related Teratogenity (20,40).

Depression, suicidality, and isotretinoin

Isotretinoin has been linked by anecdotal data to depression, psychosis, and even suicide in some patients. However, research in general has failed to establish a clear link between use of this drug and overt depression as well as suicide (41-43). Anecdotal cases of suicide in patients taking isotretinoin fuel the on-going debate. It is clear that patients with acne have increased risk for depression because of the distress that this condition can induce. It is also clear that depression and suicide are real phenomena among adolescents and young adult around the world. Separating out the role of isotretinoin as a cause of depression and/or suicide in those with severe, cystic, disfiguring acne from other factors is very difficult. Even those with so-called "mild" acne can have major distress because of negative reactions to this disorder. Clinicians should be aware of the real presence of depression and suicide in this age group and should be aware of the potentially negative effects of severe acne itself. Thus, those taking this drug and all patients with acne should receive careful and on-going screening for depression and suicidality.

Table 6. Causes of hyperandrogenemia in females with potential of severe acne*

- Genetic and familial increased androgen sensitivity
- Adrenal androgens
  - Congenital adrenal hyperplasias
    - 21-hydroxylase deficiency
      - Classic
      - Late-onset
    - 3-β hydroxysteroid dehydrogenase deficiency
      - Classic
      - Late-onset
    - 11β-hydroxylase deficiency
      - Classic
      - Late-onset
  - Adrenal tumors
    - Adrenocortical carcinoma
    - Testosterone-secreting adenoma
    - Adrenal rest adenoma and carcinoma
  - Cushing's disease
- Ovarian androgens
  - Polycystic ovary syndrome (PCOS)
    - Conditions associated with PCOS
      - PCOS with ovarian tumor
  - Pineal gland hyperplasia and diabetes
  - Congenital lipoatrophic diabetes
  - Hyperprolactinemia
  - Hyperthyroidism
  - Hypothyroidism
  - Androgen-secreting cysts and hyperplasias
    - Stromal hyperplasia and hyperthecosis
    - Solitary follicle cyst
    - Hyperreactio luteinalis of pregnancy
  - Androgen-secreting ovarian tumors
    - Arrhenoblastoma (androblastoma)
    - Thecoma-fibroma group tumors
    - Granulosa cell tumors
    - Lipoid cell tumors
    - Gynandroblastoma
    - Epithelial tumor
    - Luteoma of pregnancy
- Testicular androgens in XY females
  - 5-α reductase deficiency
  - Mixed gonadal dysgenesis
  - True hermaphroditism
  - 17-β hydroxysteroid dehydrogenase deficiency
  - Other rare intersex conditions
- Exogenous androgens
  - Medical
    - Hypoplastic anemias
    - Growth stimulation
    - Adrenal replacement
    - Danazol
    - Synthetic progestins in oral contraceptives
    - Adrenocorticotropic hormone (ACTH) therapy
  - Nonmedical
    - Bodybuilding and athletic anabolic steroids

Source: Reprinted with permission, from: Greydanus DE, Shearin RB: Adolescent Sexuality and Gynecology. Philadelphia: Lea & Febiger, 1990, p 177.

* Used with permission: Greydanus DE, Patel DR. Acne vulgaris and chronically ill adolescents. Internat J Disabil & Hum Devel 2008; 7(3): 322.

Management of acne vulgaris comorbid conditions

Another part of the overall management plan for acne is to treat underlying or co-morbid conditions. For example, acne can be very severe in disorders with increased androgens, such as congenital adrenal hyperplasia, polycystic ovary syndrome (PCOS), Cushing's disease, Syndrome X (hyperlipidemia, obesity, hypertension, and insulin resistance), and other states of hyperandrogenemia (Table 6) (1,2,20).

Acne may be the first significant sign of PCOS or adrenal hyperandrogenism. Underlying endocrine disorders should be carefully managed and appropriate medications can be very helpful in acne treatment as well; these medications include low-dose prednisone, oral contraceptives, anti-androgens (i.e., cimetidine, spironolactone, or cyproterone acetate), or even GnRH (gonadotropin-releasing hormone) agonists. Side effects of these various medications must be kept in mind; for example, adverse effects of spironolactone include menstrual irregularity, fatigue, hyperkalemia, and breast tenderness. Also, some medications can worsen acne (Table 7) and these should be discontinued if possible and alternative drugs used that do not worsen the dermatological condition.

Table 7. Medications/chemicals that worsen acne*

Androgenic steroids
Barbiturates
Bromides
Diphenylhydantoin
Glucocorticoids
Iodides
Isoniazid
Kelp and other seaweed
Lithium
Rifampin
Synthetic progestins
Vitamin B 12
Others

* Used with permission: Greydanus DE, Patel DR. Acne vulgaris and chronically ill adolescents. Internat J Disabil & Hum Devel 2008; 7(3): 323.

Management of well being in acne patients

Depression is a common aspect in human beings and also those with acne (44). Acne develops intense feelings of sadness, guilt, shame, and anger in adolescence at a time when the youth's sense of self is emerging (45-50). Approximately 25% of adolescents with acne have some scarring by late adolescence adding to their sense of distress over this disease (51,52). The development of acne is a major problem for both the adolescent as well as adult and can have immense negative impact on their psychosocial development that can last a lifetime. The art and science of managing acne patients demands that the clinician address this feature in addition to the formal and classic medical task of prescribing drugs.

Effective management of all with acne is important and its value should never be underestimated. Youth should be asked and taught about acne treatment even if the patient does not ask about management options. As noted, it is difficult to separate out depression that may occur in any person from depression worsened by the skin condition itself. It is also difficult to separate out suicidality that occurs in many youth and adults from that stimulated by acne itself. Those with acne should be evaluated for depression, suicidality, anxiety, body dysmorphic disorder, self-injury (acne excoriée—vida infra), and other mental health issues (53-56).

Successful treatment of acne includes the *sine qua non* principle that acne management is not only prescription of dermatological agents but careful and persistent attention to the psychosocial and mental health status of this patient whose feelings can be more sensitive than the acne skin (57). The emotional health of these patients should be evaluated and monitored as the acne management is developed. For example, stress can trigger and worsen acne by androgen hormone activation. Some patients may need overt mental health treatment with therapy and/or psychopharmacologic management (58-60).

Acne excoriée

Acne excoriée refers to acneform lesions on the face and other parts of the body due to deliberate self-injury on normal and/or abnormal skin. It is part of a wide range of self-induced skin diseases that includes dermatitis artefacta, neurotic self-mutilation (neurotic excoriation), self-mutilation associated with psychotic features (i.e., hallucinations or delusions), nail biting (onychophagia), Munchhausen syndrome, and acne excoriée (61). The patient may present with multiple excoriated or acne-form lesions over the face (as well as upper arms, forearms, other areas) with or without a history of previous lesions. There may be a history of mental illness such as obsessive-compulsive disorder, depression, psychosis, or other disorders. A careful medical history reveals that the patient may have an uncontrollable urge for self-mutilation and underlies the need for the clinician to know the patient carefully and not just injudiciously provide medical prescriptions (62).

The patient may not complain of these lesions even if they appear to be painful or unsightly (63). There may be lesions that do not heal despite appropriate treatment such as antibiotics and the clinician should be highly suspicious of dermatological features (including ulcers and scars) that do not conform to known patterns of physiologic illness (64). The mentally disturbed patient may develop habits that directly lead to skin trauma of various degrees that can lead to linear and stellate facial ulcers, hypertrophic scars, and other lesions (65). If treatment does not occur, the condition may continue for many years. The patient may admit to the self-injury if carefully asked and may note squeezing, rubbing, or picking at lesions. Self-destructive behavior is common in mentally retarded patients (66).

Management begins with suspicion on the part of the clinician because of lesions that do not fit known disorders and/or do not heal properly with treatment. A mental status, medical history, and careful examination are needed for all these patients. Treatment is needed for the underlying behavior/psychiatric disorder (s) and may include psychotherapy and/or psychopharmacology (61-64). As the underlying psychopathology is improved, the scars can be treated with dermatological treatments such as resurfacing (chemical peels, lasers, light therapy, cryotherapy), dermal fillers, and surgery (i.e., dermabrasion, subcision or punch excision) (14,67-69).

Acne rosacea

Acne rosacea, a condition known for centuries, is a chronic, inflammatory dermatological condition mainly observed in adults that is distinct from acne vulgaris and is characterized by flushing, central facial erythema (transient or persistent), dilated (visible) blood vessels (telangiectasias; couperosis), burning pain, comedones, papules, pustules, and/or facial skin fibrosis (10,70). There can also be ocular involvement (30% to 50%) with thickened skin and the enlargement (phymas) of the nose called rhinophyma (bulbous nose, phymatous rosacea). The cause of the bulbous nose (i.e., enlarged, bulb-shaped, erythematous) is unclear; it was erroneously linked for centuries with excess alcohol, and is now linked with being a rare part of severe rosacea. “Phyma” comes from the Greek and means mass (swelling or bulb). The nose can contain many oil glands that present a yellow or waxy appearance. The development of malignancy within rhinophyma has been reported (71,72).

The term “rosacea” denotes the facial telangiectasias with or without facial erythema and acne rosacea was separated from acne vulgaris by clinicians in the 20th century as more understanding of these conditions emerged (73). The red face has historically been used by novelists and others to denote negative traits of persons adding to the stigmata of rosacea that continues to the present (73).

Current studies present a range of epidemiologic data based on criteria used for the diagnosis. Acne rosacea classically is first noted around 30 years of age and affects 1% to 20% of the adult population to some extent (74). Though less common, acne rosacea, including ocular rosacea, can occur in children as young as one year of age (75). A positive family history and having very light skin (“Celtic” skin type) increase the risk for this disorder while the often indicted coffee and alcohol are not risk factors (74).

Four types of acne rosacea have been established based on the National Rosacea Society’s Expert Committee on the Classification and Staging of Rosacea: erythemato-telangiectatic, papulopustular, phymatous, and ocular (76-80). Other variants are noted, such as lupoid or granulomatous types, which may represent different rosacea stages or overlapping syndromes (80).

Pathophysiology

The cause of acne rosacea is unclear at this time but is currently linked to various factors such as inflammatory, genetic, environmental, vascular, and microbial (i.e., *Helicobacter pylori* and *Demodex folliculorum*) (76). Some with rosacea have a light phototype which is sensitive to various climate changes while others have genetic proclivity for primary vascular anomalies which are then influenced by a variety of factors such as ultraviolet ray exposure, skin flora, and/or climate changes (81). A precipitating factor in some may be reactive oxygen species that includes superoxide and hydroxyl radicals, hydrogen peroxide, and singlet oxygen (82).

Rosacea swelling or edema allows colonization and growth of microbes (as *Demodex folliculorum*) which can lead to inflammation that contributes to rosacea papules, pustules, and granulomas (81,83). *Demodex folliculorum* is a species of face mite that increases in amount during early adolescence due to the increase in sebaceous glands; they are found in increased concentration in the central part of the face and their food is sebaceous secretions and dead cells.

Recent research in molecular biology provides etiologic links with inflammatory and vascular factors because of immune dysfunction (77). Research also notes dysregulation of mediators and receptors involved in neurovascular as well as neuroimmune communication in early stages of rosacea; it may be a neurogenic inflammatory disorder due to sensory nerve disease because of abnormal release of key neuromediators (84). Other researchers describe acne rosacea as a disorder of cathelicidins and skin innate immunity (85). Those with rosacea have increased levels of these polypeptides called cathelicidins (vida supra) and also increased levels of stratum corneum tryptic enzymes (SCTEs). SCTEs are an important part of the desquamation process in human skin which involves production of corneocytes and their shedding from skin.

Further understanding of the pathophysiology of acne rosacea will enhance our understanding of connections between the human immune, nervous, and cutaneous vascular systems (86). For example, the development of skin fibrosis in some rosacea patients indicates a powerful link between chronic *inflammatory* mechanisms and the development of fibrosis in the skin. The vascular defects in rhinophyma can lead to local development of TGF-β1 (transforming growth factor-β1) that induces skin fibrosis and skin thickening (82). TGF-β1is a protein controlling cellular differentiation, proliferation, and other functions in most cells.

Steroid-induced rosacea (iatrosacea) is described in patients using chronic facial steroids, particularly topical steroids of class II potency which can lead to facial erythema, telangiectasias, photosensitivity, hyperpigmentation, and xerosis (87). The underlying etiology with iatrosacea is linked to steroid-induced rebound vasodilatation and proinflamatory cytokine release (87).

Management of acne rosacea

The purpose of therapy is to raise the patient's quality of life by improving this disease in which there is noticeable reduction in erythema, papules, pustules, and overt physical discomfort (77). The skin should be protected from harmful effects of sunlight and the patient should avoid known triggers for disease exacerbation (78). Triggers in some patients include ultraviolet radiation, stress, microbes, heat, cold, and/or spicy foods that can precipitate rosacea pathophysiologic mechanisms noted earlier and involve the cytokine as well as chemokine networks (88). Management of steroid-induced rosacea is stopping the topical steroid and use of topical tacrolimus and oral antibiotics (87).

Evidence-based research suggests effective results for acne rosacea can be seen with the use of acne medications such as doxycycline (40 mg) and azelaic acid (15% gel) as well as topical metronidazole. Ocular rosacea may improve with cyclosporine (0.5% ophthalmic emulsion) and 40 mg doxycycline (slow release form) (71,72,75,89,). Sodium sulfacetamide

10%-sulfur 5% (emollient foam) is also used by clinicians for acne rosacea while second-line management drugs include clindamycin, benzoyl peroxide, permethrin, and calcineurin inhibitors (77). A synergistic effect has been reported with the combination of azelaic acid as well as topical metronidazole with doxycycline (78,90). Improvement with both azelaic acid and doxycycline has been linked to the ability of these drugs to down regulate antimicrobial and proinflammatory cathelicidins (14).

Pimecrolimus is an immunomodulating topical agent (1% cream) used to treat atopic dermatitis with recent research noting some efficacy in rosacea. New products continue to be evaluated, such as brimonidine tartrate gel (0.5%), are being evaluated for rosacea; this α-2-adrenergic agonist has vasoconstrictive activity and has been shown to be efficacious in the management of rosacea (92).

Choosing the right soothing vehicle or formulation that includes cleansers, moisturizers, and facial foundation products is important to the overall management success in providing efficacy with minimal skin irritation that will increase patient compliance (93,94). It is also important to provide decongestant active ingredients and appropriate medical make-up to improve the red face appearance (95).

Oral isotretinoin is also used for phymatous rosacea and other types of acne rosacea recalcitrant to other treatments (76,78,96). Erythematous skin and telangiectasias are also managed with light-based therapies (i.e., pulsed dye laser and intense pulsed light) (78, 97). Treatment of rhinophyma is with surgery to correct the nasal appearance using laser surgery or dermabrasion (rotating brush) as well with anti-acne medications. Surgery may be requested by the patient because of cosmetic concerns, issues with airway obstruction or eating difficulty (98).

Acne variants

Table 1 lists a variety of acne variants. For example, *acne conglobata* may improve with sulfone, oral steroids, and/or oral isotretinoin. *Acne fulminans* is also called acute febrile, ulcerative, conglobate acne in which there can be an acute onset of hemorrhagic and ulcerative acne that involves the face, chest, back, and other areas. It can be the skin manifestation of SAPHO (acute fulminans with synovitis-acne-pustulosis-hyperostosis-osteitis) (99). Acne fulminans may be improved with acne measures already reviewed along with salicylates (for fever and/or muscle-joint symptomatology), oral corticosteroids (topical and systemic), dapsone (diaminodiphenyl sulfone), nonsteroidal anti-inflammatory drugs (NSAIDs), infliximab, methotrexate and/or isotretinoin (see below) (99-101). Table 1 outlines other acne variants as well as acneform disorders and outlines management concepts.

Conclusion

Acne vulgaris relates to abnormal keratinization, androgen-stimulated hormone and sebum production, follicular plug development (pilosebaceous unit obstruction), colonization with *P. acnes*, host response to inflammation, and genetic factors (102-105). Management is individualized based on disease severity, motivation of the patient for treatment, and comorbid conditions. Recommended treatment options are likely to be continued if the patient is bothered by this dermatological condition and perceives that management leads to significant improvement. Patients must be taught that treatment may take some weeks before positive results can be appreciated. Time should be spent by clinicians in explaining the cause of acne and dealing with challenging compliance issues in some patients. The time is worthwhile for the clinician and patient since acne can have lifelong negative consequences for the youth and his/her overall wellbeing in adulthood.

Fortunately, most persons can be effectively treated with a combination of topical agents (i.e., benzoyl peroxide, topical retinoids, azelaic acid, antibiotics), and oral agents (i.e., oral contraceptives, oral antibiotics) (106). Oral isotretinoin is a powerful drug for severe and/or resistant acne that is both beneficial for most but also fraught with many potential side effects including teratogenicity (107). Consultation with dermatology is necessary for dealing with situations not responsive to basic acne measures and for dealing with isotretinoin. Fortunately, most patients with acne will see improvement with currently available options. However, successful management of acne is not just prescribing dermatological agents, but includes judicious attention to the psychosocial well being of this patient who can be physically but even more seriously emotionally scarred for life by this most common of skin disorders (108). The website for treatment of acne from the American Academy of Dermatology is available at www.skincarephysicians.com/acnenet.

Acknowledgments

This paper is a revised and adapted version of an earlier publication: Greydanus DE.The acnes: Acne vulgaris, acne rosacea and acne excoritee. In: Tareen RS, Greydanus DE, Jafferany M, Patel DR, Merrick J, eds. Pediatric psychodermatology. A clinical manual of child and adolescent psychocutaneous disorders. Berlin: De Gruyter, 2013:163-92.

References

[1] Greydanus DE. Disorders of the skin. In: Hofmann AD, Greydanus DE, eds. Adolescent Medicine, 3rd edition. Stanford, CT: Appleton Lange, 1997:375-407.

[2] Greydanus DE, Patel DR. Acne vulgaris and chronically ill adolescents. Int J Disabil Hum Devel 2008;7(3):319-327.

[3] Williams HC, Dellavalle RP, Garner S. Acne vulgaris. Lancet 2012;379(9813):361-72.

[4] James WD. Acne. N Engl J Med 2005;352:1463-72.

[5] Krowchuk DP, Gelmetti C, Lucky AW. Acne. In: Schachner LA, Hansen RC, eds. Pediatric Dermatology, Fourth ed. Philadelphia, PA: Mosby, 2011:827-50.

[6] Ascenso A, Marques HC. Acne in the adult. Mini Rev Med Chem 2009;9:1-10.

[7] Friedlander SF, Baldwin HE, Mancini AJ, Yan AC, Eichenfeld LF. The acne continuum: An age-based approach to therapy. Semin Cutan Med Surg 2011;30(3 Suppl):S6-11.

[8] Schnopp C, Mempel M. Acne vulgaris in children and adolescents. Minerva Pediatr 2011;63:293-304.

[9] Bhambri S, Del Rosso JQ, Bhambri A. Pathogenesis of acne vulgaris: Recent advances. J Drugs Dermatol 2009;8:615-8.

[10] Powell FC. Rosacea. N Engl J Med 2005;252:793-803.

[11] Feinberg AN. The integument system: Skin, hair, nails. In: Greydanus DE, Feinberg AN, Patel DR, Homnick DN, eds. The pediatric examination. New York: McGraw-Hill, 2008:570.

[12] Bellew S, Thiboutot D, Del Rosso JQ. Pathogenesis of acne vulgaris: What's new, what's interesting, and what may be clinically relevant. J Drugs Dermatol 2011;10:582-5.

[13] Zouboulis CC. Modern aspects of acne pathogenesis. J Dutsch Dermatol Ges 2010;8(Suppl 1):S7-S14.

[14] Fleischer AB Jr. Inflammation in rosacea and acne: Implications for patient care. J Drugs Dermatol 2011;10:614-20.

[15] Basta-Juzbašić A. Current therapeutic approach to acne scars. Acta Dermatovenerol Croat 2010;18:171-5.

[16] Newman MD, Bowe WP, Heughebaert C, Shalita AR. Therapeutic considerations for severe nodular acne. Am J Clin Dermatol 2011;12:7-14.

[17] Szczepaniak D, Treadwell PA. Acne therapy in primary care: Comprehensive review of current evidence-based interventions and treatments. Adolesc Med 2011;22:77-96.

[18] Zaenglein AL, Thiboutot DM. Expert committee recommendations for acne management. Pediatrics 2006;118(3):1188-99.

[19] Baldwin HE, Friedlander SF, Eichenfield LF, Mancini AJ, Jan AC. The effects of culture, skin color, and other nonclinical issues on acne treatment. Semin Cutan Med Surg 2011;30(3 Suppl):S12-5.

[20] Krowchuk DP. Disorders of the skin. In: Greydanus DE, Patel DR, Pratt HD, eds. Essential adolescent medicine. New York: McGraw-Hill, 2006:411-43.

[21] Haider A, Shaw JC. Treatment of acne vulgaris. JAMA 2004;292:726-35.

[22] Layton AM. Optimal management of acne to prevent scarring and psychological sequelae. Am J Clin Dermatol 2001;2(3):135-41.

[23] Dutil M. Benzoyl peroxide: Enhancing antibiotic efficacy in acne management. Skin Therapy Lett 2010;15:5-7.

[24] Fakhouri T, Yentzer BA, Feldman SR. Advancement in benzoyl-peroxide-based acne treatment: Methods to increase both efficacy and tolerability. J Drug Dermatol 2009;8:657-61.

[25] Thiboutot DM, Gollnick HP. Treatment considerations for inflammatory acne: Clinical evidence for adapalene 0.1% in combination therapies. J Drugs Dermatol 2006;5:785-94.

[26] Eady EA, Cove JH, Joanes DN. Topical antibiotics for the treatment of acne vulgaris: A critical evaluation of their clinical benefit and comparative efficacy. J Dermatol Treat 1990;1:215-20.

[27] Ozolins M, Eady EA, Avery AJ, et al: Comparison of five antimicrobial regimens for treatment of mild to moderate inflammatory acne vulgaris in the community: randomized controlled trial. Lancet 2004;364:2188-95.

[28] Monk E, Shalita A, Siegel DM. Clinical applications of non-antimicrobial tetracyclines in dermatology. Pharmacol Res 2011;63:130-45.

[29] Garner SE, Eady EA, Popescu C, Newton J, Li WA. Minocycline for acne vulgaris: efficacy and safety. Cochrane Database Syst Rev 2003;(1):CD002086.

[30] Redmond GP, Olson WH, Lippman JS. Norgestimate and ethinyl estrodiol in the treatment of acne vulgaris: A randomized, placebo-controlled trial. Obstet Gynecol 1997;89:615-20.

[31] Rosen MP, Breitkopf DM, Nagamani M. A randomized controlled trial of second versus third generation oral contraceptives in the treatment of acne vulgaris. Am J Obstet Gynecol 2003;188:1158-60.

[32] Guerra-Tapia A, Sancho Pérez B. Ethinylestradiol/chlormadinone acetate: dermatological benefits. Am J Clin Dermatol 2011;12(Suppl 1):3-11.

[33] Katsambas A, Dessinioti C. New and emerging treatments in dermatology: Acne. Dermatol Ther 2008;21:86-95.

[34] Kim RH, Armstrong AW. Current state of acne treatment: highlighting lasers, photodynamic therapy, and chemical peels. Dermatol Online J 2011;17:2-5.

[35] Bowe WP, Logan AC. Acne vulgaris, probiotics and the gut-brain-skin axis—back to the future? Gut Pathol 2011;3:1-4.

[36] Gold MH. Photodyamic therapy. Curr Probl Dermatol 2011;42:181-92.

[37] Abel EA. Isotretinoin (Accutane) therapy for acne vulgaris for adolescents. Adolesc Med 1990;1(2):315-24.

[38] Goldsmith LA, Bolognia JL, Callen JP. American Academy of Dermatology Consensus Conference on the safe and optimal use of isotretinoin: summary and recommendations. J Am Acad Dermatol 2004;50:900-6.

[39] Rigopoulos D, Larios G, Katsambas AD. The role of isotretinoin in acne therapy: why not as first line therapy? Facts and controversies. Clin Dermatol 2010;28:24-30.

[40] Krowchuk DP. Managing adolescent acne: A guide for pediatricians. Pediatr Rev 2005;26:250-61.

[41] Hull PR, D'Arcy C. Isotretinoin use and subsequent depression and suicide: presenting the evidence. Am J Clin Dermatol 2003;4:493-505.

[42] Wysowski DK, Pitts M, Beitz J. An analysis of reports of depression and suicide in patients treated with isotretinoin. J Am Acad Dermatol 2001;45:515-9.

[43] McGrath EJ, Lovell CR, Gillison F, Darvay A, Hickey JR, Skevington SM. A prospective trial of the effects of isotretinoin on quality of life and depressive symptoms. Br J Dermatol 2010;163:1323-9.

[44] Yentzer BA, Hick J, Reese EL, Uhas A, Feldman SR, Balkrishnan R. Acne vulgaris in the United States: a descriptive epidemiology. Cutis 2010;86:94-9.

[45] Smith JA. The impact of skin disease on the quality of life of adolescents. Adolesc Med 2001;12(2):343-54.

[46] Simić D, Situm M, Letica E. Psychological impact of isotretinoin treatment in patients with moderate and severe acne. Coll Antropol 2009;33(Suppl 2):15-19.

[47] Uhlenhake E, Yentzer BA, Feldman SR. Acne vulgaris and depression: a retrospective examination. J Cosmet Dermatol 2010;9:59-63.

[48] Féton-Danou N. Psychological impact of acne vulgaris. Ann Dermatol Venereol 2010;137(Suppl 2):S62-5.

[49] Rapp DA, Brenes GA, Feldman SR, Fleischer AB Jr., Graham GF, Dailey M, et al. Anger and acne: Implications for quality of life, patient satisfaction and clinical care. Br J Dermatol 2004;15:183-9.

[50] Mallon E, Newton JN, Klassen A. The quality of life in acne. Br J Dermatol 1999;140:672-6.

[51] Yan AC. Current concepts in acne management. Adolesc Med Clin 2006;17:613-37.

[52] Fried RG, Wechsler A. Psychological problems in the acne patient. Dermatol Ther 2006;19:237-40.

[53] Misery L. Consequences of psychological distress in adolescents with acne. J Invest Dermatol 2011;131:290-2.

[54] Halvorsen JA, Stern RS, Dalgard F, Thoresen M, Bjertness E, Lien L. Suicidal ideation, mental health problems, and social impairment are increased in adolescents with acne: a population-based study. J Invest Dermatol 2011;131:363-70.

[55] Saitta P, Keehan P, Yousif J, Way BV, Grekin S, Brancaccio R. An update on the presence of psychiatric comorbidities in acne patients, part I. Overview of prevalence. Cutis 2011;88:33-40.

[56] Saitta P, Keehan P, Yousif J, Way BV, Grekin S, Brancaccio R. An update on the presence of psychiatric comorbidities in acne patients, part 2. Depression, anxiety, and suicide. Cutis 2011;88:92-7.

[57] Niemeier V, Kupfer J, Gieler U. Acne vulgaris—psychosomatic aspects. J Dtsch Dermatol Ges 2006;4:1027-36.

[58] Niemeier V, Kupfer J, Gieler U. Acne vulgaris—psychosomatic aspects. J Dtsch Dermatol Ges 2010;8(Suppl 1):S95-104.

[59] Greydanus DE, Calles J, Patel DR, eds: Pediatric and adolescent psychopharmacology: A practical manual for pediatricians. Cambridge, England: Cambridge University Press, 2008.

[60] Greydanus DE, Calles JL, Patel DR, Nazeer A, Merrick J, eds. Clinical aspects of psychopharmacology in childhood and adolescence. New York: Nova Science Publishers, 2012.

[61] Broniarczyk-Dyla G, Pajor A. Skin injuries in psychodermatological aspect. Wiad Lek 2011;64(2):142-6.

[62] Kent A, Drummond LM. Acne excoriée—a case report of treatment using habit reversal. Clin Exp Dermatol 1989;14:163-4.

[63] Shama H. Psychogenic excoriation responding to fluoxetine: a case report. J Indian Med Assoc 2008;106:245-7.

[64] Shah KN, Fried RG. Factitial dermatoses in children. Curr Opin Pediatr 2006;18:403-9.
[65] Chuh A, Wong W, Zawar V. The skin and the mind. Aust Fam Physician 2006;35:723-5.
[66] Dimoski A, Duricić S. Dermatitis artefacia, onychophagia and trichotillomania in mentally retarded children and adolescents. Med Pregl 1991;44:471-2.
[67] Gupta MA, Gupta AK. Olanzapine may be an effective adjunctive therapy in the management of acne excorée: a case report. J Cutan Med Surg 2001;5:25-7.
[68] Bowes LE, Alster TS. Treatment of facial scarring and ulceration resulting from acne excoriée with 585-nm pulsed dye laser irradiation and cognitive psychotherapy. Dermatol Surg 2004;30:934-8.
[69] Jansen T, Podda M. Therapy of acne scars. J Dtsch Dermatol Ges 2010;8(Suppl 1):S81-8.
[70] Van Zuuren EJ, Kramer S, Carter B, Graber MA, Fedorowicz Z. Interventions for rosacea. Cochrane Database Sys Rev 2011;16;(3):CD003262.
[71] Lazzeri D, Colizzi L, Licata G, Pagnini D, Proietti A, Ali G, Maseri P, et al. Malignancies within rhinophyma: report of three new cases and review of the literature. Aesthetic Plast Surg 2012;36(2):396-405.
[72] Scheinfeld N, Berk T. A review of the diagnosis and treatment of rosacea. Postgrad Med 2010;122:139-43.
[73] Cribier B. The red face: art, history and medical representations. Ann Dermatol Venereol 2011;138(Suppl 2):S116-23.
[74] Chosidow O, Cribier B. Epidemiology of rosacea: updated data. Ann Dermatol Venereol 2011;138(Suppl 2):S124-8.
[75] Léoni S, Mesplié N, Aitali F, Chamailliard M, Boralevi F, Marques da Costa C, et al. Metronidazole: alternative treatment for ocular and cutaneous rosacea in the pediatric population. J Fr Ophthalmol 2011;34(10):703-10.
[76] Buechner SA. Rosacea: an update. Dermatology 2005;210:100-8.
[77] Elsaie ML, Choudhary S. Updates on the pathophysiology and management of acne rosacea. Postgrad Med 2009;121:178-86.
[78] Kennedy Carney C, Cantrell W, Elewski BE. Rosacea: A review of current topical, systemic and light-based therapies. G Ital Dermatol Venereol 2009;144:673-88.
[79] Crawford GH, Pelle MT, James WD. Rosacea: I. Etiology, pathogenesis, and subtype classification. J Am Acad Dermatol 2004;51:327-41.
[80] Jansen T. Clinical presentations and classification of rosacea. Ann Dermatol Venereol 2011;138(Suppl 2):S138-47.
[81] Cribier B. Physiopathology of rosacea. Redness, telangiectasia, and rosacea. Ann Dermatol Venereol 2011;138(2):S129-37.
[82] McAleer MA, Lacey N, Powelll FC. The pathophysiology of rosacea. G Ital Dermatol Venereol 2009;144:663-71.
[83] Forton FM. Papulopustular rosacea, skin immunity and Demodex: pityriasis folliculorum as a missing link. J Eur Acad Dermatol Venereol. Epub 2011 Oct 24.
[84] Schwab VD, Sulk M, Seelinger S, Nowak P, Aubert J, Mess C, et al. Neurovascular and neuroimmune aspects in the pathophysiology of rosacea. J Investig Dermatol Symp Proc 2011;15:53-62.
[85] Yamasaki K, Gallo RL. Rosacea as a disease of cathelicidins and skin innate immunity. J Investig Dermatol Symp Proc 2011;15:12-5.
[86] Steinhoff M, Buddenkotte J, Aubert J, Sulk M, Novak P, Schwab VD, et al. Clinical, cellular, and molecular aspects in the pathophysiology of rosacea. J Investig Dermatol Symp Proc 2011;15:2-11.
[87] Bhat YJ, Manzoor S, Qayoom S. Steroid-induced rosacea: A clinical study of 200 patients. Indian J Dermatol 2011;56:30-2.
[88] Gerber PA, Buhren BA, Steinhoff M, Horney B. Rosacea: the cytokine and chemokine network. J Investig Dermatol Symp Proc 2011;15:40-7.
[89] Pfeffer I, Borelli C, Zierhut M, Schaller M. Treatment of ocular rosacea witih 40 mg doxycycline in a slow release form. J Dtsch Dermatol Ges 2011;9:904-7.
[90] Del Rosso JQ, Bhatia N. Azelaic acid gel 15% in the management of papulopustular rosacea: A status report on available efficacy data and clinical application. Cutis 2011;88:67-72.

[91] Kim MB, Kim GW, Park HJ, Chin HW, Kim SH, Kim BS, et al. Pimecrolimus 1% cream for the treatment of rosacea. J Dermatol Epub 2011;38(2):1135-9..

[92] Fowler J, Jarratt M, Moore A, Meadows K, Pollack, A, Steinhoff H, et al. Once-daily topical brimonidine tartrate gel 0.5% is a novel treatment of moderate to severe facial erythema of rosacea: results of two multicenter, randomized and vehicle-controlled studies. Br J Dermatol 2011; 165(5):111-115.

[93] Jackson JM, Pelle M. Topical rosacea therapy: the importance of vehicles for efficacy, tolerability and compliance. J Drugs Dermatol 2011;10:627-33.

[94] Levin J, Miller R. A guide for the ingredients and potential benefits of over-the-counter cleansers and moisturizers for rosacea patients. J Clin Aesthet Dermatol 2011;4:31-49.

[95] Guerrero D. Dermocosmetic management of the red face and rosacea. Ann Dermatol Venereol 2011;138(Suppl 2):S163-6.

[96] Park H, Del Rosso JQ. Use of oral isotretinoin in the management of rosacea. J Clin Aesthet Dermatol 2011;4:54-61.

[97] Dahan S. Laser and intense pulsed light management of couperose and rosacea. Ann Dermatol Venereol 2011;138(Suppl 2):S167-70.

[98] Sadick H, Riedel F, Bran G. Rhinophyma in rosacea: what does surgery achieve? Hautarzt 2011;62:834-41.

[99] Iqbal M, Kolodney MS. Acne fulminans with synovitis-acne-pustulosis-hyperostosis-osteitis (SAPHO) syndrome treated with infliximab. J Am Acad Dermatol 2005;52(5 Suppl 1):S118-20.

[100] DeSouza A, Solomon GE, Strober BE. SAPHO syndrome associated with hidradenitis suppurativa successfully treated with infiximab and methotrexate. Bull NYU Hosp Jt Dis 2011;69:185-7.

[101] Azevedo VF, Dal Pizzol V, Lopes H, Coelho SP, Czeczko LE. Methotrexate to treat SAPHO syndrome with keloidal scars. Acta Rheumatol Port 2011;36:167-70.

[102] Bergler-Czop B. The aetiopathogenesis of acne vulgaris-what's new? Int J Cosmet Sci 2014;36(3):187-94.

[103] Kircik LH. Evolving concepts in the pathogenesis of acne vulgaris. J Drugs Dermatol 2014;13(6):s56.

[104] Harvey A, Huynh TT. Inflammation and acne: putting the pieces together. J Drugs Dermatol 2014;13(4):459-63.

[105] Rocha MA, Costa CS, Bagatin E. Acne vulgaris: an inflammatory disease even before the onset of clinical lesions. Inflamm Allergy Drugs Targets 2014 Jun 6.

[106] Bowe W, Kober M. Therapeutic update: acne. J Drugs Dermatol 2014;13(3):235-8.

[107] Nickle SB, Peterson N, Peterson M. Updated physician's guide to the off-label uses of oral isotretinoin. J Clin Aesthet Dermatol 2014;7(4):22-34.

[108] Mooney T. Preventing psychological distress in patients with acne. Nurs Stand 2014; 29(22):42-8.

In: Pediatric and Adolescent Dermatology
Editors: D Greydanus, A Feinberg and J Merrick
ISBN: 978-1-63321-853-6

Chapter 6

Atopic dermatitis

Ruqiya S. Tareen, MD*
Department of Psychiatry,
Western Michigan University Homer Stryker MD School of Medicine,
Kalamazoo, Michigan, United States of America

Atopic dermatitis (AD) is a very common, multifactorial skin disease affecting about 20% of children. It usually starts in the early formative years, having a relapsing remitting course throughout the childhood and in about 3% of cases, persists throughout their life. Atopic dermatitis provides us with a model of a psychophysiologic disorder with delicate interactions between various factors including genetic predisposition, environmental triggers, acute and chronic psychosocial trauma as well as stress in addition to its impact on the developing immune system, and endocrine system as well as peripheral and central neuromodulators. Atopic dermatitis ultimately results in dermatologic and psychiatric manifestations. This discussion aims to elucidate some of these complex phenomena and how they impact the course and management of atopic dermatitis.

Introduction

Coca et al (1) first described the term "atopy" in literature in 1923 while classifying the states of hypersensitiveness. Atopy is defined as an inherited preponderance to increased production of IgE immunoglobulin antibodies, which predisposes that person to certain "atopic diseases" including asthma, hay fever, and atopic dermatitis. Atopic dermatitis is a multifaceted disease with an onset before age 5 years and with a chronic sometimes a lifelong relapsing remitting course. It was approximately 50 years ago that attention was focused on a possible link between the psychological stress and atopic dermatitis. Since then our understanding of the

* Correspondence: Ruqiya Shama Tareen MD, Associate Professor, Department of Psychiatry, Western Michigan University Homer Stryker MD School of Medicine, 1000 Oakland Drive, Kalamazoo, Michigan 49008-1284, United States. E-mail: shama.tareen@med.wmich.edu

intertwining of the emotional state and expression of atopy has improved significantly with increasing evidence pointing towards a psychophysiological origin of atopic dermatitis.

Epidemiology

Atopic diseases (AD) in general and atopic dermatitis in particular appear to have rising prevalence in children born after 1980 in European countries. The prevalence rates differ from country to country but generally hover between 10-20% in different parts of Europe. Much higher prevalence rates of up to 35% were found in northern parts of Scandinavia at about 69 N latitude. In United States lifetime prevalence was found to be around 17.2% in Oregon in children born during 1987 to 1991 (2). Prevalence rates in countries of Africa were about 11.1%. In Japan prevalence rate was quite different between the two cities studied ranging from 9.5 to 24% among children of age 5-12 years. In the continent of Australia the lifetime prevalence was about 18.7 to 31.9% depending on the type of the area studied. AD can occur at any age but 65% of patients develop atopic dermatitis in the first year of their life (2) .

Pathophysiologic factors

Genetic predisposition is considered the most important risk factor in atopic dermatitis with 77% concordance in monozygotic twins and 15% in dizygotic twins (3). The genetic transmission is quite complex, as atopic dermatitis does not have a Mendelian inheritance pattern with an identifiable gene locus. Twin studies has proven the high genetic link but it appears that genetic susceptibility is the first hit and having a genotype may or may not result in full expression of phenotype unless other risk factors plays a role of second hit. Various candidate genes have been identified but no definitive associations are found. Maternal transmission is much stronger then paternal indicating a possibility of genomic transmission, by suppressing the paternal genes (3). Atopic dermatitis is 2.6 times more common in girls than in their age matched counterparts (4).

Socio-economic status

Atopic dermatitis, similar to other atopic diseases, tends to favor the upper socioeconomic strata. A stepwise progression in the prevalence was reported by Freeman in United States and duplicated by many other studies in England, Germany, and Spain (2)

Family size

An inverse relationship has been reported with the number of the siblings and atopic dermatitis. Having three or more siblings was found to be protective against atopic dermatitis (4).

Food allergens

Unlike other atopic diseases atopic dermatitis is not directly related to food allergens, but a temporal relationship with certain food allergens is reported in up to 15 to 40% of patients with atopic dermatitis according to different studies. Most common food allergens associated were egg, soy, peanuts, wheat, fish, and cow's milk (4).

Psychoneuroimmunologic factors

Atopic dermatitis is considered as a neurogenic, cutaneous inflammation resulting from a dysregulated immune system. It is hypothesized that exposure to early life stressors (such as neglect, abandonment, inconsistent care giving, or even high family stress) can sensitize the child's immune system. It all starts with over-activation of hypothalamic-pituitary axis, causing excessive release of cortisol and catecholamine. This in turn leads to production of the T lymphocyte helper cells (T_H cells), more specifically of T_H2 cells, causing an imbalance of T_H1 and T_H2 cells ratio. T_H2 cells are found in abundance in atopic lesions and are responsible for a cascade of events including release of several cytokines, increase production of mast cells, augmentation of eosinophils and B lymphocyte cells production that in turn produce IgE immunoglobulin.

Newborns who have a genetic predisposition to atopic disease are found to have up to 70% higher levels of IgE in their cord blood. Compared to only 3% of controls, about 10.5% of the genetically predisposed infants developed atopic dermatitis during the first 18 months of life (5). Although IgE seems to be the predominant immunoglobulin in atopic dermatitis, deficiency of IgA in early few months of infancy allows easy absorption of allergens and primes the subject to produce more IgE in response (6). Various neuropeptides (such as substance P, vasoactive intestinal peptides, neurokinin, leukotriene, neurotensin, and neuropeptide Y) are some of the well known mediators of inflammation released in response to emotional stress causing neurogenic inflammation (6).

Breast feeding

The efficacy of breast-feeding in preventing atopic dermatitis (AD) has been proven by several large community based studies. In a study in Belarus of over 1,600 infants, prevalence rate of AD was 3.3% in breast fed infants in comparison to 6.3% in formula fed infants. Some hypoallergenic formulas are also reported to decrease the incidence in infants who had no genetic predisposition to atopic dermatitis (4).

Environmental allergens

Degree of sensitivity to environmental allergens (especially house dust mites) has been shown to have a positive correlation with severity of atopic dermatitis (AD). Conflicting results were reported from different studies about the negative impact of having a furry pet in the household. Having small rodents, rabbits, and guinea pigs in household were found to be associated with increased risk of developing AD in school-aged children. Contradictory to this finding more recent studies have reported that exposure to animal allergen (especially cat and dog dander) may in fact be protective against developing atopic dermatitis (4). Being raised at a farm has been shown to have a protective effect against atopic respiratory disease but the correlation was not well established in AD. Several aeroallergens are found to increase the risk of atopic dermatitis including living near high traffic area and volatile organic exposure (especially toluene and tobacco exposure); this is particularly increased if the mother smoked during pregnancy and the lactation period (4).

Psychophysiological aspects of atopic dermatitis

Psychological undercurrents in atopic dermatitis still remain somewhat less clearly defined than some of the other aspect of the disease. For a better understanding of this topic atopic, dermatitis is discussed under four main categories: impact of stress on the immunological system, psychoanalytic hypothesis, biopsychosocial model, and psychological dysregulation due to atopic dermatitis.

Impact of stress on the immunological system

Skin touch is the very first and most important way of communication for the neonate. Most of the neonatal introduction to the world occurs though the tactile communication with others via their skin. A soft touch, a warm cuddle, a comforting lap, and a nestle against the mother's breasts, all are some of the earliest experiences which shapes an infant's impression of the world outside of mother's womb. Animal studies and behavior studies in premature infants have shown that tactile communication plays an important role in neuronal cell growth and maturation (8).

Histamine, one of the main mediators of the itch and scratch cycle, was released in guinea pigs in response to classical conditioning in response to repeated stress (8). The relationship of stress to atopic dermatitis is bidirectional. Psychological stress, especially early on in infancy is known to cause an indelible mark on the still evolving neuronal, hormonal, and immunological systems. The first response to any stress is the activation of the sympathetic system with release of catecholamine resulting in increased production of prostaglandins, leukotrienes, and histamine, triggering pruritus and an inflammatory response (9,10). This understanding of neuroimmunological response to stress has been strengthen by the finding that CD8 lymphocyte counts increase in response to psychological stress and stay elevated one hour after the initial stressful event in patient with AD, suggesting a heightened autonomic arousal in response to stressful events (10).

Sieffert et al (9) measured this psycho-reactivity in a study of atopic dermatitis patients during acute exacerbations of eczema and then during disease free states; in this study several psychophysiological markers of stress were compared with normal controls. This research failed to confirm that there was a higher psychophysiological response to mental stress in patients with atopic dermatitis; however, it did show that AD patients had higher levels of psychophysiological activation regardless of whether they were in a relapse of atopic dermatitis or were free of their AD. Patients with atopic dermatitis showed higher heart rates and lower rates of heart rate variability, confirming a baseline sympathetic system overstimulation. The atopic dermatitis patients in this study also demonstrated a higher level of anxiety and depression; this is a finding that has been reported by other studies (11,12).

The sensory and autonomic nerves in the epidermis and dermis, when stimulated by exogenous stimuli (such as environmental allergens) or by internal stimulus (such as stress) release a number of neuropeptides (i.e., histamine, tryptase, TNF-α, leukotrienes, and β-endorphins). These mediators exert their inflammatory responses through their specific receptors located on primary afferent neurons (13).

Psychoanalytic hypothesis

The skin is the largest organ in human body and plays a unique role in our earliest understanding of our world (see chapter 2). The sense of being touched and caressed promotes a sense of attachment and bonding in the neonate to its primary care giver or object, which in the majority of cases is the mother. The physical contact with the mother is a soothing experience for infants due to the pleasant sensation they derive from tactile, thermal, and pressure senses. A study of mother's behavior towards their atopic children by Rosethental et al (14) showed that mothers of atopic children were less likely to pick up their children when they cried, in comparison to mothers of non-atopic children. Other studies have proposed that mothers of children with atopic dermatitis are conflicted in terms of whether their touch is going to be soothing or will cause more discomfort to the already irritated skin in the case of active disease; also, there could be a sense of repulsion due to the skin condition, however, at a subconscious level.

Psychoanalytic perspective proposes that infants who are not given this soothing physical contact go on to develop a predisposition to atopic dermatitis. Miller et al studied the impact of earliest psychological trauma in the form of a "rejecting mother" and its impact on expression of atopic disease. The rejecting mother was defined as "one whose behavior toward the child is such that she consciously or unconsciously has a desire to be free from the child and considers it a burden." They followed 63 infants with atopic dermatitis with possibility of being rejected by their mother and found that 98.4% had atopy in comparison to only 24.3% of control group of children with no atopy (15). A coexisting overprotection by mothers followed by earlier rejection was seen in 57% of infants with atopic dermatitis compared to 10.8% of children with no atopic condition (15).

Object relation theory is a modern take on the Freudian term of *object*. According to this theory the infant arrives in this world in an infantile autistic state where a presence of a nurturing, comforting, reliable external object (i.e., a primary caregiver, most likely the mother) is necessary. The infant, when nurtured by this object, proceeds to internalize that primary object to create awareness about self and the surrounding world in context of this object. When object constancy is achieved successfully, it leads to a coherent sense of self. The infant is completely dependent on this object for meeting its needs, and unavailability of this object or even inconsistent fulfillments of the infant's needs may give rise to feelings of abandonment, rejection, anger, and even hostility which it projects back towards the object. Adequate physical care provision by the mother to the infant along with reassurance and comfort by touch and caressing during this crucial period of development of self enables the infant to regulate its biological function and immunological system. This also allows these systems to not be over burdened in times of stress and thus, subsequently impact the disease susceptibility in a positive manner (16).

Biopsychosocial model

This contemporary model of mind-body relationship also takes into account various systems surrounding the dyad of mother and baby. This mother-child interaction is impacted by an interactional system that exists between mother and child and this system that interacts with the immediate surrounding system (such as father and siblings, and other family members) as well as how their interaction with broader systems of structural, financial, spiritual, cultural, and medical systems occurs. The theory proposes that a good relationship with the caregiver is the fundamental determinant of the child's ability to acquire normal physical and emotional health. This theory also takes into account the biological predisposition to disease such as atopic dermatitis and other predisposing and perpetuating factors along with the psychological stress in pathogenesis of atopic dermatitis (16).

Psychological dysregulation due to atopic dermatitis

Having a young child with atopic dermatitis (AD) creates many complex emotions in the child but also evokes many mixed emotions in parents. An infant with AD needs the physical contact, reassurance by touch of parents more so than infants without AD. On the other hand, the same soft caress can be painful and uncomfortable or perceived in a distorted way by the inflamed and excoriated skin, leading the child to feel being punished or attacked by the mother or care giver. Since these early sensory perceptions are how the infant perceives him or her sense of self, this unpleasant or bad perception of self could be internalized.

On the other hand, parents perceive infants with atopic dermatitis as somewhat defective as the sense of joy and pride of parenthood is tarnished by the visible skin lesions, constant itching, crying, and discomfort associated with it. The complex interaction between an infant with atopic dermatitis who tends to be more demanding, irritable, and less consolable and the parent who feels resentful, embarrassed, and powerless creates a cycle of negative emotions on both sides.

Parents may withdraw from care provision resulting in an infant with unmet needs who may develop a sense of "bad fit" and resort to self-soothing with self-stimulation of skin by excessive scratching. The parent, when finally identifying the unconscious withdrawal from the infant, becomes anxious and guilty and then frantically try to correct the neglect by showering too much attention; in addition, the parent become overprotective towards the child, resulting in another cycle of unhealthy patterns of interaction, where the child becomes excessively demanding, clinging, whining, and taking control of parent-child relationship (17).

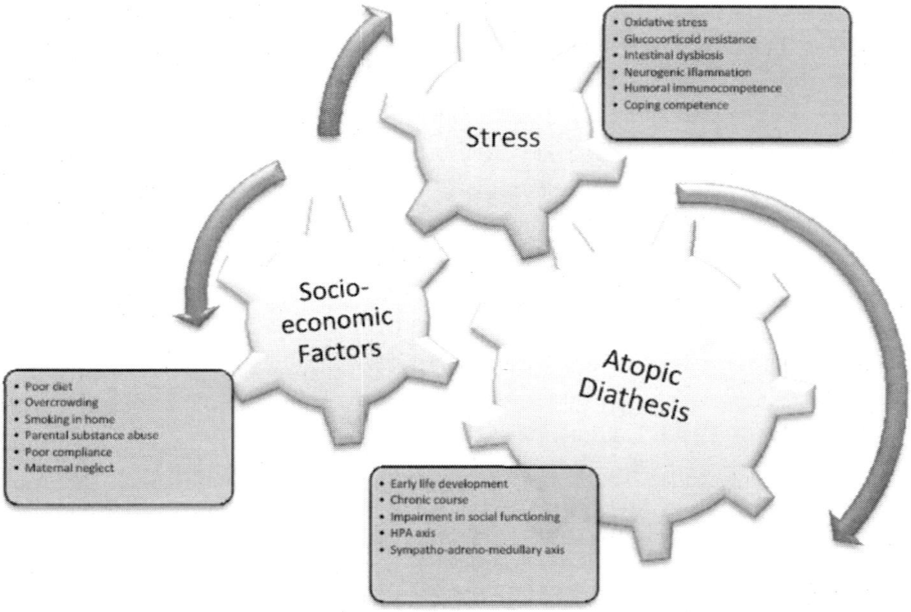

Figure 1. Bidirectional interaction of different factors contributing to psychological issues.

Clinical features

Atopic dermatitis (AD) is characterized by development of an erythematous, papulovesicular rash that initially is weeping and crusting but later on becomes lichenified, maculopapular patches due to constant scratching. Atopic dermatitis can involve all of the body, but it typically follows a characteristic distribution according to age of pediatric patient. In *infantile* eczema which occurs in those less than two years of age, erythematous, exudative lesions first appear on the face (especially cheeks, forehead, and scalp); lesions then progress to the trunk and extensor surfaces of extremities, sparing the diaper area. In the *childhood* phase, which is from 2 to 11 years of age, lesions are more localized to the flexural surfaces of the limbs and tend to be dry. Perioral region lesions and cheilitis are common, though the rest of the face is usually spared. Hand involvement is common and can be very troublesome for these children. The *adolescent* phase from 12 years onward usually presents with lichenified, macular lesions involving face, neck, upper trunk, and flexures aspects of the extremities. In adolescent girls the first and only manifestation of the AD can be the highly pruritic hand eczema (18).

Diagnosis

Atopic dermatitis can be difficult to diagnose because of its varied morphologic features and the fact that it lacks a definite laboratory marker. The Hanifin-Rajka Diagnostic Criteria was developed in 1980 to help this difficulty and consists of a set of 4 major and 23 minor criteria for the diagnosis of atopic dermatitis. Since its inception, the Hanifin-Rajka Diagnostic Criteria is still the most widely tool used to diagnose atopic dermatitis (19). Several other studies examined the Hanifin-Rajka Diagnostic Criteria and recommended some modifications in minor criteria based on their findings (19). Several of the minor criteria were considered less specific and these include nipple eczema, ichthyosis, cheilitis, anterior subcapsular cataracts, keratoconus, food intolerance, hypopigmented patches (pityriasis alba), and anterior neck folds (19). A simplified diagnostic guideline was introduced by a working group of United Kingdom (UK) dermatologists in 1990 which included most of the main diagnostic criteria from Hanifin-Rajka Diagnostic Criteria (19). This set of diagnostic criteria was used in epidemiological studies and showed 74% to 84% sensitivity as well as 97% to 99% specificity in community settings in the United Kingdom (19). Although when the same criteria were used to study school aged children in Australia, the sensitivity was found to be much lower at 43% but specificity remained high at 95% (2).

Table 1. Hanifin-Rajka diagnostic criteria

Major Criteria **Must meet three or more of the major criteria**	• Pruritus • Flexural involvement and lichenification in older children and adolescents and facial and extensor involvement in infants and young children • Chronically relapsing dermatitis • Personal and or family history of atopic dermatitis and other atopic disorders
Minor Criteria **Must meet 3 or more of the minor criteria**	**Typical Skin Manifestations** • Xerosis • Cheilitis • Ichthyosis, keratosis pilaris, palmar hyperlinearity • Nipple eczema • Perifollicular accentuation • Facial pallor or erythema • Pityriasis alba • Anterior neck folds • Pruritus with sweating • Dermographism, delayed blanching • Nonspecific hand or foot dermatitis **Immune System Related Features** • Immediate (type I) skin test reactivity • Elevated serum IgE • Impaired cell immunity (propensity for skin infections esp. Herpes simplex and Staph aureus) • Food intolerance • Wool and lipid intolerance **Ophthalmic and Periorbital Features** • Keratoconus • Anterior subcapsular cataracts • Recurrent conjunctivitis • Infraorbital fold (Dennie-Morgan) • Orbital darkening **Early age of onset** **Course of disease affected by emotional and environmental factors**

Ref: Larsen FS, Hanifin JM. Epidemiology of atopic dermatitis. Immunol Allergy Clin North Am 2002;1:1-24.

Table 2. UK Working Party Refinement of Hanifin and Rajka Criteria

Mandatory criteria (must meet)
• **A self report of itchy skin condition** *or*
• **Parental report of scratching, or rubbing noticed in a child**
Plus at least 3 of the following criteria
1. Involvement of flexural folds of elbow, knees, ankles, neck (cheeks in children under 10 years of age)
2. Personal history of another atopic disease like asthma or hay fever *or* Family history of an atopic disease in children under age 4 years
3. History of general dry skin in past year
4. Visible signs of eczema at typical flexural sites *or* Eczema on cheeks, forehead or outer aspects of extremities in children under 4 years of age
5. Age of onset under age of 2 years (not used if child is 4 years of age)
Minor Criteria
Must meet 3 or more of the minor criteria

Ref: Larsen FS, Hanifin JM. Epidemiology of atopic dermatitis. Immunol Allergy Clin North Am 2002;1:1-24

Allergy testing

Skin prick test (SPT)

Mast cell-bound IgE medicated food allergy can be diagnosed by introduction of food allergens via skin prick testing; the resulting atopic reaction is found to be 100% predictive of a particular food allergy. A positive reaction is identified in children over 2 years of age, when exposed to cow's milk if they develop a SPT weal diameter >8 mm and under 2 years of age with an SPT weal of >6 mm in diameter. However, SPT is found to be not reliable when used in infants (20).

Atopy patch test (APT)

The atopic patch test (APT) is useful in the diagnosis of aeroallergens and food allergies that involve T cell and dendritic cell mediated inflammatory processes. APT can increase the accuracy of the diagnosis substantially when used in combination with SPT. APT is especially useful in identifying late phase clinical reactions with a specificity of 95%. APT has higher specificity, up to 92% compared to SPT with a 53% and IgE level with 64%. The European Task Force on Atopic Dermatitis (ETFAD) has developed a protocol to standardized APT administration, using 5,000 to 7,000 PNU/g in adults and proposes its use with half of this concentration in children. ETFAD supports using 12 mm diameter chambers, and does not advocate use of any pretreatment. Some reaction may be observed in 48 hours but maximal response may not be observed until 72 hours (20).

Double blind placebo controlled food challenge (DBPCFC)

Regarded as a gold standard in early studies, the Double Blind Placebo Controlled Food Challenge (DBPCFC) still remains the most definitive test for food allergy. Reasons for limited use of DBPCFC include the inherent risk involved in exposure to potentially life threatening allergic reactions, the amount of resources needed to undertake this test, and the development of SPT testing (20).

Differential diagnosis

The differential diagnosis of atopic dermatitis is outlined in Table 3.

Table 3. Differential aiagnosis of atopic dermatitis

Condition	Clinical Features	Pruritus	Common Sites
Atopic Dermatitis	May be associated with asthma and allergic rhinitis.	+++	Flexor aspects of limbs. Face, scalp and trunk in children under 2 years.
Contact Dermatitis	History of contact with irritant, exposed surfaces	+++	
Seborrheic Dermatitis	Reddish pink, greasy, punctate lesions coalesces to form diffuse lesions	+/-	Scalp, scalp, skin folds, behind ears
Psoriasis	Discrete, raised reddish pink lesions with fine silver scales	+	Extensor surfaces of extremities
Icthyosis vulgaris	Generalized dry skin, positive family history	++	Extensor surfaces of limbs
Scabies	Crowded conditions, burrows	+++	Interdigital spaces

Management

Prevention of relapse

Avoidance of the offending irritants and allergens is the first step in the management of atopic dermatitis (AD). Taking a thorough history and identifying the offending agents are the most important components of a successful treatment plan (21).

Food allergens

About 30% to 50% of children with AD have defined food allergies which perpetuates the atopy (20). Some of the most common food allergens are cow milk, peanuts, eggs, fish, soy, wheat, and nuts (21). Exhaustive protection from food allergens has not been proven to be very effective and overzealous attempts to avoid food allergens may lead to nutritional deficiencies, complicating the clinical presentation (20). It is not prudent to attempt challenging exposure to allergens to establish food allergy as in the case of severe allergies which may lead to severe reactions, such as anaphylaxis. In high risk infants, recommendations to delay or even prevent the onset of atopic dermatitis include postponing the introduction of solid food until 6 months of age, feeding completely on breast milk, and when breast feeding is not possible, using hydrolyzed hypoallergenic formula (20).

Aeroallergens

House dust with thirteen species of identified dust mites is known to be the most common aeroallergen implicated in atopic disease. High levels of Der p1 specific antibodies were detected in 95% of AD patients and correlated well with the severity of the disease (22). Bedding, overstuffed furniture, carpets, and other items provide the perfect breeding ground for these fomites (22). Covering of mattresses, diligent vacuuming, and removal of carpets can significantly improve the prognosis of the atopic dermatitis.

Optimizing epidermal barrier (EB)

The epidermis is the first line of defense against any percutaneous invasion of allergens, infective agents, irritants, chemicals, and other substances. The epidermal skin barrier is a protective shield that is located in the deeper part of stratum corneum. The efficacy of this barrier in resisting the penetration of these molecules depends on the thickness of stratum corneum. There are wide inter-individual variations in the efficacy of epidermal barrier (EB) according to different areas of body as well as intra-individual variations. Many enzymes are needed to maintain the integrity of the EB and these enzymes are pH dependent (23). Any disruption of the normal skin pH of 7.0 can cause increase in the activity of enzymes (such as proteases) that can lead to thinning of stratum corneum and impairment of the epidermal barrier (23). Commonly used soaps and other agents to cleanse skin can disrupt this pH, and repeated use can cause significant thinning of the EB. Avoidance of soap and detergents as well as use of emollient wash products (such as hyroxyurea, soft paraffin, mixture of soft and liquid paraffin, and mineral oils with or without any active ingredients) can be key factors in successful treatment of atopic dermatitis. See Box 1.

Box 1. Commonly used emollients used for maintaining epidermal barrier

Emollients
E45 Cream ®
Hydromol products ®
Lipobase ®
Oilatum Plus ®
Balneum Plus ®
Aquaphor®
Eucerine ®
Petroleum Jelly®

Hydration therapy

Due to the damaged epidermal barrier and decreased levels of ceramide in their skin, children with atopic dermatitis have a tendency to have low skin water content leading to excessive dryness of skin or xerosis, leading to a relapse of the atopic dermatitis (24). Keeping the skin hydrated to prevent a relapse or to improve healing during an acute episode of atopic dermatitis is very important. Soaking baths are beneficial although showers can be used in milder cases. Soaking baths in lukewarm water followed by gentle pat drying and applying an occlusive sealer (such as petroleum jelly or a urea containing moisturizer) to seal the water in the epidermis is the best way to optimize hydration of skin. In cases of localized atopic dermatitis, the affected body area, such as an arm or leg, can be soaked in a water basin (24).

Management of pruritus

Pruritus or itch is almost synonymous with atopic dermatitis, affecting almost 100% of the patients with atopic dermatitis. The unrelenting itch and scratching further damages the skin, exacerbating dermatitis as well as perpetuating an unending "itch-scratch" cycle. Pruritus is particularly troublesome at night. Several mechanisms are at interplay behind this cycle of itch and scratch including peripheral mediators of itch such as histamine, various neuropeptides, acetylcholine, tryptase, cytokines, neurotphin-4, eosinophils, platelet aggravating factor, cannabinoids, opioids peptides, interferon gamma vanilloids, and calcineurin inhibitors (25).

Since the mechanism of the pruritus is so complex it is of no surprise that traditional remedies such as antihistamines are often not effective. The current approach is to focus on the reduction of inflammation in the skin and thus decrease the intensity of the pruritus. The most commonly used and effective anti-inflammatory agents are topical corticosteroids. Recently immunomodulatory agents inhibiting calcineurin (such as tarcolimus and pimecrolimus) has been shown to abort the acute attacks of atopic dermatitis by decreasing pruritus, and stopping the itch-scratch cycle (25).

Other inhibitors of mediators of pruritus (such as interferon gamma, capsaicin, opiate receptors antagonists, and leukotriene antagonists) have also been shown to decrease the pruritus along with overall favorable impact on the atopic dermatitis. Systemic treatment with immunomodulators (such as cyclosporine, glucocorticoids, tarcolimus, and pimecrolimus) has been used in treating refractory atopic dermatitis; however, topical therapy is the mainstay of treatment (25).

Topical corticosteroids

Since the discovery of hydrocortisone in the 1950s, the glucocorticoids are the most important medical discovery in the history of dermatologic therapies. Later, the development of halogenated corticosteroids opened the door for even more potent agents. When used inappropriately corticosteroids can induce various systemic side effects and this has led to a serious debate about which corticosteroids for which part of body and for how long should they be used without causing any deleterious lifelong adverse effects.

Corticosteroids are lipophilic and are easily absorbed from the epidermis; after entering the cells they bind to the DNA binding glucocorticoid receptors, causing down or up-regulation of gene expression. The genes that are expressed encode various enzymes leading to four main mechanisms of actions of corticosteroids: immunomodulation, vasoconstriction, anti-inflammation, and anti-proliferation (26). Any decision in regards to initiation of treatment with corticosteroids and which ones to use depend on various factors discussed below.

Age

The younger the child, the greater is the absorption of the corticosteroids from the epidermis. This along with the relative larger body surface area that young children have, readily predisposes them for serious local and systemic side effects. Thus, in infants and younger children, first all the alternative treatment options should be employed and only when all other measures fail, should use of corticosteroids (steroids) be considered.

When indicated the lowest potency corticosteroid should be used, although moderate potency agents (such as methylprednisolone acetate or prednicarbate) can be used as they have a better side effect profile if used for a limited time. The relapsing, remitting nature of atopic dermatitis requires the treating physician to be mindful that the need for a course of corticosteroids (steroids) may arise multiple times during the course of disease; however, great care should be taken that individual courses of corticosteroid treatment should not be longer than 3 weeks at a time (27,28).

Potency of corticosteroids

Corticosteroids are divided in seven classes based on their potency on vasoconstrictor assay, class 1 being the most potent. As a general rule the use of potent corticosteroids in children is reserved only for very severe, recalcitrant disease that has not responded to other forms of treatment. When a decision is made to use a potent corticosteroid**,** the effort should be made to use it for the minimal effective period to avoid topical and systemic side effects. Children have a low body volume to skin surface area ratio which can predispose them to higher rates of steroid absorption and this effect when combined with a higher potency steroid application, can produce deleterious side effects even in short term therapy (27,28). See Table 4.

Table 4. Classification of topical corticosteroids by potency

Class	Corticosteroid	Strength
I	Betamethasone dipropionate	0.05%
	Clobestol propionate	0.05%
	Diflorasone diacetate	0.05%
	Halobetasol propionate	0.05%
II	Amcinonide	0.1%
	Betamethasone dipropionate	0.05%
	Desoximetasone	0.05%
	Desoximetasone	0.25%
	Fluocinonide	0.05%
	Halcinonide	0.1%
	Mometasone furoate	0.1%
	Triamcinolone acetonide	0.5%

Table 4. (Continued)

Class	Corticosteroid	Strength
III	Amcinonide	0.1%
	Betamethasone valerate	0.1%
	Diflorasone diacetate	0.05%
	Fluticasone propionate	0.005%
	Clocortolone pivalate	0.1%
	Triamcinolone acetonide	0.1%
IV	Betamethasone valerate	0.12%
	Flucinolone acetonide	0.025%
	Flurandrenolide	0.05%
	Hydrocortisone valerate	0.2%
	Mometasone furoate	0.1%
V	Hydrocortisone butyrate	0.1%
	Hydrocortisone probutate	0.1%
	Prednicarbate	0.1%
VI	Alcometasone dipropionate	0.05%
	Desonide	0.05%
	Flucinolone acetonide	0.01%
VII	Dexamethasone	0.1%
	Hydrocortisone	0.25%
	Hydrocortisone	0.5%
	Hydrocortisone	1%
	Hydrocortisone acetate	0.5%
	Hydrocortisone acetate	1%

Site of topical application

Penetration and absorption of steroids is much more rapid and complete from the sites where the skin is thinner—such as the face, eyelids, forehead, axillae, and genital area. Use of high to medium high potency corticosteroids (class 1-5) should be avoided in such areas. Lowest potency of steroids and shorter treatment time can reduce the risk of topical side effects such as skin thinning and atrophy (27,28).

Frequency of application

The stratum corneum serves as a reservoir that can release the active ingredient over time; thus, once daily application may be sufficient in most cases while highly active disease may require twice daily application. Frequency of application should be tapered gradually until stopping the medication in order to prevent any rebound of the atopic dermatitis (27,28).

Type of application

It is important to select the right medium of delivery for the steroid being prescribed to optimize the therapeutic effects. Ointments are most viscous as they are oil based and are the best choice to provide occlusion of the dry xerotic type of lesions. Creams, being less viscous, have more acceptance from patients and care givers. Creams are well suited for the lesions that are wet and oozy. Lotions and gels are water based and are generally not suited for dry lesions or xerotic skin but can be of use in areas where creams and ointments cannot be used, such as scalp or other hairy areas (27,28).

Amount of application

Generally used "fingertip unit" (FTU) is a reliable and effective way of gauging the amount to be applied. One FTU is considered enough to treat an area of skin twice the size of an adult's hand. It is estimated that 2 FTU are approximately equal to 1 gram of corticosteroid. Recommended maximal dose in grams depends on patient age, the amount of the body surface area covered with atopic dermatitis, the site of lesions, disease severity, and steroid potency. As a general rule a corticosteroid prescription should not exceed 50 grams at one time. Close monitoring and frequent visits are keys in avoiding the longterm local and systemic side effects in children requiring frequent corticosteroid prescriptions (26-28).

Topical immunomodulators

Calcineurin inhibitors (such as tarcolimus and pimecrolimus) act by binding to cytosolic immunophilin receptors and inhibiting calcineurin; this action results in decreasing inflammation by down regulation of inflammatory mediators such as interleukins (IL-2, IL-4, & IL-8), along with tumor necrosis factor alpha (TNFα), interferon gamma (INFγ), lymphocytes (TH1, T_H1 and T_H2) and granulocyte –macrophage colony stimulating factor.

Tarcolimus

The efficacy of tarcolimus alone or in combination with steroids has been shown by multiple studies. Tarcolimus ointment (0.03% and 0.1%), when used twice daily in pediatric patients age 2-15 years of age, was shown to be more effective than 1% hydrocortisone (29). Tarcolimus has also shown superiority when compared to 0.005% fluticasone pivalate ointment in the pediatric population (29). Tarcolimus (0.1% ointment) has been shown to be effective and safe for up to 12 months to 3 years of treatment in those aged 2-15 years (27). The most common side effect, reported in 29.9% of children, was a burning sensation at the site of application followed by transient pruritus in 23%; which improved in few days (29).

Pimecrolimus

When pediatric patients 2-17 years old with mild to moderate atopic dermatitis were treated with pimecrolimus 1% cream twice daily for 6 weeks, 34.8% became clear or almost clear of atopic dermatitis (27). Pimecrolimus was effective when used in those 3-23 months of age, and others 2-17 years of age.

Infants with atopic dermatitis showed 61% improvement at week 6 and >80% improvement at 12 months when pimecrolimus was applied twice daily along with a moderately potent corticosteroid. After the active treatment period ended, fewer infants had a relapse when compared to the control group. It was also reported that pimecrolimus seems to be more effective in treating lesions on the face. About 2.5% of infants and 10.5% children reported burning sensation at the site of application that improved in 1-3 days (27,29).

Systematic treatment of atopic dermatitis

Antihistamines

Histamine is the most well known mediator of cutaneous inflammation. It is released from mast cells in response to an atopic challenge causing pruritus, vasodilation, and edema. Most atopic effects are mediated by H_1 receptors and all antihistamine used in atopic conditions works at H_1 receptors. The first generation antihistamine readily crosses the blood brain barrier, thus causing side effects such as sedation, daytime drowsiness, motor incoordination, and others. The main concern when using histamine in pediatric populations is the paradoxical irritability and hyperactivity that can occur after the immediate sedative effects wear off. Diphenhydramine is the first antihistamine introduced in 1947 followed by chlorpheniramine, promethazine, cyproheptadine, and hydroxyzine. Second generation of antihistamine became popular after they came on market in the 1980s due their low penetration of blood brain barrier, making them comparatively non-sedative. Loratadine, desloratadine, cetirizine, and fexofenadine are beneficial especially when there are other comorbid atopic conditions. Fexofenadine has shown an edge in this group of antihistamines in terms of reduction in pruritus due to atopic dermatitis (30).

Phototherapy

Ultraviolet B (UVB) therapy with a wavelength of 290-320 nm has been used effectively in the treatment of atopic dermatitis for many years. Phototherapy doses are defined as minimal erythema doses (MED) and 0.5-1 MED is considered effective (31). UVB works by causing apoptosis of T lymphocytes, immunosuppression by its effect on cytokines and interleukin, and by its antimicrobial action as well as possible thickening of epidermis enhancing the EDB. Clayton et al in a 6 years retrospective review of children with AD treated with narrow band UVB (NB-UVB), showed a response rate of 40% with improvement sustaining at 3 months follow up. However, the children were also using emollients and topical steroids during active treatment (32).

Combination UVA and UVB (UVA/B) has shown effectiveness against atopic dermatitis; however, when NB-UVB was used in combination of UVA, it resulted in more than 90% reduction in atopic dermatitis symptoms. When NB-UVB/A was used in combination with topical corticosteroids, the need for UVB dose decreased without affecting the overall response and remission rates (33). There is a risk of developing cataracts in children with severe atopic dermatitis that peaks between 15-25 years of age; thus, a slit lamp examination is necessary to rule out any cataracts before the initiation of phototherapy and optimal use of eye protection gear during treatment is necessary (34). Concomitant use of any topical immunosuppressant is contraindicated due to the increased risk of skin malignancies (34).

Antibiotics

Atopic dermatitis skin is highly susceptible to colonization with *Staphylococcus aureus* resulting in frequent secondary infections. Widespread infection will require systemic antibiotics. For example, a 7-10 day course of cephalosporin and synthetic penicillin are usually effective. For penicillin allergic patients, fusidic acid and clindamycin are effective alternatives (35).

Systemic corticosteroids

The literature is quite sparse in terms of use of systemic steroids in children. Two randomized clinical trials of short-term use of high potency systemic steroids showed modest improvement. No clinical studies are available for use of prednisone in children. Due to the concerns about the systemic side effects (especially the suppression of hypothalamic-pituitary-adrenal axis), systemic corticosteroids should only be used to control severe flare ups at the smallest effective dose and for the shortest duration possible in order to optimize positive results (35).

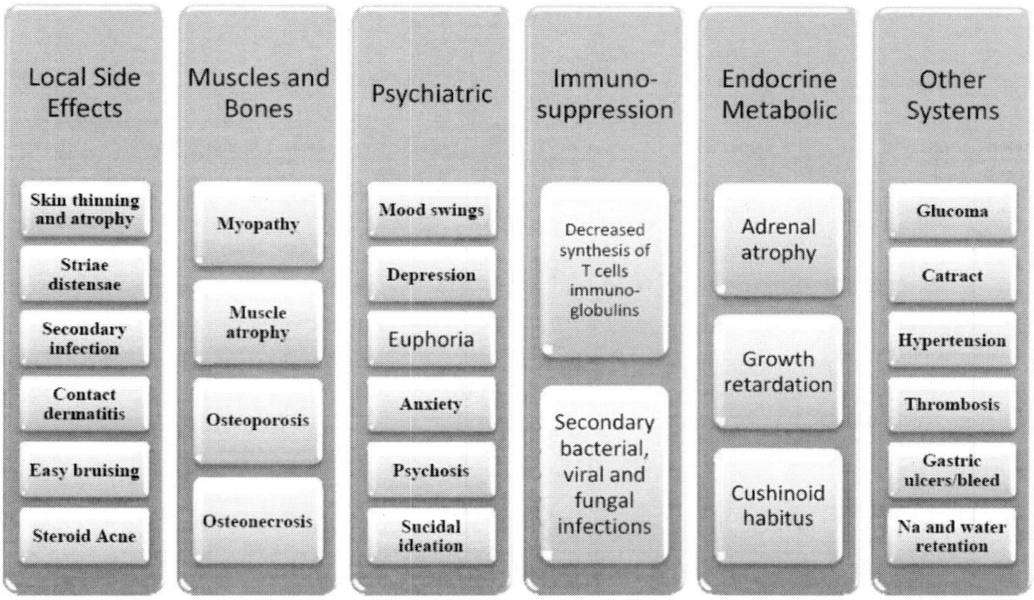

Figure 2. Local and systemic side effects of corticosteroids.

Immunomodulators

The majority of pediatric patients respond well to topical treatments; however, a very small percentage of children with severe recalcitrant atopic dermatitis may require systemic treatment with such agents as immunomodulators. As systemic treatment carries the risk of some very serious long-term side effects, the decision to embark on such therapy has to be weighed very carefully in terms of benefits of symptom improvement and gain in quality of life versus risks of immunosuppression, renal insufficiency, and malignancy. Sexually active female adolescents should be screened for pregnancy. In general, such treatment should only be used in difficult-to- treat or recalcitrant cases and only with the lowest effective dose for the shortest possible time frame in addition to close monitoring by appropriate specialists (35,36).

Cyclosporine

The very first calcineurin inhibitor, cyclosporine, is a non-cytotoxic immunosuppressant, which acts by inhibiting lymphocyte activation. Careful selection of patients is necessary to exclude ones with any contraindication to cyclosporine including any renal insufficiency, uncontrolled hypertension, history of hepatitis B or C or any malignancy. Patients 2-16 years of ages have been treated with doses of up to 5 mg/kg/day; this was well tolerated and was efficacious in studies both in short term cases of 12 weeks and in long term continuous treatment of up to 12 months (35,36). Quality of life improvement was seen in both short term and long term treatment at 12 weeks (35,36). Cyclosporine is the only systemic treatment with convincing evidence to support its use in children with severe treatment refractory atopic dermatitis (35,36).

Azathioprine

An inhibitor of purine synthesis and subsequently of cellular DNA and RNA, azathioprine is shown to be effective in severe atopic dermatitis. Before using this medication, it is necessary to get such screening tests as a complete blood count, liver function tests, and assay of thiopurine methyltransferase (TPMT) to assess for bone marrow function at base line; this is followed by continued monitoring weekly for the first 6 weeks and then at 3 months intervals (37). When used in doses of 2 -3.5 mg/kg/day in patients 6-16 years old, good response was seen in 41 out of 48 children in 2-6 weeks (37). Adverse events include gastrointestinal upset, transient elevation of liver function, anemia, thrombocytopenia, hypersensitivity phenomenon and increased risk of lymphoreticular malignancy (37).

Infliximab

Infliximab is a monoclonal antibody that neutralizes the tumor necrosis factor α (TNF α) and is found to be effective in other atopic disorder such as asthma; however, its use in atopic dermatitis is relatively new and appears to be promising (35).

Interferon-γ

Interferon γ (INF γ) causes inhibition of IgE production that theoretically should restore immune balance in patients with atopic dermatitis who show a deficiency of INF γ. There is lack of good controlled trials to support the use of INF γ at this time unless the patients are not eligible for other proven systemic therapies (35).

Leukotriene inhibitors

Since patients with atopic dermatitis produce leukotrienes in abundance, which are strong inflammatory mediators; thus, the idea of using a leukotriene antagonist to counter this proinflammatory response and potentially diminishing atopy is appealing. One study of pediatric patients 6-16 years of age with moderate to severe atopic dermatitis who were treated with montelukast for 4 weeks at a dose of 5 mg daily showed a significant reduction in severity of atopic dermatitis; however another study failed to replicate these positive results (35).

Psychiatric comorbidities

Atopic dermatitis, due to its early manifestation in life in addition to severity and course of illness, tends to cause everlasting temperamental and psychological changes in both younger and older children. The dilemma of a child with atopic dermatitis is not that he or she is not getting enough attention by parents but that the attention and at times too much attention is received, which can be misguided or even negative in some situations. Most of the attention is focused on the skin and its care at the cost of neglecting the emotional and developmental needs of the child (16). Also, providers may be mainly focused on treating the skin disorder based on the severity of its lesions and never attempt to go deeper than the skin to take care of the emotional and psychosocial wounds contributing to the atopic dermatitis.

Several psychiatric disorders are found to have higher prevalence in children with any atopic diseases. Children with atopic dermatitis are more prone to develop depression as well as various nonspecific psychosomatic symptoms when compared to age matched controls (38). Behavioral problems are also an issue in these children. A study of school aged children in the United Kingdom found a twofold risk of having psychological problems in children with atopic dermatitis in comparison to the children without this dermatological condition (39).

Family dynamics

The strain on any family unit dealing with a child with atopic dermatitis is challenging, and when you add other psychosocial stressors (i.e., associated economic burdens) it can become overwhelming. Families with low socioeconomic levels can be overburdened with the caregiving more quickly, leading to unhealthy coping styles and negative parenting; these results can have damaging long term psychological impact on the child during the most important formative years of his or her life when the foundation for personality, temperament, and coping mechanisms are being laid down (39).

Internalizing and externalizing behaviors

All atopic conditions are known to be associated with internalizing behaviors and to a lesser degree with externalizing behaviors. Lien et al conducted a base line survey of 3,674 high school Norwegian students who were 15 to 16 years of age and followed them up at age 18 to 19 years (39). Internalizing behaviors were identified as feeling panicky, anxious, dizzy, feeling tense, sadness, sleeplessness, worthless, blaming oneself, feeling hopeless, and finding everything a burden. Externalizing factors were restlessness and hyperactivity, inattention, peer relationship problems, conduct problems, and being more comfortable with adults than age appropriate peers.

Children with atopic dermatitis were found to have more likelihood of developing internalizing behaviors but findings were not as robust as in asthma. No clear relationship was found between atopic conditions and externalizing behaviors (39). The study also showed an increase in internalizing behaviors at three years follow-up. Schmitt et al conducted a 10 years follow up of 2,252 children first identified with atopic dermatitis in infancy. They found that infants who were diagnosed with this skin disorder prior to age two years had a preponderance for developing emotional problems at age 10. Infant-onset atopic dermatitis was also found to be associated with conduct problems, and a trend was seen for these children to develop attention deficit hyperactivity disorder (40).

Anxiety and depression

The most prevalent co-morbid diagnosis in patients with atopic dermatitis appears to be a heightened anxiety state that can even lead to development of an overt anxiety disorder. Adolescents with atopic dermatitis have lifetime rates of anxiety and depression that are increased over controls. Studies have reported 46% of adolescents with atopic dermatitis having anxiety and 17% suffering from depression (41). Anxiety levels tend to decrease with the improvement in skin condition only to revert back to the high levels after the relapse. Linnet et al reported higher levels of state and trait anxiety in children with atopic dermatitis that correlated well with severity of illness (42). Association of atopic dermatitis with depression has not been as robust as it has been seen in other chronic dermatologic conditions, as for example, psoriasis and acne. When depression is seen in children with atopic dermatitis, it is more likely comorbid with heightened anxiety especially related to social situations (43).

Personality traits

An atopy-specific personality has been proposed for children suffering from atopic disorders. It has been postulated that an infant with atopic dermatitis who is irritable due to skin lesions needs physical contact from a parent for reassurance and comfort; also, a parent's feelings of disappointment and failure along with reluctance to touch in fear of aggravating the illness leads to a sense by the infant of being rejected by the mother. This leads to elevated anxiety and hostility in the infant or child giving rise to the foundation of some specific personality traits. The atopic personality is said to have traits of hypersensitivity, aggressiveness, sense of inferiority, insecurity, mood labiality, and cognitive rigidity. These individuals have difficulty dealing with anger and hostility in interpersonal relationships. Further studies have failed to agree on such specific personality disorders and there is concern that these personality traits are not atopic dermatitis- or atopic disease-specific but is more of a representation of chronic illnesses such as autoimmune disorders or cancers.

Management of mental health issues

Multidisciplinary approach

Chronic dermatologic diseases, as for example atopic dermatitis, are best served with a multidisciplinary approach. The team should aim to include professionals from different areas of healthcare to provide a comprehensive interdisciplinary approach to management aiming to reduce the frequency and severity of relapses as well as avoid complications from this complex skin disorder. A typical team should include a clinical social worker, psychologist, and psychiatrist to address psychosocial and psychiatric issues. The dermatologist or the primary care physician leads the team with an ability to convene the team or consult with individual professionals as needed. Some major concerns in maintaining a multidisciplinary team are turf as well as territory issues, conflict communication, and organizational constraints (44).

Psychoeducation

Psychoeducation of the child, adolescent, and the family should be the integral part of a multidisciplinary treatment plan of a child or adolescent with atopic dermatitis. Psychoeducation can play a major role in situations with more frequent and severe relapses which are difficult to manage by particularly focusing not only on a good understanding of the physiologic and pathologic factors at play in their illness in terms understood by family members, but also by improving some understanding of the role of stress and its negative interactions. Education on specific techniques (such as relaxation, assertive communication, self-control of itching and scratching, and stress management) can lead to improved disease outcome (45).

Psychosocial assessment

A thorough psychosocial assessment is necessary to understand the family interaction and dynamics. Gustaffson et al proposed a family interaction evaluation using standardized family testing comprising of tasks related to skills of decision making, conflict resolution, cooperation, and differences of opinion about likes and dislikes among family members. Social network and support system assessment was also conducted asking parents to list individuals outside of the immediate family, their availability, geographic proximity, and the importance of their relationship with that particular individual; this was done to outline a weak versus healthy social support network (46).

Evaluation of socioeconomic status is also important as low income levels along with other associated factors (i.e., overcrowded living conditions, poor nutrition, negative family interactions, substance abuse, smoking by parents, and non adherence to the treatment plan) can adversely impact the prognosis (46).

Psychiatric symptoms review

It is imperative to assess children and adolescents with atopic dermatitis for any comorbid psychiatric conditions because of the high incidence of associated general anxiety, social anxiety, depression, and personality traits. Many psychometric scales are available which can be readily used in different clinical settings with high reliability in identifying comorbid illnesses.

Quality of life assessment

Children with atopic dermatitis are shown to have a significant reduction in quality of life (QoL) when compared to their age matched counterparts (see chapter 4). QoL impact all domains of their life including family interaction, school performance, ability to engage in extracurricular activities, participation in physical contact sports, as well as interpersonal and social relationships. QoL research has shown that children with atopic dermatitis have much higher impairment in this regard not only when compared to patients suffering from other chronic dermatologic conditions but also when compared with those suffering from other chronic illnesses such as malignancies (11).

Psychodynamic therapy

It is important to help patients with atopic dermatitis understand the unrecognized and unconscious meaning of their illness and its impact on their understanding about themselves and their interaction with others (see chapter 23). Children, based on their level of development, may not be able to engage in any in-depth psychodynamic therapy; however, such therapy may be beneficial to adolescents with atopic dermatitis. Psychodynamic-based group therapy is more beneficial where working on neuroticizing and pathological relationships, issues of transference, and counter transference that can be worked out in a group setting (11).

Cognitive behavioral therapy

Exploring the negative schema the patients have developed over many years about self, care givers, and the world itself as well as attempting to change these issues in a positive direction will help develop a better understanding of their illness, compliance with treatment, and ultimate disease outcomes. The aim of therapy is to help children and adolescents with atopic dermatitis recognize automatic negative thoughts, dysfunctional assumptions about self-image, self-depreciatory as well as blaming attitudes; therapy then replaces them with more positive attitudes. This approach will give rise to a more balanced understanding of self and illness which will help the patient develop improved coping skills and decrease the social phobia, depression, and anxiety along with other avoidance behaviors.

Behavioral modifications

Relaxation techniques are shown to have some effectiveness in decreasing the itch and scratch cycle; these techniques include progressive muscle relaxation, autogenic training, electromyographic (EMG) biofeedback training, and cue controlled relaxation (11) (see chapter 23). Strategies to teach more self control and scratch avoidance led to these children being symptom free for prolonged periods; these strategies include rewarding children for not scratching and ignoring the scratching behavior (11).

Psychotropic medications

Use of psychotropic medication will be necessary in a small number of pediatric patients with severe anxiety spectrum or depressive disorders who have failed to respond to psychotherapeutic approaches. *Selective serotonin reuptake inhibitors* (SSRIs) are now considered the first line medications for the management of anxiety and depression in these patients. In terms of efficacy all of the available SSRIs are considered equal but only a few are officially approved for use in the pediatric population. At present fluoxetine is approved for use in those ≥8 years for depression and in those ≥7 years for obsessive compulsive disorder (OCD). Fluvoxamine is approved in patients ≥8 years, sertraline in patients ≥ 6 years, and escitalopram for adolescents ≥12 years for OCD.

Tricyclic antidepressants (TCAs) are the older antidepressants that are less commonly used in this early part of the 21st century mostly because of their unfavorable side effects profile and also because of better tolerability and lesser drug-drug interactions of SSRI antidepressants. In fact, TCAs are very effective antidepressants; doxepin and imipramine are approved for OCD in those ≥12 years of age for depression and clomipramine in patients ≥10 years of age for OCD (47).

How one decides to choose an SSRI depends on various factors such as: the specific side effect profile, whether this medication has been used with good results in this patient before or has shown a good response in a family member, any contraindications, availability as an acceptable formulation (i.e., solution or suspension), and medication costs. In order to improve patient compliance, prescribing a medication with daily dosing is usually preferable to two or three times a day dosing (47).

The United States Food and Drug Administration (FDA) has issued an advisory and black box warning about emergence of suicidal ideation during the initial phase of SSRIs treatment; this development has changed the prescribing behaviors of many primary care physicians and pediatricians in recent years leading to a reluctance in some to prescribe SSRIs. It is, however, recommended that the use of SSRIs in children and adolescents should be taken in consideration in situations where it is really indicated and these pediatric patients should be followed closely, especially in the earlier phase of treatment, to monitor for any suicide risk.

Conclusion

Atopic dermatitis is a chronic, relapsing, remitting disease starting in very early childhood and 20-40% of those afflicted continue to suffer throughout their life. It affects every aspect of these patients' lives with resultant decrease in their quality of life. The impact of illness extends beyond the skin management alone and can lead to neglecting other aspects of disease especially the known psychophysiologic and psychoneuroimmunologic links with psychiatric disorders. A comprehensive multidisciplinary approach is necessary including a psychiatric perspective to enhance the success of any treatment plans for atopic dermatitis.

Acknowledgments

This paper is a revised and adapted version of an earlier publication: Tareen RS. Atopic dermatitis: A psychocutaneous review. In: Tareen RS, Greydanus DE, Jafferany M, Patel DR, Merrick J, eds. Pediatric psycho-dermatology. A clinical manual of child and adolescent psychocutaneous disorders. Berlin: De Gruyter, 2013:119-46.

References

[1] Coca AF, Cooke RA. On the classification of phenomena of hypersensitiveness. J Immul 1923;8:163-82.
[2] Larsen FS, Hanifin JM. Epidemiology of atopic dermatitis. Immunol Allergy Clin North Am 2002;1:1-24.
[3] Larsen FS. Clinical genetics of atopic eczema. Handbook of Atopic Eczema, 2nd ed. 2006.
[4] Schäfer T, Ring J, Epidemiology of atopic eczema. In: Ring J, Przybilla B, Ruzicka T, eds. Handbook of atopic eczema, 2nd ed. Berlin: Springer, 2006: 21-30.
[5] Croner S, Kjellman NIM, Erikkson B, Roth A. IgE screening in 1701 newborn infants and the development of atopic disease during infancy. Arch Dis Child 1982;57:364-8.
[6] Chapman RH, Parish WE. Atopic dermatitis. In: Chapman RH, Burton JL, Ebling FJ, eds. Textbook of dermatology. London: Blackwell,1992;5:589-610.
[7] Novak N, Bieber T. The pathogenesis of atopic dermatitis. In: Reitamo S, Lugar TA, Steinhoff M. Textbook of atopic dermatitis. London: Informa Healthcare, 2008:210-20.
[8] Schneider G. Psychosomatic aspects and psychiatric conditions. In: Misery L, Ständer S. Pruritus. Berlin: Springer, 2010: 211-5.
[9] Arndt J, Smith N, Tausk F. Stress and atopic dermatitis. Curr Allergy Asthma Rev 2008,8:312-7.
[10] Seiffert K, Hilbert E, Schaechinger H. Psychophysiological reactivity under mental stress in atopic dermatitis. Dermatology 2005;210:286–93. Original Text
[11] Gieler U, Ehlers A, Hohler T, Burkard G. The psychosocial status of patients with endogenous eczema: a study using cluster analysis for the correlation of psychological factors with somatic findings. Hautarzt 1990;41:416–23.
[12] Faulstich ME, Williamson DA, Duchmann EG, Conerly SL, Brantley PJ. Psychophysiological analysis of atopic dermatitis. J Psycho-Som Res 1985;29:415–7.
[13] Steinhoff A, Steinhoff M. Neuroimminuology of atopic dermatitis. In: Granstein RD, Luger TA, eds. Neuroimmunology of skin: basic sciences to clinical practice. Berlin: Springer, 2008:197-07.
[14] Rosenthal MJ. Psychosomatic study of infantile eczema: I. Mother child relationship. Pediatrics 1952;10:581-91.

[15] Miller H, Baruch DW. Psychosomatic studies of children with allergic manifestations: I Maternal rejection; a study of 63 cases. Psychosom Med 1948;10:275-88.

[16] Howlett S. Emotional dysfunction, child–family relationships and childhood atopic dermatitis. Br J Dermatol 1999;140:381–4.

[17] Marmor J, Ashley M, Tabachnik N, et al. The mother-child relationship in the genesis of neurodermatitis. Arch Dermatol 1956;74:599-605.

[18] Jones SM, Buchanan A, Burke AW. Atopic dermatitis. In: Lieberman P, Anderson JA. Current clinical practice: allergic diseases: diagnosis and treatment, 3rd ed. Totowa, NJ: Humana Press, 2007:217-47.

[19] Rothe MJ, Grant-Kels JM. Diagnostic criteria for atopic dermatitis. Lancet 1996;348:769-70.

[20] Heine RG, Hill DJ, Hosking CL. Role of food allergens in atopic dermatitis. In: Reitamo S, Lugar TA, Steinhoff M, eds. Textbook of atopic dermatitis. London: Informa Healthcare, 2008:85-99.

[21] Peterson JD, Chan LS. A comprehensive management guide for atopic dermatitis. Dermatol Nurs 2006;18(6):531-42.

[22] Mrabet-Dahbi S, Renz H. Role of inhalant allergens in atopic dermatitis. In: Reitamo S, Lugar TA, Steinhoff M, eds. Textbook of atopic dermatitis. London: Informa Healthcare, 2008;101-15.

[23] Cork MJ, Danby S, Vasilopoulos Y. Epidermal barrier dysfunction in atopic dermatitis. In: Reitamo S, Lugar TA, Steinhoff M, eds. Textbook of atopic dermatitis. London: Informa Healthcare, 2008;35-58.

[24] Boguniewicz M, Nicol N. General management of patients with atopic dermatitis. In: Reitamo S, Lugar TA, Steinhoff M, eds. Textbook of atopic dermatitis. London: Informa Healthcare, 2008;147-164.

[25] Ständer S, Lugar TA, Steinhoff M. Itch –pathophysiology and treatment. In: Reitamo S, Lugar TA, Steinhoff M, eds. Textbook of atopic dermatitis. London: Informa Healthcare, 2008;117-29.

[26] May E, Zollner T, Schäcke H. Mode of action of glucocorticoids. In: Reitamo S, Lugar TA, Steinhoff M. Textbook of atopic dermatitis. London: Informa Healthcare 2008:165-79.

[27] Paller, AS. The 2004 process of care: treatment options for the management of atopic dermatitis. New York: Millennium CME Institute, 2004.

[28] Peterson JD, Chan LS. A comprehensive management guide for atopic dermatitis. Dermatol Nurs 2006;18(6):531-42.

[29] Reitamo S, Van Leent EJ, Ho V, et al. Efficacy and safety of tacrolimus ointment compared with that of hydrocortisone acetate ointment in children with atopic dermatitis. J Allergy Clin Immunol 2002;109:539–46.

[30] Maurer M, Worm M, and Zuberbie T. Antihistamines in atopic dermatitis. In: Reitamo S, Lugar TA, Steinhoff M, eds. Textbook of atopic dermatitis. London: Informa Healthcare, 2008;210-20.

[31] Grundmann SA, Beissert S. Phototherapy of atopic dermatitis. In: Reitamo S, Lugar TA, Steinhoff M, eds. Textbook of atopic dermatitis. London: Informa Healthcare, 2008:187-95.

[32] Clayton TH, Clark SM, Turner D, Goulden V. The treatment of severe atopic dermatitis in childhood with narrowband ultraviolet B phototherapy. Clin Exp Dermatol 2007;32:28-33.

[33] Valkova S, Velkova A. UVA/UVB phototherapy for atopic dermatitis revisited. J Dermatol Treat 2004;15:239–44.

[34] Holmes SA, Anste AV. Phototherapy and PUVA photochemotherapy in children. Photodermatol Photoimmunol Photomed 2004;20:69–75.

[35] Ricci G, Dondi A, Patrizi A. Systemic therapy of atopic dermatitis in children. Drugs 2009;69(3):297-306.

[36] Harper JI, Ahmed I, Barclay G. Cyclosporin for severe childhood atopic dermatitis: short course versus continuous therapy. Br J Dermatol 2000;142(1):52-8.

[37] Murphy LA, Atherton D. A retrospective evaluation of azathioprine in severe childhood atopic eczema, using thiopurine methyltransferase levels to exclude patients at high risk of myelo-suppression. Br J Dermatol 2002;147:308–15.

[38] Hashiro M, Okumura M. Anxiety, depression and psychosomatic symptoms in patients with atopic dermatitis: comparison with normal controls and among groups of different degrees of severity. J Dermatol Sci 1997;14:63-7.

[39] Lien L, Green K, Thoresen M. Atopic conditions and mental health problems: a 3-year follow-up study. Eur Child Adolesc Psychiatry 2010;19:705–13.

[40] Schmitt J, Apfelbacher C, Chen CM. Infant-onset eczema in relation to mental health problems at age 10 years: Results from a prospective birth cohort study (German Infant Nutrition Intervention plus) J Allergy Clin Immunol 2010;125(2):404-10.

[41] Slatter MJ, Hetzel S, Essex MJ. Anxiety and depression in adolescents with atopic dermatitis. Brain Behav Immunity 2009;23:25–6.

[42] Linnet J, Jemec A. An assessment of anxiety and dermatology life quality in patients with atopic dermatitis. Br J Dermatol 1999;140:268–72.

[43] Gupta MA, Gupta AK. Depression and suicidal ideation in dermatology patients with acne, alopecia areata, atopic dermatitis and psoriasis. Br J Dermatol 1998;139:846–50.

[44] Lewallen JP, Tuturro CT, Turturro A. Working with other healthcare providers. In: Norman RA, ed. Preventive dermatology. London: Springer, 2010;47-56.

[45] Habib S, Morrissey S. Stress management for atopic dermatitis. Behav Change 1999;16(4):226–36.

[46] Gustafsson PA, Kjellman N-IM, Bjorksten B. Family interaction and a supportive social network as salutogenic factors in childhood atopic illness. Pediatr Allergy Immunol 2002;13:51–7.

[47] Kamboj MK, Tareen RS. Management of nonpsychiatric medical conditions presenting with psychiatric manifestations. Pediatr Clin North Am 2011;58:219–41.

In: Pediatric and Adolescent Dermatology
Editors: D Greydanus, A Feinberg and J Merrick
ISBN: 978-1-63321-853-6

Chapter 7

Psoriasis

Sandra Ros*

Department of Dermatology, Hospital de la Santa Creu i Sant Pau,
Barcelona, Spain

Psoriasis is one of the most important dermatological inflammatory diseases in children and adolescents. Its appearance in this pediatric age group has considerable psychological effects on the patient as well as the family. This chapter reviews these issues and provides recommendations for management. Basic areas of intervention involve focusing on facilitating and managing stress, developing self-control skills, improving self-esteem, strengthening adaptive features of each child or adolescent, stabilizing the psycho-emotional condition of the child and providing or facilitating problem solving and social skills.

Introduction

Psoriasis is one of the most important dermatological inflammatory diseases in children and adolescents. Psoriasis is an inflammatory inherited dermatosis, characterized by erythematous scaly papules and plaques that usually follow a chronic fluctuating course with flares of variable duration and severity. Psoriasis is a multifactorial genetic disorder triggered by several environmental factors such as trauma, infections, or stress. (1-3). Childhood psoriasis is a well-recognized entity, but its true prevalence is not known and the studies carried out yield various percentages.

There is not much literature on the impact of psoriasis in children and adolescents compared with that found in adults; in spite of this, our experience shows that considerable emotional vulnerability exists in the pediatric population, which has been extensively studied in other diseases such as oncological processes (4).

* Correspondence: Sandra Ros, Psychologist, Dermatology Department, Hospital de la Santa Creu i Sant Pau.,C. Sant Antoni Mª Claret 167. 08025, Barcelona, Spain. E-mail: SRos@santpau.cat.

In order to understand the scope that psoriasis has on the child or adolescent, we must not only measure and treat the physical damage of psoriasis, but we must also assess how this disease affects the child's emotional development and his vital areas such as social development, family health, and education (5-6). Psoriasis can affect physical appearance and growth, resulting in reduced activity, pain, itching, the need for regular therapy, and sometimes, unpleasant procedures as well as possible loss of school attendance.

For this purpose, in this discussion we will emphasize the relationship between psoriasis and stress, the aspects derived from the visibility of lesions, the child's psycho-emotional aspects (e.g., body image and self-esteem) and, finally, the relationship with his family environment. The latter will partly determine how the child lives and faces this disease and its treatment. It is important to remember that because of the chronicity of this disorder, health education, family support, and coping strategies will help these children to a better acceptance of a disease which they have not chosen. For this reason, patients with childhood psoriasis as well as their families require special attention.

Epidemiology

Psoriasis in childhood is not uncommon (7-12). The prevalence in the general adult population ranges from 1-3% (13), but the exact prevalence of psoriasis in childhood is unknown, largely because diverse age definitions have been used in different studies (14-17). Furthermore, psoriasis may be underdiagnosed in childhood. Psoriatic diaper rash may be diagnosed as diaper dermatitis and inverse, scalp psoriasis may be confused with infantile seborrheic dermatitis.

In the prevalence study carried out by Gelfand *et al.* in the United Kingdom, the data show an estimate of psoriasis of 0.6% in children from 0-9 years old and 1.4% in those between 10-19 years old (18). Other results are those obtained by the group of Augustin in Germany, who found a prevalence of 0.71% in pediatric patients under 18 years old (3). Farber and Nall reported that in the United States, 35% of patients with psoriasis had the disease onset before the age of 20 (2% in infants, 8% in childhood, and 25% in adolescence) (15). Overall, it may be said that at least one third of psoriatic patients develop the disease during childhood (10). Congenital psoriasis has been reported, but it is rare (19-21). It has been postulated that based upon age of onset, psoriasis vulgaris can be divided in two groups: early onset psoriasis, presenting before the age of 40, and late onset psoriasis presenting after the age of 40 (10, 22). Clinical features seem also to support this classification (7,10).

Childhood psoriasis seems to be more prevalent in girls than in boys, approaching a 2:1 ratio (14,17). This female preponderance has not been confirmed by others (11,16). Among the infant population (0-18 years old), the mean age of psoriasis onset ranges between 7 and 10 years old (23-25).

Swanbeck et al. found that the lifetime risk of inheriting psoriasis, if no parent, one parent or both parents have psoriasis is 4%, 28%, and 65%, respectively (26). If there is already one affected child in the family, the corresponding risks are 24%, 51%, and 83%, respectively. Family history of psoriasis also predicts an early disease onset (27-28). Spontaneous remissions are more frequent in children (17).

Clinical features

The lesions of psoriasis consist in well-demarcated erythematous, scaly papules and plaques. The scales have a characteristic silvery aspect and the so- called Auspitz's sign is seen after removing them by scratching punctate hemorrhages. This phenomenon is useful for diagnosis. Another useful clinical sign is the presence of erythema and/or fissuring at the intergluteal fold (Brunsting's sign).

The distribution is frequently symmetric. The areas of predilection are the scalp and extensor surfaces of the extremities. Psoriasis tends to develop in areas of previous trauma (Koebner phenomenon). Psoriatic plaques, although usually asymptomatic in adults, may be pruritic in a high percentage of children (16,17). Several clinical sub-types of psoriasis have been described both in adults and children: plaque-type, guttate, erythrodermic, pustular, inverse psoriasis, and arthropatic psoriasis. The clinical aspects depend also on the location. Therefore, further topographic variants may also be defined: scalp, facial, napkin, palmo-plantar, nail, fingertip, and folicular psoriasis.

Plaque psoriasis

Plaque psoriasis is the most common variant in children (11,16). Plaques of psoriasis in children tend to be thinner, with finer scales than in adults, and may be confused with eczematoid lesions. Erythematous, squamous plaques of different sizes appear most commonly on extensor aspects of the extremities, knees, elbows, and scalp. The face is very often affected in children.

Guttate psoriasis

Guttate psoriasis is characterized by the sudden appearance of small, teardrop, erythematous, scaly papules and plaques on the trunk and proximal extremities. The face may also be affected. It may be the only and initial manifestation of psoriasis, or may develop on pre-existing plaque-type psoriasis. Guttate psoriasis commonly occurs one or two weeks after an upper respiratory tract infection, usually streptococcal pharyngitis. Triggering by streptococcal perianal dermatitis has been also described (29-30).

Guttate psoriasis responds rapidly to treatment with either antistreptoccocal antibiotics or phototherapy. Even without treatment it resolves spontaneously in several months, after which the child may remain in remission for several years. In children in whom there is a streptococcal infection triggering the disease, it is common to see a bout of guttate psoriasis every time the child has pharyngitis (16).

Erythrodermic psoriasis

Psoriasis can progress to involve the entire skin with erythema and exfoliation. This form of psoriasis is exceedingly rare in children (7, 31). Precipitating factors in children with pre-existing psoriasis include certain drugs (such as antimalarials, gold therapy, and lithium), stress, phototoxicity, and sudden withdrawal of corticosteroid treatment. A few congenital cases have been reported; these congenital forms are usually very severe, respond poorly to treatment, and commonly develop arthropathy at a later age (11,32).

Pustular psoriasis

Pustular psoriasis is an uncommon form of psoriasis that represents about 1% of childhood psoriasis (7,11,32). It can be divided into generalized and localized forms (33-34). Generalized pustular psoriasis is further subdivided in generalized pustular psoriasis (Von Zumbush type), circinate, or annular pustular psoriasis (Bloch-Lapiére type), and localized forms of generalized pustular psoriasis (not acral or palmoplantar). Mixed forms may also occur. Localized pustular psoriasis can be subdivided in palmoplantar pustulosis of Barber and acrodermatitis continua of Hallopeau, affecting the distal aspect of one or two fingers.

In generalized pustular psoriasis Von Zumbush type, there are widespread, 1 to 2 mm sterile pustules of abrupt onset. Individual pustules may coalesce to form lakes of pus. Mucous membranes lesions are common and geographic tongue has been described (33,36,37). During the acute flares, the patients are often ill, with high fever, malaise, and pain, secondary to their exfoliating skin. Individual lesions resolve within 3 to 4 days, with recurrent flares of inflammation. The conversion to psoriatic erythroderma is possible (37). This form of pustular psoriasis tends to occur more commonly in infants and toddlers. Some of them go on to develop psoriasis vulgaris at a later age (7,32,35).

Generalized pustular psoriasis has been described in children with non bullous congenital erythroderma (7,32,38) and rare congenital cases have been reported (7). Several provocative factors have been recognized in children with generalized pustular psoriasis. Infection, not only streptococcal, seems to be the most common trigger (32). Other factors include irritating local treatment with coal tar or anthralin, sun exposure or drugs.

Annular pustular psoriasis (Bloch-Lapiére) is a milder generalized variant characterized by gyrate, annular lesions with a pustular border. Onset and clinical course is often subacute and affects children of older age (32,34). Systemic symptoms may be present although they are usually less severe than in the Von Zumbush form. Annular pustular psoriasis may follow acute von Zumbush forms. Localized forms of generalized pustular psoriasis include those plaques of psoriasis not acrally located that develop pustules on top (psoriasis with pustules). This may be seen after local treatment with anthralin or coal tar. Diaper psoriasis may also develop pustules in instances of secondary candida infection.

Localized acral pustular psoriasis, both Barber type or acrodermatitis continua of Hallopeau, have been considered exceptional in children. However, in a recent pediatric series, acral pustular psoriasis was seen in 5% of patients (11). In palmoplantar pustular psoriasis of Barber there are recurrent crops of pustules, 2-4 mm in diameter, on normal appearing skin of the palms and soles. Older pustules become dark brown in color and are finally shed. The eruption is usually symmetric and the preferred sites of occurrence are the thenar and hypothenar eminences on the palms and the insteps on the soles. Palmoplantar pustulosis may coexist with sternocostoclavicular arthritis and chronic recurrent multifocal osteomyelitis (39).

Achrodermatitis continua of Hallopeau may be slightly more common than palmoplantar pustulosis . In this form, pustules develop on the tips of one or two fingers or toes. Pustulation of the nail bed and nail folds leads to progressive nail destruction. Psoriatic-form scaling develops upon desiccation of pustules. Bony changes may occur with progressive tapering of the finger tips. The disease remains localized to the same finger for months or years.

Psoriatic arthritis

Psoriatic arthritis is one of the well-known complications of psoriasis (40-42). Arthritis and psoriasis appear in about 2% to 4% of children with chronic arthritis (43). Skin manifestations, usually mild, most commonly precede or occur simultaneously with articular symptoms, which are diagnostically useful. Nail changes are more common in children with arthritis than in those without it.

Five different clinical subsets have been recognized in psoriatic arthropathy: 1) predominant distal interphalangeal (DIP) joint involvement; 2) arthritis mutilans; 3) symmetric polyarthritis similar to rheumatoid arthritis (but seronegative); 4) asymmetric oligoarthritis, and 5) ankylosing spondylitis. Mixed forms may also occur (44). A joint pattern with asymmetric arthritis of large and small joints and a high rate of dactylitis (sausage finger) is prototypical for the disease (43). Children with psoriatic nail disease have higher incidence of distal interphalangeal joints (DIP) involvement. Fortunately, in juvenile psoriatic arthritis, systemic manifestations are extremely rare.

Inverse psoriasis

In some patients psoriasis may almost exclusively affect skin folds such as the inguinal, axillary, suprapubic, and intergluteal folds. Psoriatic diaper dermatitis is a particular form of inverse psoriasis that is very common in infants. Small folds such as the retroauricular folds, interdigital folds, the external canthi, lip comissure, and the periumbilical area may also be affected. Due to the natural maceration of the skin in those areas, inverse psoriasis lacks scaling, and is thinner and of a brighter red than in other areas.

Psychological aspects

The relationship between psycho-emotional factors, psycho-social impact, and psoriasis in adults has been extensively described by different authors (45-49). However there is little scientific literature regarding its involvement in childhood and adolescence (4,5,50,51). Although certain factors can be extrapolated to children and adolescents, there are some differentiated features due to disease impact on an emotional level in leisure time activities being reduced as well as less time spent in other areas (i.e., at school, in social relationships, in sleeping); also, there are other inconveniences caused by the symptoms and treatments in this population. We will highlight some of the most representative and relevant aspects such as the role of the family, the role of stress, and the visibility of the lesions. Our experience shows that the diagnosis of a chronic disease such as psoriasis in children and adolescents can cause a strong emotional impact on the child and his familial environment. This is why special attention to features of the child's familial environment has to be drawn.

The family plays a vital role in the course of the disease, whether or not there are family members affected with psoriasis. In a first stage it will be important to understand how the family experiences the diagnosis, because it can help to mitigate the emotional impact of the disease on the child or adolescent, or on the contrary, create a situation of overprotection, anxiety and stress. Later, the family involvement will influence how the parents and/or caregivers live the child's disease. We must take into account that the deterioration of health that involves a chronic disease and the visibility of lesions typical of psoriasis in children can create clinical conditions of anxiety and depression in parents that will probably require psychological treatment. The family also will have a crucial role in the child's treatment which may be complex due to the time spent on treatment, the disease perseverance, the financial difficulties in paying the medical services as well as treatments, and the changes in certain routines and family habits (5).

Stress is another factor to consider when we talk about childhood psoriasis. In the same line of what happens in adults, stress plays an important role in the adaptive system overload of the body, accelerating the onset of psoriasis, and exacerbating their symptoms. However, we must also highlight that the disease itself is creating a stressful situation in the child or adolescent.

Due to nervous-psychic genesis of psoriasis stress situation, it initiates the cascade of biochemical and immunological reactions leading to a psoriasis focus. The stress situations in children can be generated by family situations, school problems, and difficulties in the relationship with the parents or siblings. The beginning and exacerbations of these dermatoses depend on many psycho-social risk factors in children (6). The psychotherapeutic treatment of stress in children and adolescents will facilitate a better management of stressful situations, whether they are derived from psoriasis or exogenous situations.

The body image disturbance suffered by children and adolescents with psoriasis due to the visibility of their lesions is one of the characteristic aspects of the psoriasis which makes it different from other chronic diseases. Thus, we find studies which demonstrate that children with psoriasis have a worse quality of life than children with diabetes or epilepsy (see chapter 23). Visibility of the lesions may result in a child's sense of differentiation from his close environment, feeling that his skin is different; also, in some cases, psoriasis limits his or her participation in games, sports, and even at school. This sense of differentiation and the limitations can affect the child's self-esteem and his emotional development. The role of the family is fundamental to mitigate and face these situations, which are not only confronted by the child, but the parents, who have to accept the visible disease of their child. However, we must consider that young children do not feel ashamed about their image, although eventually and as they grow, such negative feelings will appear (52).

Adolescence is more vulnerable (53). It is a life stage in which the body image is really important. The adolescent begins to go outside leaving aside the family protection and a visible disease such as psoriasis seriously affects the development of the self-concept, self-image, and self-esteem. It is a life stage in which social relationships play a leading role. The adolescent with psoriasis may show fear of rejection, social isolation and inhibition, and shame due to the psoriasis. All of this may have its psychopathological correlate: some teens may present symptoms of anxiety and depression reactive to psoriasis and even medical conditions that can be diagnosed by criteria from the American Psychiatric Association's Diagnostic and Statistical Manual of Mental Disorders (DSM IV-R). The presence of this emotional distress can affect the academic performance (i.e., concentration problems due to anxiety). Difficulties in the sleep area due to psychopathology or also due to certain disease symptoms such as itching are also common (5,54). The presence of this psychopathology can also affect family unity, in a time of life where the parent-child relationship is highly sensitive.

It would be interesting to perform a psychological profile of pediatric patients with psoriasis, yet it is not possible because we can not forget that every patient, every child, and every adolescent is different, as well as the familial, social, and educational environment. The premorbid psychopathological characteristics and personality traits of children or adolescents will also be protective and risk factors may exert a modulatory role in this network. Therefore, to generalize attitudes, feelings about the disease, fears, frights, and concerns, seem an unattainable task. There will be so many profiles of children and adolescents with psoriasis equivalent to existing children and adolescents.

The psycho-emotional support to face this situation is vital for the adaptation to the disease situation. However, an assessment focused on two aspects is necessary: the first one, unmistakably focused on the child or adolescent to determine potential emotional damage, levels of anxiety, depression, and stress; also important is the detection of internalizing behavior problems (i.e., anxious, depressive, and overcontrolled) or externalizing (i.e., aggressive, hyperactive, noncompliant, and undercontrolled), and the self-esteem. The second aspect will be the family. An extensive analysis of familial relationships and how parents and siblings are living the disease and the changes occurred at the familial level since the diagnosis, is very helpful to establish an effective psychological intervention.

Differential diagnosis

The diagnosis of psoriasis is usually made by clinical appearance. In children, some other diseases may be considered and in case of doubt, a skin biopsy would be necessary. Guttate psoriasis may be confused with pityriasis rosea and chronic pityriasis lichenoides. In pityriasis rosea there is a herald patch, the lesions are oval as well as distributed along skin lines, and usually have a shorter duration. In chronic pityriasis lichenoides, papules are brownish with a central crust or scale.

Follicular psoriasis on the elbows and knees as well as scalp psoriasis may be confused with pityriasis rubra pilaris, frictional dermatitis or lichen spinulosus. The constant involvement of the palms and soles and the typical salmon hue of the lesions may differentiate pityriasis rubra pilaris. Napkin psoriasis may be very difficult to differentiate from seborrheic dermatitis. Psoriatic diaper rash is usually brighter red, better demarcated and shinier than seborrheic dermatitis, and lacks the yellow scale. Candidiasis should also be ruled out; satellite pustules and peripheral scaling are highly suggestive of Candida infection.

Eczema of the palms and soles may be impossible to differentiate from psoriasis. In many cases there is a true overlap of both diseases. If vesicles are present, it is highly suggestive of eczema as vesicles are not a feature of psoriasis. Palmoplantar psoriasis in children may manifest with glazed erythema of the palms and soles as in juvenile plantar dermatitis.

Hyperkeratotic eczema is very difficult to differentiate. Nummular eczema may be considered in the differential diagnosis of plaque type psoriasis.

Acral pustular psoriasis has to be differentiated from acropustulosis of infancy, scabies, and tinea pedis. In acropustulosis, each crop of lesions resolves spontaneously in a few days, while pustular psoriasis is more persistent. Tinea pedis is usually asymmetric and a direct potassium hydroxide examination allows a rapid differentiation in case of doubt. Scabies usually shows lesions elsewhere and scraping helps to establish the diagnosis. Erythrodermic psoriasis, especially if congenital, is very difficult to differentiate from other forms of erythroderma such as icthyosis, metabolic disorders or immunodeficiencies. Skin biopsy may not be useful in these situations and only observation over time will confirm the correct diagnosis.

Psychotherapeutic intervention

It is clinically challenging to provide psychological care to children and adolescents with psoriasis who present with various psycho-emotional difficulties. These difficulties are mainly due to two barriers: the lack of specialized professionals connected to dermatology departments and the resistance shown by the families of children and adolescents because of the stigma associated with the psychological treatment. It is important to note that contributing to the family resistance barrier is that many parents feel that they are being blamed for not managing the child's condition well enough. The last aspect can be redirected by giving the family support and information about the difficulties and the potential stress at the family level in the care of a child with a chronic, visible disease such as psoriasis.

In order to improve the knowledge on psoriasis, treatments and expectations will be of vital importance in this first stage. It is important to explain to the family, especially the parents, that the multidisciplinary approach utilized by the dermatologist and psychologist can help the child achieve a better coping mechanism with resultant adaptation to the disease and to situations generated by childhood psoriasis, and a reduction of the associated psychopathology (i.e., anxiety and sadness). This makes it easier for the parents to understand and appreciate the necessity for this type of treatment without the feeling of being judged in any way.

We must not forget to explore the relationships established at the familial level of the onset and course of psoriasis which will be very helpful for future psychotherapeutic interventions. The attitude of the family regarding the child may be permissive, inducing a dependent behavior, or overprotective, inducing infantile behaviors that can prevent social autonomy and hinder the adherence to self-care (i.e., skin hydration). Difficulties in mother-child relationships could emerge, as for example, negative attitudes from the parents focused on the disease and the symptoms, distancing from other family members, and psychopathology in the closest family environment.

Another point of vital interest in our psychotherapeutic intervention should be focused on how parental stress and anxiety directly affect the child. For this reason, the programs with pediatric patients should also be oriented to the parents to achieve two main objectives:

a) to reduce stress, depressive and anxiety symptoms, or the medical condition (anxiety and mood disorders). The presence and intensity of psychopathological factors will determine the father-child relationship and may even facilitate the appearance of these symptoms in the pediatric patient.

b) to teach the parents procedures to help their children and themselves cope with the disease. We know that the diagnosis of psoriasis creates a start up of coping mechanisms and important adjustments in family dynamics. Psoriasis is a disease that even if not disabling, involves a chronicity, visibility, as well as social stigma that can severely affect ones self-esteem. Therefore, an inadequate coping of the psoriasis by the parents can lead the family to become a risk factor and not a protector factor against the potential psycho-emotional involvement of the child. The psychotherapeutic treatment needs to reduce anxiety and stress of parents. Therapy in group or individual format will correct some of the maladaptive behaviors of parents towards the child, improving the quality of life of parents, and ensuring the emotional bonding with the child.

When performing a psychotherapeutic intervention in children with psoriasis, we must have the child's age in mind. In younger pediatric population, the intervention is focused on the family and the child. In older pediatric population, the intervention will be focused on the adolescent, clearly separating the psychotherapeutic space of the patient from the psychotherapeutic space of the family (55-56). In our clinical practice the psychotherapeutic intervention in the pediatric patient is focused on two constructs: progressive relaxation techniques and psychotherapy.

In progressive relaxation techniques (i.e., autogenic and progressive muscle relaxation), the objective is to train children in different relaxation techniques to learn how to manage and/or reduce the tension produced by daily events of life, associated with psoriasis as well as stressful situations that may arise in their environments. Through them, we teach the child or adolescent to control his body physically through progressive relaxation and to identify the stressful situations. We know, as we mentioned above, the important role of stress as it can precipitate or exacerbate outbreaks. Through the progressive relaxation technique adapted to children, we can provide our patients with a useful and necessary tool to feel able to regulate their levels of anxiety.

Psychotherapy

Pediatric patient-oriented psychotherapy starts with the psychological interview in which the clinician assesses, in addition to an existing psychopathology, the cognitive abilities, personal resources, and protective factors, such as family support and in the case of adolescents, social support (see chapter 23). Children with emotional and behavioral problems prior to psoriasis, with pediatric psychiatric disorders and history of psycho-social maladjustment as well as a tendency to anticipatory fears, can show the clinician or clinician team certain vulnerability to maladjustment when facing new situations. An early intervention when detecting these potential risk factors can help to minimize the impact of psoriasis later in life even when we do not detect psycho-emotional alterations due to a skin disease.

The objectives of psychotherapy is to identify the stressful situations related to the psoriasis perceived by the adolescent as, for example, avoidance behavior, social isolation, and even the anticipation to social rejection. At such a vital stage of personal development in which the adolescent walks towards socialization and emotional autonomy, adolescents with psoriasis face a situation of vulnerability linked to the visibility of psoriasis, different treatments, and distressing physical symptoms. These three variables will affect most of our patients as stress generators.

In psychotherapy, it is a priority to analyze each of these factors through a comprehensive dialogue with the adolescent, creating a safety climate which promotes the active involvement of the patient; there is a space in which the adolescent may freely express all those situations that generate anxiety and fear. Although every patient is unique in his or her innermost core, it is true that certain similar stressful situations are commonly perceived in this population. Stressful situations comprise social avoidance behaviors due to fear of rejection together with a cognitive anticipation of social rejection. Hiding the lesions by using specific clothes also causes a stressful situation in the adolescent with psoriasis. In the case of lesions not affecting exposed areas, we can identify this constant anticipatory anxiety, focused on the thought that it may affect those exposed areas or the fear of being discovered.

The physical limitations generated by the symptoms of psoriasis (i.e., skin tension, bleeding lesions, itching, and pain) will necessarily modify some daily activities as sport or leisure of our patients, generating for them more tension, stress, and rejection because of the disease. Physical symptoms may alter the sleep area: frequent awakenings occur during the night and these symptoms hinder the normal resting cycle of adolescents or children, thus facilitating more emotional distress and irritability.

All this factors may facilitate social isolation or withdrawal of adolescents because of the fear of being discovered and thus being isolated from their environment. Expressing all these situations in a therapeutic environment, as a catharsis, helps the adolescent to be aware of his or her emotional state. Often on the first visit the adolescent unconsciously denies having any suffering. The goal of psychotherapy is to be able to work on these situations at both cognitive and behavioral levels, so that the adolescent can generate coping tools that help him or her deal with the stressful situation.

At the cognitive level, the therapist works on the identification, expression, and confrontation of the feelings generated by psoriasis in adolescents. Fear of worsening of the disease, physical imperfection feelings induced by not following the current aesthetic canons, rejection of one's own body image, and maladaptive thoughts that accompany this feelings directly influence the presence of symptoms of anxiety and depression. These symptoms can emerge as a result of personal insecurity; these involve feelings of stigmatization mentioned above and alteration of the socialization process, and are the key to the psychotherapeutic approach and to the prevention of authentic clinical diagnosis according to classification by the American Psychiatric Association's DSM-IV-R.

The last aspect on which we have to focus the psychological intervention is to differentiate the identity of the patient from the disease. Adolescent patients often do not feel like teenagers with a chronic disease, but they feel like "psoriatic". This establishes limits because everything in their life revolves around the disease. This is certainly the most intimate and committed process in psychotherapy. The therapeutic relationship with adolescents having psoriasis should indeed be intense, in order to be able to work out this differentiation aspect between "I" and "psoriasis".

The establishment of the positive and valuable aspects of every adolescent and his strengths at the personal and social level are important to establish. Also, it is helpful to strengthen those personality characteristics that are favorable at the relational level; this will allow him to see by himself the negative aspects (of his own and of the disease) in which until now he has based his reality, but also his own positive and adaptative aspects which until this moment have been ignored.

In order to understand and respect the difficulty and hostility that the acceptance of a chronic disease as psoriasis represents for the adolescent, it will help us as professionals to understand the nature of the disease and to facilitate the adolescent's assumption of psoriasis as part of his or her life and person instead of an acceptance of a disease that has been imposed. Therefore, it is necessary to encourage the positive and negative feelings that these patients experience.

Helping the adolescent to develop coping strategies with the disease and the typical situations that every adolescent (with or without a chronic disease) faces in this stage of life probably is the last step of psychotherapy. At this point the therapist works on the autonomy of the adolescent and the active involvement in the treatment of psoriasis. This facilitates the adolescent to express to the dermatologist the difficulties that the treatment involves and which can reduce the treatment adherence.

In summary, psychotherapy focuses on generating an adequate space without prejudice where the therapist and the adolescent can work together, facilitating the expression of the feelings caused by psoriasis, either internalizing (fears, anxious-depressive symptoms, withdrawal, low self-concept) or externalizing disorders (failure, challenges, irritability, self-harm), as well as facilitating the adaption to the disease and the management of emotions generated by psoriasis in this population of patients who are so vulnerable at this moment of their lives.

In patients in whom psoriasis appears at a younger age, the intervention focuses on these issues: facilitating the adoption of active coping mechanisms to psoriasis; the adjustment to a new family situation due to the appearance or the course of psoriasis in the pediatric patient; the prevention and/or treatment of the potential psychopathological symptoms that could appear in parents or caregivers of the child because of the emotional overload that represents the appearance of the chronic disease as well as the treatments and the loss of the child's health; and the strategies to promote necessary self-care in psoriasis tailored to each pediatric patient age.

Conclusion

We know that the diagnosis of psoriasis can cause a strong psychological impact on any stage of life and involves a large variety of psychological adjustments in the individual who suffers from it. When this chronic and visible skin disease appears in childhood and adolescence, it involves both the family and the child or adolescent. Finally, it can be said that the complete therapeutic approach aims to facilitate a process of normalization of the different members of the family throughout the course of the disease. However, we know that each situation is different, that psoriasis can enhance or worsen certain pre-existing aspects, and that each family will find a variety of strategies to accept the situation of the disease in the most optimal manner.

The basic areas of intervention in pediatric patients primarily focuses on facilitating and managing stress as well as self-control skills, improving self-esteem, strengthening adaptive features of each child or adolescent, stabilizing the psycho-emotional condition of the child and providing or facilitating problem-solving as well as social skills. Finally, it is important not to forget that each of our pediatric patients is unique and understand as well as respect each of their situations.

Acknowledgments

This paper is a revised and adapted version of an earlier publication: Ros S, Baselga E. Psoriasis and children: A psycological approach. In: Tareen RS, Greydanus DE, Jafferany M, Patel DR, Merrick J, eds. Pediatric psycho-dermatology. A clinical manual of child and adolescent psychocutaneous disorders. Berlin: De Gruyter, 2013:147-61.

References

[1] Baselga E, Mascaro JM. Dermatosi infiammatorie: La psoriasis nell'età pediatrica. In: Abrizi G, ed. Dermatologia pediatrica. Milano: Masson, 2003;367-80. [Spanish]
[2] Gudjonsson JE, Elder JT. Psoriasis: Epidemiology. Clin Dermatol 2007;25:535-46.
[3] Augustin M, Krüeger K, Radtke MA, et al. Disease severity, quality of life in health care in plaque psoriasis: a multicenter prospective cross-sectional study in Germany. Dermatology 2008;216:366-72.
[4] Beattie PE, Lewis-Jones MS. A comparative study of impairment of quality of life in children with skin disease and children with other chronic childhood disease. Br J Dermatol 2006;155:145-51.
[5] Ganemo A, Wahlgren CF, Svensson A. Quality of life and clinical features in Swedish children with psoriasis. Pediatric Dermatol 2011;28:375-9.
[6] Nyfors A, Lomholt K. Psoriasis in children. A short review of 245 cases. Br J Dermatol 1975;72:437-42.
[7] Beylot C, Puissant A, Bioulac P, Saurat JH, Pringuet R, Doutre MS. Particular clinical features of psoriasis in infants and children. Acta Derm Venerol 1979:Suppl 87:95-7.
[8] Farber EM, Mullen RH, Jacobs AH, Nall L. Infantile psoriasis: a follow-up study. Pediatr Dermatol 1986;3:237-43.
[9] Farber EM, Nall L. Childhood psoriasis. Cutis 1999;64:309-14.
[10] Swanbeck G, Inerot A, Martinsson T, Wahlstrom J, Enerback C, Enlund F, et al. Age at onset and different types of psoriasis. Br J Dermatol 1995;133:768-73.
[11] Morris A, Rogers M, Fischer G, Williams K. Childhood psoriasis: a clinical review of 1262 cases. Pediatr Dermatol 2001;18:188-98.
[12] Verbov J. Psoriasis in childhood. Arch Dis Child 1992;67:75-6.
[13] Farber EM, Nall L. Epidemiology: natural history and genetics. In: Roenigk HH, Maibach HI, Eds. Psoriasis. New York: Marcel Dekker, 1998:107-57.
[14] Al Fouzan AS, Nanda A. A survey of childhood psoriasis in Kuwait. Pediatr Dermatol 1994;11:116-9.
[15] Farber EM, Nall ML. The natural history of psoriasis in 5600 patients. Dermatologica 1974;148:1-18.
[16] Nanda A, Kaur S, Kaur I, Kumar B. Childhood psoriasis: an epidemiologic survey of 112 patients. Pediatr Dermatol 1990;7:19-21.
[17] Raychaudhuri SP, Gross J. A comparative study of pediatric onset psoriasis with adult onset psoriasis. Pediatr Dermatol 2000;17:174-8.
[18] Gelfand JM, Weinstein R, Porter SB, et al. Prevalence and treatment of psoriasis in the United Kingdom: a population-based study. Arch Dermatol 2005;141:1537-41.
[19] Lehners-Weber C, de la Brassine BM, Dezfoulian B, Richert B, Bonardeaux C, Willemaers V. Congenital psoriasis following the lines of Blaschko. Pediatr Dermatol 1996;13:219-21.
[20] Lerner MR, Lernr AB. Congenital psoriasis: report of three cases. Arch Dermatol 1972;105:598-601.
[21] Chang SE, Choi JH, Koh JK. Congenital erythrodermic psoriasis. Br J Dermatol 1999;140:538-9.

[22] Henseler T, Christophers E. Psoriasis of early and late onset: characterization of two types of psoriasis vulgaris. J Am Acad Dermatol 1985;13:450-6.

[23] Fan X, Xiao FL, Yang S, et al. Childhood psoriasis: a study of 277 patients from China. J Eur Acad Dermatol Venereol 2007;21:762-5.

[24] Seyan M, Coskum BK, Saglam M, et al. Psoriasis in childhood and adolescence: evaluation of demographic and clinical features. Pediatr Int 2006;48:525-30.

[25] .Kumar B, Jain R, Sandhu K, et al. Epidemiology of childhood psoriasis: a study of 419 patients from northern India. Int J Dermatol 2004;43:654-8.

[26] Swanbeck G, Inerot A, Martinsson T, Enerback C, Enlund F, Samuelsson L, et al. Genetic counselling in psoriasis: empirical data on psoriasis among first-degree relatives of 3095 psoriatic probands. Br J Dermatol 1997;137:939-42.

[27] Altobelli E, Petrocelli R, Marziliano C, et al. Family history of psoriasis and age at disease onset in Italian patients with psoriasis. Br J Dermatol 2007;156:1400-1.

[28] Henseler T, Christophers E. Disease concomitance in psoriasis. J Am Acad Dermatol 1995;32:982-6.

[29] Herbst RA, Hoch O, Kapp A, Weiss J. Guttate psoriasis triggered by perianal streptococcal dermatitis in a four-year-old boy. J Am Acad Dermatol 2000;42:885-7.

[30] Patrizi A, Costa AM, Fiorillo L, Neri I. Perianal streptococcal dermatitis associated with guttate psoriasis and/or balanoposthitis: a study of five cases. Pediatr Dermatol 1994;11:168-71.

[31] Prystowsky JH, Cohen PR. Pustular and erythrodermic psoriasis. Dermatol Clin 1995;13:57-770.

[32] Zelickson BD, Muller SA. Generalized pustular psoriasis. A review of 63 cases. Arch Dermatol 1991;127:1339-45.

[33] Tay YK, Tham SN. The profile and outcome of pustular psoriasis in Singapore: a report of 28 cases. Int J Dermatol 1997;36:266-71.

[34] Baker H, Ryan TJ. Generalized pustular psoriasis: a clinical and epidemiological study of 104 cases. Br J Dermatol 1968;80:771-93.

[35] Judge MR, McDonald AM, Black MM. Pustular psoriasis in childhood. Clin Exp Dermatol 1993;18:97-9.

[36] Langtry JA, Carr MM, Ive FA, Gordon P, Hunter JA, Harper JI. Ichthyosiform erythroderma associated with generalized pustulosis. Br J Dermatol 1998;138:502-5.

[37] Juanqin G, Zhiqiang C, Zijia H. Evaluation of the effectiveness of childhood generalized pustular psoriasis treatment in 30 cases. Pediatr Dermatol 1998;15:144-6.

[38] Langtry JA, Carr MM, Ive FA, Gordon P, Hunter JA, Harper JI. Ichthyosiform erythroderma associated with generalized pustulosis. Br J Dermatol 1998;138:502-5.

[39] Job-Deslandre C, Krebs S, Kahan A. Chronic recurrent multifocal osteomyelitis: five-year outcomes in 14 pediatric cases. Joint, Bone, Spine 2001;68:245-51.

[40] Scarpa R, Mathieu A. Psoriatic arthritis: envolving concepts. Curr Opin Rheumatol 2000;12:274-80.

[41] Southwood TR, Petty RE, Malleson PN, Delgado EA, Hunt DW, Wood B, et al. Psoriatic arthritis in children. Arthritis Rheum 1989;32:1007-13.

[42] Shore A, Ansell BM. Juvenile psoriatic arthritis--an analysis of 60 cases. J Pediatr 1982;100:529-35.

[43] Hafner R, Michels H. Psoriatic arthritis in children. Curr Opin Rheumatol 1996;8:467-72.

[44] Scarpa R, Lubrano E, Cozzi R, Ames PR, Oriente CB, Oriente P. Subcorneal pustular dermatosis (Sneddon-Wilkinson syndrome): another cutaneous manifestation of SAPHO syndrome? Br J Rheumatol 1997;36:602-3.

[45] Gupta MA, Gupta AK. Depression and suicidal ideation in dermatology patients with acne, alopecia areata, atopic dermatitis and psoriasis. Br J Dermatol 1998;139:846-50.

[46] Kimball A, Jacobson C, Weiss S, Vreeland MG, Wu Y. The psychosocial burden of psoriasis. Am J Clin Derm 2005;6:383-92.

[47] Ginsburg IH, Link BG. Psychosocial consequences of rejection and stigma feelings in psoriasis patients. Int J Dermatol 1993;32:587-91.

[48] Gupta MA, Gupta AK, Watteel GN. Perceived deprivation of social touch in psoriasis is associated with a greater psychologic morbidity: an index of the stigma experience in dermatologic disorders. Cutis 1998;61:339-42.

[49] Vardy D, Besser A, Amir M, et al. Experiences of stigmatization play role in mediating impact of disease severity on quality of life in psoriasis patients. Br J Dermatol 2002;147:736-42.

[50] de Jager ME, van der Kerkhof PCM, de Jong EMGJ, Seyger MMB. Br J Dermatol 2010;163:1099-1101.

[51] Bilgic A, Bilgic Ö, Akış HK, Eskioğlu F, Kılıç EZ. Psychiatric symptoms and health-related quality of life in children and adolescents with psoriasis. Pediatr Dermatol. 2010;27:614-7.

[52] Walters E. Problems faced by children and families living with visible difference. In: Lansdown R, Rumsey N, Bradbury E, Carr T, Oartrudge J, Eds. Visibly different: coping with disfigurement. Oxford: Butterworth-Heinmann, 1997.

[53] Smith JA. The impact of skin disease on the quality of life of adolescents. Adol Med 2001;12:343-353.

[54] Weisshaar E, Seeliger S, Diepgen TL, et al. Pruritus in childhood. A diagnostic and therapeutic challenge. Haurtarzt 2004;55:855-68.

[55] Rauch PK, Jellinek MS. Pediatric dermatology: developmental and psychological issues. Adv Dermatol 1989;4:143-56.

[56] Czyzewski DJ, Lopez M. Clinical psychology in the management of pediatric skin disease. Pediatric Dermatol 1998;3:619-29

In: Pediatric and Adolescent Dermatology
Editors: D Greydanus, A Feinberg and J Merrick

ISBN: 978-1-63321-853-6

Chapter 8

Dermatology: Intellectual and developmental disabilities

Arthur N Feinberg*[*], *MD
Department of Pediatric and Adolescent Medicine,
Western Michigan University Homer Stryker MD School of Medicine,
Kalamazoo, Michigan, United States of America

The goal of this chapter is to formulate a framework of reference for the clinician to appreciate dermatologic manifestations in people with intellectual and developmental disability (IDD). Because of the common ectodermal origin of skin, hair, nails and neural tissue, we emphasize the importance of this association. First we provide an overview of dermatologic manifestations in general, and present a table of these descriptors, with which conditions causing developmental disability are associated. Then we present an overview of these conditions classified by pattern of inheritance, highlighting their other manifestations. Although these conditions are generally well-known, the main goal of the chapter is to provide a ready reference to help the clinician to develop an organized approach to dermatologic manifestations in patients with IDD. The clinician should be able to develop a strong knowledge base regarding dermatologic manifestations in these patients so that he/she can not only identify, diagnose and manage them, but also provide anticipatory guidance to caregivers who may well be apprehensive of future developments. Since children and adolescents with IDD are equally, and sometimes even more subject to all the common dermatologic conditions of the population at large, e. g. infection (bacterial, viral, fungal), infestation, allergy, eczema, seborrhea, we conclude with a discussion of management of some common dermatologic conditions that are problematic in these children.

[*] Correspondence: Professor Arthur N Feinberg, MD, Department of Pediatric and Adolescent Medicine, Western Michigan University Homer Stryker MD School of Medicine, 1000 Oakland Drive, D48G, Kalamazoo, MI 49008-1284 United States. E-mail: arthur.feinberg@med.wmich.edu.

Introduction

First, it is important to appreciate the association between intellectual and developmental disability (IDD) and dermatologic manifestations based on embryology. Melanocytes, the pigment producing cells of the body have their origin in the ectodermal neural crest cells. Thus, many disorders of ectodermal development may have associated neurologic findings. The table below outlines dermatologic findings and the neurodevelopmental conditions with which they are associated (1).

The classical description of dermatologic conditions is based on configuration, color, pattern and distribution (2). We limit the list of descriptors to those that are inherent in conditions associated with IDD.

Configuration:

- Macules
  Flat, circumscribed, non-palpable
- Papules, plaques and lichenifications
  Papules are raised lesions ≤ 1cm in diameter.
  Plaques are raised papules > 1 cm in diameter.
  Lichenifications are extensive areas of dried plaques
- Nodules
  Nodules are elevated lesions located deeper than papules and do not attach to the overlying dermis or epidermis.
- Vesicles and bullae
  Vesicles are sharply marginated collections of fluid in the epidermis and are ≤ 1 cm in diameter
  Bullae are large vesicles > 1 mm in diameter
- Scales
  Dried fragmentations of dead skin
- Erosions
  Well-demarcated losses of superficial epidermis usually due to rupture of a vesicle
- Crusts
  Dried exudates that consist of serum, pus, dried blood or scales
- Ulcers
  Depressed lesions with loss of both epidermis and dermis
- Scars and indurations
  These are both hardening of the skin. Scars involve formation of new connective tissue whereas indurations and sclerosis are thickening of skin.
- Excoriations
  Areas of irritation secondary to scratching

Color:

- Red
  Indicates blood flow
- Purple

Indicates blood flow with more venous stasis or extravasation

- Brown or black
  Pigment deposit
- Blue
  Pigment deposit or vascular collection
- Yellow
  Fat or sebum deposit
- White
  Depigmentation or keratin deposits
- Flesh-colored
  Lesion with normal overlying skin

Pattern:

- Linear
- Annular
- Round, oval or irregularly shaped
- Reticular
- Variable

Distribution:

- Dermatomal
- Lines of Blashko
- Sun-exposed areas
- Extremities
- Facial

Dermatologic descriptors associated in persons with intellectual disability

Table 1 correlates dermatologic descriptors with diagnoses involving IDD (3). As hair and nails are also derived from ectoderm, table 2 correlates IDD with these descriptors.

Table 1. Dermatologic descriptors in patients with neurodevelopmental disorder

Descriptor	Neurodevelopmental Condition
Macules	
A. Hyperpigmented	Café-au-lait macules (CALMs): Neurofibromatosis (NF), Tubereous sclerosis (TS), Cowden, Banniyan-Riley-Rubalcava, Noonan, Carney complex, Russell-Silver Pigmented macules: Xeroderma Pigmentosum (XP), Epidermal Nevus syndrome with linear nevi (EN), LEOPARD syndrome, Neurocutaneous melanosis (giant

Table 1. (Continued)

Descriptor	Neurodevelopmental Condition
	nevus) Dyskeratosis congenita (DC), Cockayne, Bloom, Costello, Fanconi
B. Hypopigmented	Partial: Waardenberg, TS, DC, EN General: Albinism, Phenylketonuria (PKU), Menke's, Prader-Willi, Ectrodactyly-Ectodermal Dysplasia-Clefting syndrome (EEC)
C. Cap hemangioma	Beckwith-Weidemann (BW), Roberts, Bloom, I-Cell
Papules and plaques	
A. Vascular	Mucopolysaccharidosis (MPS) Hunter's, TS (angiofibroma), Proteus, Multiple Carboxylase Deficiency, PKU, Darier, Dubowitz
B. Eczematoid	EN
Scales/ichthyosis/hyperkeratosis	Sjogren-Larsson, Conradi-Hunerman, Tyrosinemia II, Trisomy 21, Trichothiodystrophy, XP, Cockayne, KID syndrome, Cardio-Facial-Cutaneous, CHILD, MPS (Hurler) I-Cell, Costello, Pachonychia Congenita, EEC, Clouston
Excoriations	Lesch-Nyhan (LN), Hereditary Autonomic & Sensory Neuropathy (HASN)
Vesicles and bullae	Rothmund-Thompson (RT), XP, DC, Hartnup
Ulcerations	Focal Dermal Hypoplasia (Goltz), Adams-Oliver (AO), Homocystinuira, L N, HASN
Atrophy/aplasia	Goltz, AO, DC, Cockayne, XP, MIDAS
Vascular	
A. Port wine stain	Sturge-Weber, Klippel-Trenaunay
B. Telangiectasia	Ataxia-telangiectasia, Bloom, Goltz, DC, RT, XP
C. Capillary malformation	EN, Rubinstein-Taybi
D. Livedo reticularis	Homocystinuria
E. Cutis marmorata	Cornelia-DeLange, AO, Trisomy 21, Trisomy 18
Photodistribution	XP, RT, Hartnup, Cockayne
Dermatomes and Lines of Blaschko	Incontinenta Pigmenti, Hypomelanosis of Ito, Goltz
Scars	Rubinstein-Taybi, AO, Fetal varicella, LN, HASN
Yellow nodules	Goltz , Niemann-Pick (xanthomas), Proteus

Chromosomal abnormalities

Down syndrome

This is the most common trisomy with an incidence of 1 in 733 live births. Its main characteristics are hypotonia, intellectual disability (mild-moderate), flat facies, brachycephaly, upward-slanted palpebral fissurs, epicanthal folds, flat nasal bridge, protruding tongue, congenital cardiac lesions (endocardial cushion, septal defects, PDA), joint hyperextensibility, single palmar creases, widened gap between first and second toes, increased incidence of gastrointestinal anomalies (duodenal atresia, annular pancreas, T-E fistula Hirschprung disease and imperforate anus). Most common skin manifestations are hyperkeratosis, seborrhea, xerosis and folliculitis (4).

Table 2. Hair and nail descriptors in patients with neurodevelopmental disorders

Descriptors	Neurodevelopmental condition
Hair:	
A. Hair loss	Focal Dermal Hypoplasia (Goltz): sparse, brittle, patchy alopecia Conradi-Hunerman: coarse hair with patchy alopecia Aplasia Cutis Congenita: divots of alopecia on scalp Trisomy 13: divots of alopecia on scalp Dyskeratosis Congenita (DC): alopecia, scalp, eyelashes and eyebrows Rothmund Thompson (RT): alopecia, scalp, eyelashes and eyebrows Menkes: brittle "steel-wool" hair, pili torti, sparse eyebrows and eyelashes Trichothiodystrophy: short, brittle sparse hair on scalp, eyebrows and eyelashes Multiple Carboxylase Deficiency: sparse hair to total alopecia Homocystinuria: sparse hair Cardio-Facial-Cutaneous (sparse curly hair, absent eyebrows and lashes)
B. Hypertrichosis	Clouston: sparse hair, deficiency of eyelashes and eyebrows Cornelia De Lange: low hairline, synophrys, long eyelashes
C. Hirsuitism	Rubinstein-Taybi (RT): heavy arched eyebrows, long eyelashes Hajdu-Cheney (HJ): coarse hair, prominent eyebrows RT, Cornelia De Lange, Mucopolysaccharidoses (Hurler), Trisomy 18
Nails:	
A. Absence, hypoplasia or dystrophy	Chondroectodermal Dysplasia (Ellis-Van Creveld), Goltz, DC, RT, Trichothiodystrophy, Robinow, Ectrodactyly-Ectodermal Dysplasia-Clefting syndrome HJ: short nails, distal clubbing Coffin-Siris: hypoplastic to absent 5th finger and toenails
B. Other	Darier (longitudinal bands, V-shaped nicking , subungual hyperkeratosis) Pachonychia Congenita (thickened nails, pinched margins) Tuberous Sclerosis (peri-ungual fibroma)

Trisomy 13

This trisomy occurs in 1 in 10,000 live births and it features cleft lip and palate, flexed fingers with post-axial polydactyly, ocular hypotelorism (as severe as Cyclops), microcephaly, holoprosencephaly, severe cardiac and gastrointestinal malformations. It carries 91% mortality by age one year. Developmental delay is severe. Skin manifestations are capillary hemangiomas and localized scalp defects (4).

Trisomy 18

This occurs in 1 in 6,000 live births and is characterized by low birthweight, a characteristic positioning of the hand (closed fist with overlapping 2nd and 3rd fingers and 4th and 5th fingers), short sternum, rocker-bottom feet, microcephaly, and prominent occiput, severe cardiac and renal malformations. Mortality rate is 95% in the first year and developmental delay is profound. The main skin manifestations and hair are cutis marmorata and hirsutism (4).

Monogenetic abnormalities

Autosomal dominant

P-Ten inheritance (Cowden, Banniyan-Riley Ruvalcaba)
The P-Ten (Phosphatase and tensin homolog) genes involve cell proliferation, cycle progression and apoptosis and is felt to be a tumor-suppressor gene. Cowden syndrome is associated with macrocephaly, and multiple hamartomas. Its main skin manifestations are trichilemmmas, oral fibromas and punctuate palmar keratoses. There is a high incidence of polyps and cancers including breast, endometrial thyroid, colorectal and kidney. Developmental delay occurs in 12% of patients and there is a higher incidence of autism in this population. Banniyan-Riley-Ruvalcaba syndrome consists of multiple subcutaneous lipomas, gastrointestinal polyps, macrocephaly, macrosomia vascular abnormalities and penile pigmentation in boys. There is not a high an incidence of cancer as in Cowden syndrome (5).

Hereditary hemorrhagic telengiectasia (Weber-Osler-Rendu)
These are multiple arteriovenous malformations (AVM) located in mucosal areas of the lungs, gastrointestinal tract, liver and brain. There are recurrent episodes of epistaxis and gastrointestinal bleeding causing iron deficiency anemia. Intracranial bleeds can cause a wide range of neuro developmental disability (6).

Gorlin syndrome
This condition consists of craniofacial anomalies, mainly macrocephaly and frontal bossing, thoracic anomalies and short metacarpals. Skin manifestations are mainly nevoid basal cell carcinomas mainly over the trunk and face and palmar-plantar pitting. There are ectopic

calcifications. Developmental delay occurs when there are brain malformations such as agenesis of the corpus callosum and hydrocephalus, or intracerebral calcifications (7).

LEOPARD syndrome

LEOPARD is a mnemonic for lentigines, EKG abnormalities (hypertrophic cardiomyopathy, aortic stenosis, pulmonic stenosis, and arrhythmias), ocular hypertelorism, pulmonic stensois, abnormalities of genitalia, retardation of growth and deafness. About 25% have learning disabilities. Lentigines are located mainly on the neck and trunk, but may be present anywhere (1,3).

KID syndrome

KID is a mnemonic for keratitis, congenital icthyosios and neurosensory deafness. It is a rare disorder which also includes alopecia, palmoplantar keratoderma, dystrophic nails and diminished sweating. Educational difficulties stem mainly from loss of vision and hearing (8).

Clouston syndrome

This is a rare condition consisting of hydrotic ectodermal dysplasia, hyperkeratosis of the palms and soles, nail dystrophy and hair defects (fine, sparse and brittle). This may be associated with visual problems, hearing loss and mild mental dullness (3,8).

Cornelia de Lange syndrome

Characteristics of this condition are growth deficiency, intellectual disability in all ranges, autistic behavior, hypertonicity, microbrachycephaly, bushy eyebrows and synophrys. Also there are nasal anomalies (anteverted nostrils, depressed bridge) down-turned thin lips, micromelia and other limb abnormalities. The main dermatologic manifestations are hirsuitism, cutis marmorata and perioral cyanosis (1,3).

Costello syndrome

This includes mild to moderate intellectual disability, several craniofacial abnormalities including macrocephaly, coarse facies, epicanthal folds, downslanting palpebral fissures, low-set ears, depressed nasal bridge, short bulbous nose and full cheeks. Cardiac abnormalities may include various congenital defects, hypertrophic cardiomyopathy and arrhythmias. The major dermatologic problems are skin pigmentation, cutis laxa, abnormalities of the palms and soles (hyperkeratosis, deep creases), thick eyebrows, and sparse hair and teeth anomalies). There is an association with childhood cancers, especially rhabdomyosarcoma (3,9).

Beckwith Wiedemann syndrome

This well-known condition is associated with more severe intellectual disability if cue to chromosomal origin (11p15 region), but any degree of intellectual disability is possible, due to hypoxia (enlarged tongue) or hypoglycemia. The main hallmarks of Beckwith-Weidemann syndrome are macrosomia, macroglossia, organomegaly (particularly enlarged adrenals, pancreas and kidneys). Other hallmarks noted in the neonatal period are polycythemia, hypoglycemia and omphalocoele. Major dermatologic manifestations are capillary hemangiomas, especially on the face (3,10).

Ectrodactly ectodermal dysplasia clefting syndrome (EEC)

Ectrodactyly (lobster claw) has been known to be associated with cleft lip, but appreciation of ectodermal abnormalities came later. These include: fair thin skin with mild hyperkeratosis, light sparse hair and teeth anomalies. Approximately half will have genitourinary abnormalities. Intellectual disability occurs in about 7%, but abnormalities in hearing (14%) can lead to further educational challenges (3).

Adams Oliver syndrome

This condition consists mainly of aplasia cutis congenital and variable degrees of terminal transverse defects of the limbs including very short fingers and toes and their respective nails. In the small number of those with associated neurologic defects such as encephalocoele, arrhinencephaly, and defects of neuronal migration, intellectual disability occurs. The major skin problem is cutis marmorata (3,8).

Autosomal recessive

Dubowitz syndrome

The main hallmark of this condition is very short stature, microcephaly, sloping of forehead, multiple eye abnormalities and malformed ears. Approximately ¾ have intellectual disability in all ranges along with co-morbid ADHD. The main dermatologic manifestations are eczema and sparseness of scalp and lateral eyebrow hair (3).

Cockayne syndrome

This condition involving abnormal DNA repair is often first noted because of its senile-like appearance with profound growth deficiency and microcephaly. From an ectodermal standpoint there are brain malformations and multiple ocular and dental abnormalities. There is autonomic dysfunction including decreased sweating and lacrimation. About half have sensorineural hearing loss. Intellectual disability is common, but usually does not become apparent until the age of two years. Main skin manifestations are photosensitivity dermatitis with dryness and scales (3,11).

Rothmund-Thompson syndrome

This condition has multiple ectodermal manifestations mainly poikiloderma (telangiectasia, progressing to scarring with both hyper and hypo-pigmentation, referred to as "marbled hypoplasia). About 35% of these are due to photosensitivity. Eye abnormalities include mainly cataracts in about half the patients. There are teeth abnormalities in 40% and the hair is generally sparse and prematurely gray. Nails can be dystrophic. Occasional findings are cryptorchidism and predisposition to certain cancers (osteosarcoma) (1,3).

Roberts syndrome

This rare syndrome is most often associated with intrauterine or very early demise. Its main characteristics are severe midline facial defects and hypomelia. The hair is sparse and often silvery-blond in those who survive. Growth and mental deficiency are profound.

Fanconi syndrome

This condition is known mainly because of pancytopenia, radial and thumb anomalies, ptosis and genitourinary abnormalities. However, 64% may manifest brownish pigmentation and 25% have some degree of mental deficiency (3).

Ataxia telangiectasia (Louis-Bar syndrome)

The earliest manifestation of this condition is ataxia, followed by telangiectasia in early to mid childhood. The telengiectasia usually present first on the bulbar conjunctivae and then progress to other areas of the face. The neurologic status progressively deteriorates and mental deficiency becomes more prominent in late childhood and adolescence. These patients are both humoral and cellular immune-deficient and have a predilection for many carcinomas (1,3).

Bloom syndrome

This condition, with a high incidence in the Ashkenazi Jewish population is associated with in-vitro chromosomal breakage. Its earliest manifestations are growth deficiency and relative mild craniofacial abnormalities. After the first year, facial telangiectatic erythema appears due to photosensitivity, but this may improve with age. Cafe-au-lait spots also occur. Although mental deficiency is not common, there is a very high incidence of learning disabilities. There is a strong predilection to various cancers, especially leukemia (3,13).

Xeroderma pigmentosum

This is due to inability of cells to repair DNA damage when exposed to ultraviolet radiation. Its main dermatologic manifestations are sunlight sensitivity, erythema, telengiectasias, freckling and bullae with eventual atrophy and scaling especially around the mouth and lips. There is a high risk of all types of skin cancer. There are ocular manifestations including photophobia and keratitis. There is slowly progressive overall neurologic degeneration including intellectual disability (1,3).

Hereditary autonomic and sensory neuropathy

Although there are five types of hereditary autonomic and sensory neuropathy, the more frequently occurring types are Riley-Day syndrome and congenital indifference to pain (type 4). Type 4 also demonstrates anhydrosis and skin manifestations are primarily due to self-mutilation (12).

Mucopolysaccharidoses (Hurler, I-Cell disease)

Hurler syndrome is due to an absence of the enzyme αL-iduronidase in lysosomes and presents usually during the first year of life, initially with coarsening of facies and skeletal abnormalities such as joint stiffness, rib-flaring and gibbus deformity. As the mucopolysaccharides accumulate in parenchymal tissue, there is progressive hearing loss blockage of the respiratory tree and intimal thickening of blood vessels. Developmental delay is very significant and life expectancy is only through mid childhood. The major skin manifestation is hirsutism. I-cell disease is due to deficient lysosomal enzyme activity in leucocytes and skin fibroblasts, but increased activity in blood, cerebrospinal fluid and urine. They also have coarse facies similar to Hurler syndrome with anteverted nostrils and a long philtrum. Developmental delay is significant, starts slowly and plateaus at about 18 months. Life expectancy is poor with death usually around age 5. Main skin manifestations are tight skin, more during infancy and cavernous hemangioma (3)

Phenylketonuria

This condition, famous for the inception of newborn screening is due to deficiency of the enzyme tyrosine hydroxylase. The main neurodevelopmental problems are seizures, hyperreflexia and delay. Because this enzyme is in the pathway of melanin synthesis, the patients are characteristically blond-haired and blue-eyed and fair skinned. They also have eczematoid rashes frequently (1).

Multiple carboxylase deficiency

Biotin synthesized with the enzyme biotinidase, is an important co-factor for the carboxylase enzymes to function. Thus carboxylases may be deficient primarily, or be deficient because of the absence of biotin. Biotinidase deficiency, from a neurologic standpoint presents with optic atrophy and high tone hearing loss, whereas primary deficiency usually presents with hypotonia, seizures, vomiting and acidosis. The skin manifestations of both conditions are peri-oral facial dermatitis and sparse to absent hair (1).

Hartnup disease

This is a rare disorder of transport of neutral amino acids in the intestine and kidney, particularly tryptophan. Tryptophan is integral in the production of Niacin, thus, dermatologic findings are similar to those of niacin deficiency (pellagra) with photodermatitis and looking like severe eczema. Neurologically, there are bouts of ataxia. Mental deficiency is variable and often absent (1,14).

Tyrosinemia II (Richner-Hanhart)

This is due to an absence of the enzyme tyrosine aminotransferase and is referred to as tyrosinemia type II. There is palmo-plantar keratoderma and hyperkeratosis of elbows and knees. There is intellectual disability and keratitis with photophobia and eventual blindness (1).

Fatty aldehyde dehydrogenase (Sjögren-Larsson)

This presents with severe generalized icthyosis and erythroderma worse in flexural areas and very pruritic. Intellectual disability is both cognitive and linguistic. There are motor disabilities which present similarly to severe cerebral palsy. There are severe eye manifestations with macular degeneration and retinal crystals (1,15).

Sphingomyelinase deficiency (Niemann-Pick)

This lipidosis is due to absence of sphingomyelinase and sphingomyelin deposits everywhere causing mainly hepatosplenomegaly, muscle weakness, lymphadenopathy, progressive neurologic deterioration, blindness, deafness. Skin manifestations include xanthomas and yellow-brown indurations on exposed surfaces (1).

GM1 Gangliosidosis

This is a deficiency of the enzyme β-galactosidase depositing in neural and visceral cells. It presents with hepatosplenomegaly, progressive seizures and progressive psychomotor retardation and blindness (50% have a cherry-red macula) and deafness. The major skin manifestation is angiokeratoma. Death usually occurs by 3-4 years of age (16).

X-Linked dominant

Incontinentia pigmenti

In this condition, skin lesions present in four stages along the developmental lines of Blaschko. The stages are: 1) Vesicular at or near birth, 2) Verrucous from 2-6 weeks, 3) Pigmented from 12-36 weeks and 4) Depigmented from early teens to adulthood. Other ectodermal changes are hair (alopecia of vertex, agenesis of brows and lashes), nails (pitting, ridging, subungual keratotic tumors) and teeth (pegged, coned). From the CNS standpoint there are seizures, intellectual disability, ataxia, spasticity and various brain anomalies (1).

Goltz syndrome

Also called focal dermal hypoplasia, it presents as linear areas of hypoplasia, with telangiectasia, ulceration and protrusion of fatty deposits. The nails are thin, hair is sparse and there is enamel hypoplasia of the teeth. Frequently there are skeletal anomalies (adactyly, syndactyly and lobster claw) and various eye malformations with strabismus. Mental deficiency is usually present in those with associated microcephaly (8).

Conradi-Hunermann syndrome

This condition demonstrates limb shortness, stippled epiphyses, and flat facies with down slanting palpebral fissures. Skin manifestations are erythema and icthyosis in the newborn period resolving in large skin pores resembling orange peel. Hair is coarse, yet sparse with patchy areas of alopecia. Also present can be scoliosis and cataracts. Mental deficiency can be mild to moderate (1,3).

MIDAS syndrome

A hamartosis, MIDAS is the acronym for microophthalmia, dermal aplasia and sclerocornea. Dermal involvement is of the face, neck, scalp and occasionally the upper thorax and it leaves residual hyperpigmented areas. Intellectual disability falls in all ranges, and may be a function of more of the concomitant visual disability.

X-linked recessive

Lesch-Nyhan syndrome

This condition is due to a metabolic block causing an excess of uric acid formation. Its clinical hallmarks are pyramidal and extra-pyramidal movement disorders mental deficiency and self-mutilating behavior causing multiple excoriations and skin ulcers.

Menkes kinky hair disease

This condition, a disorder of copper transport, is characterized by feeding difficulty, failure to thrive, thin hypopigmented sparse yet kinky hair which is described as "steel wool." Eyebrows and eyelashes are also sparse. The skin is hypopigmented and described as "doughy." Neurologic involvement is severe with progressive deterioration, seizures, hypertonia and hypothermia. Death is usually in infancy (1,3).

Mucopolysaccharidosis (Hunter)

Hunter disease mucopolysaccharidosis 2, due to deficiency of iduronate sulfatase presents similarly to Hurler syndrome, but less severely so. It is differentiated by presence of clear corneas, less gibbus deformity lack of presentation in females. Characteristic skin findings are firm white or flesh colored nodular lesions over the scapular area and the posterior axilla.

Combined inheritance

Robinow Syndrome (Autosomal dominant and autosomal recessive)

Also known as the fetal face syndrome, the features are mainly craniofacial, consisting of macrocephaly, frontal bossing, hypertelorism, prominent eyes small up-turned nose, downward angles of the mouth, and others. Limbs are short with small hands and axial skeletal manifestations are hemivertebrae and rib anomalies. The major skin manifestation is nevus flammeus in about ¼ the cases and intellectual disability and seizures are occasional in 18% (3).

Waardenberg Syndrome (Autosomal dominant and autosomal recessive)

The hallmark of this condition is defective migration of neural crest cells leaving areas of depigmentation or hyperpigmentation of the skin and eyes. There are four distinct genetic types of Waardenberg syndrome, three of which are autosomal dominant with variable penetrance. Other common manifestations are sensorineural hearing loss and a white forelock of hair. Although often discovered when noticing a white forelock in an infant, this finding is present in only about half the cases. Any child suspected of having this syndrome should have a thorough audiologic evaluation. Although deafness and mutism are common, intellectual disability independent of this has been reported (1).

Dyskeratosis congenita (Autosomal recessive and X-linked recessive)

This condition has many dermatologic manifestations including Reticulate hyper and hypo-pigmentation with telangiectasia and atrophy, palmoplantar keratoderma, friction bullae and hyperhydrosis. Hair is thinned on the scalp, lashes and brows and nails may be dystrophic, atrophic or absent. There are numerous eye problems including blepharitis, conjunctivitis, lacrimal duct obstruction and ectropion. Mental deficiency is mild to moderate. This may also be associated with a Fanconi-like pancytopenia (1).

Unknown inheritance

Sturge-Weber

This well-known hamartosis presents as a port wine stain in the trigeminal nerve distribution, noted at birth. It is unilateral with a sharp cut-off at the midline. Only patients with a distribution in the ophthalmic branch of the trigeminal nerve are subject to neuro-ocular complications. This is associated with other secondary ophthalmic problems especially glaucoma. There are associated capillary malformations particularly of the pia and arachnoid mater, but not necessarily in the trigeminal distribution often occurring in the parieto-occipital areas. Eventually, these malformations will calcify, but often not until after the first year of life. The infants may be asymptomatic at birth, but most will eventually develop seizures. Intellectual disability seems to correlate with the earliness of seizure onset. Klippel Trenaunay Weber syndrome also features port wine stains, but involvement is more of the extremities with concurrent hypertrophy due to proliferative angiogenesis. This condition is not generally associated with mental deficiency (3,17).

Hypomelanosis of Ito

These are swirled hypopigmented patches that follow the lines of Blaschko. They also may be plaque-like. There is variable internal involvement, but when present in the CNS will cause profound developmental delays. Hair and teeth are involved and present with alopecia or hypertrichosis and dental hypoplasia. There may also be associated eye and facial abnormalities (1,3).

Neurocutaneous melanosis

This melanocytic hamartosis presents as the well-known "bathing trunk" nevi, very large and subject to malignant degeneration. There are often associated smaller nevi, and when present, carries a greater association with neurocutaneous melanosis. Serious neurological complications occur when there is an association with leptomeningeal melanoma. These can cause seizures and cranial nerve palsies in and of themselves, or due to secondary hydrocephalus due to blockage of CSF flow by the tumor. When a melanoma occurs, the prognosis is extremely poor.

Epidermal nevus syndrome

This falls under the rubric of "Nevus sebaceous of Jadassohn." Typically, a single linear oblong waxy verrucous lesion in the parietal area presents in the newborn period and is isolated. The only concern in this situation is to observe for potential malignant degeneration (basal cell epithelioma) in about 15-20%. However, if the sebaceous nevi are midline or diffuse there is a very high incidence of seizures and mental deficiency (3,18).

Proteus syndrome

A hamartosis, it is named after the Greek God Proteus, known for changing shapes. Infants may be normal at birth, but soon develop abnormal irregular growth with generalized thickening of the skin which develops epidermal nevi, lipomas and vascular malformations, more on the thorax and upper abdomen. There are skeletal abnormalities including hemi hypertrophy and hyperostosis. Moderate mental deficiency occurs in about 20% of cases (3).

Rubinstein-Taybi syndrome

This syndrome has a large constellation of symptoms, the most frequent of which are growth deficiency, hypoplastic maxilla with narrow palate, downward slanted palpebral fissures, prominent beaked nose with short columella, broad thumbs and great toes, sometimes with other finger involvement and cryptorchidism. Skin manifestations include capillary hemangioma and keloid malformation. Hair abnormalities include hirsutism, heavy arched eyebrows and long eyelashes. Mental deficiency is significant with moderate to severe delay (3).

Russell-Silver syndrome

The hallmark of this condition is intrauterine growth restriction. Immature skeletal developmental progression including delayed closure of the fontanelles and limb asymmetry soon become evident in early infancy. The facies are typically triangular with frontal prominence and there is micrognathia with a down-turned mouth. Although mental deficiency may not be present, about 25% have learning disability. The major cutaneous manifestation is café-au-lait spots (3).

Cardio facial cutaneous syndrome

This relatively rare condition consists of cardiac problems, principally atrial septal defect and pulmonic stenosis. Craniofaical manifestations are macocephaly, frontal bossing, bi-temporal narrowing, hypertelorism, prominent philtrum and others. Skin manifestations are severe atopic dermatitis progressing to an icthyosis pattern. Hair abnormalities are sparse slow-growing curly hair and lack of eyebrows and eyelashes. Mental deficiency is highly prevalent along with hypotonia, nystagmus and strabismus. Developmental anomalies of the brain are seen with imaging studies (3).

Coffin-Siris syndrome

This condition is associated with intrauterine growth restriction. There are many craniofacial manifestations including microcephaly, coarse facies, wide mouth with full lips, flat nasal bridge and long philtrum. Limbs demonstrate hypoplastic fingers and toes, especially the fifth digits. Joints are lax with frequent dislocations. Hair manifestations include generalized hirsutism, but sparse scalp hair. There is delayed dentition. General performance is in the mild-moderate mental deficiency range and there are frequent vision and hearing problems.

Common dermatologic conditions in individuals with IDD and their management

Children and adolescents with IDD are particularly prone to common dermatologic conditions such as infections, infestations, dermatitis and trauma. We present a brief discussion of their management. Because of difficulties in maintaining skin hygiene in children with developmental disability they are more prone to infection than the normal population. Common bacterial infections include folliculitis, impetigo, furunculosis and carbuncles. Fungal infections include Tinea (corporis, captits, cruris) and may involve the nails as well (onychomycosis).

Bacterial

Folliculitis

This is a simple infection of the hair follicle and is usually bacterial, Staphylococcus aureus, although may also be fungal (Majocchi's granuloma), viral or inflammatory in cases of immunodeficiency. They occur most frequently in hair-bearing areas that are also exposed to increased friction and sweating. Lesions are typically pustular, but may be papular or nodular if located more deeply. Treatment is preferably topical antistaphylococcal medication (Mupirocin, Erythromycin, Clindamycin), but oral antibiotics such as first-generation cephalosporins or trimethoprim-sulfamethoxazole (for MRSA) may be necessary for deeper infections. Folliculitis may also be due to gram negative organisms such as Pseudomonas, or

Klebsiella, especially if the patient with IDD is exposed to water from hydrotherapy. Treatment of "hot-tub folliculitis" is primarily symptomatic with acetic acid applications (1,19).

Furunculosis

This is a skin infection that has gone deeper beyond the follicular unit that contains pus. It may be firm or fluctuant and is almost always painful. Causative organisms are similar to those in folliculitis and treatment is principally by incision and drainage, if the lesion is >5 mm in diameter (1,19).

Fungal

Tinea corporis (commonly ringworm) presents as a circular lesion initially which then undergoes central clearing. There are scales present, which are denser on the lateral aspect of the lesion. The diagnosis is usually clinical, but may be confirmed by viewing hyphae on a KOH preparation, or if necessary, a fungal culture. Lesions caused by genus Microsporum may fluoresce under a Woods lamp. However, most lesions are due to genus Trycophyton which will not fluoresce. Treatment is with local antifungal agents such as Miconazole or Ketoconazole (1,19).

Tinea capitis is an infection involving the scalp and may present as a discrete lesion or sometimes more diffusely with scalp flaking. Discrete lesions may be non-inflamed, have initially a scaly appearance followed by hair loss and diffuse "black dots" (residual stubble) throughout. Some lesions do become secondarily inflamed with a boggy feeling to them (kerion). Treatment of Tinea capitis is always with oral medications, usually Griseofulvin, a dose of 20 mg/kg/day in one dose for a 30 day period. There may be hepatoxicity associated with this, but it is rare and dose-related so routine liver function tests are no longer recommended unless treatment has to be extended for >30 days. Other oral antifungals that may be used include Terbenafine and Itraconazole. Kerions should be treated with oral corticosteroids (1,19).

Tinea cruris may occur more frequently in those with IDD because of difficulty in keeping the area clean due to obesity, need for diapers, and inherent problems with cooperation on the part of the patient. The diagnosis may be confused with intertrigo due to Corynebacterium, seborrhea, or to a candidal infection which is more pinkish with satellite lesions. Treatment is with topical antifungals mentioned above (1,19).

Onychomycoses are more common in patients with IDD, particularly in Down syndrome. Frequent touching objects and placing of fingers in the mouth may predispose to this condition. The lesions are described by location (base of nail, lateral aspect). Depending on the depth of the lesion splitting of the nail (onycholysis) may occur with subsequent thickening. Treatment is with oral antifungals (Griseofulvin, Terbenafine, Itraconazole, Fluconazole) (1,19).

Infestations

Because patients with IDD are more likely to live group home settings, and more prone to sharing items, mainly out of naïveté to privacy issues, they can be more likely to acquire head lice or scabies. It is important to keep in mind adolescents with IDD, just like their normal counterparts are sexual beings and are subject to Pediculosis pubis as well.

Head lice (*Pediculosis capitis*)

Diagnosis is made by direct visualization of a louse. If nits are discovered they should be <1/4inch from the scalp and even with this, a diagnosis is only reliable 1/3 of the time. Treatment is with Permethrin 1% left for 10 minutes in the hair and then rinsed out. A second treatment in 10 days is recommended. Avoid the use of Lindane if there are any excoriations on the skin (1,19).

Scabies

This may be seen more frequently in those with IDD due to sharing of beds in institutional settings. The classical presentation is diffuse burrowing lesions with concentration on the web areas of the fingers and toes as well as in the groin region. It is highly pruritic and causes significant excoriations, especially in IDD patients who may have less impulse control. Treatment is with 5% Permethrin cream over affected areas, washed off after 8-12 hours. Other medications include Malathion and Ivermectin (1,19).

Dermatitis

Dry skin is prevalent in children with IDD, particularly Down syndrome, along with consequent eczematous dermatitis. Seborrhea is also common in Down syndrome.

Dry skin

This common condition is prevalent in the entire population. It may predispose to subsequent eczema and may excoriate due to frequent scratching. Skin moisteners are effective if used preemptively. Ointments are more effective than creams, which are more effective than lotions. Ammonium Lactate may also be used in more difficult cases (1,19).

Eczematous dermatitis

Eczema may be due to scratching of dry skin, or may be atopic in nature. Treatment can be difficult in patients with IDD because of increased scratching. The four mainstays of treatment involve management of skin dryness (emollients, occlusive dressings), itching (antihistamines), inflammation (topical steroids) and secondary complications such as infection. Successful treatment requires significant teamwork involving physician, patient and caregiver.

Seborrhea

Although called "cradle cap" in infants, the distribution of the yellowish greasy-appearing lesions is typically over the scalp, eyebrows, post-auricular area, skin creases (axilla, groin, crural area) nasolabial folds and umbilicus. IDD patients who may tend to be obese will have more difficulty with this condition in the skin fold areas. Treatment consists of a mild potency corticosteroid applied locally or selenium sulfide lotion or shampoo applied twice weekly (1,19).

Trauma

Traumatic skin conditions are prevalent in those with IDD and occur as a consequence of immobility (decubitus ulcers) obesity associated with Down or Prader-Willi syndrome (lesions due to rubbing, intertrigo) and self inflicted skin lesions.

Decubiti

Pressure ulcers are common in IDD patients, particularly those with physical disability and immobility. The four basic causes are pressure, shearing forces, friction and moisture. Present thinking indicates that shearing forces, friction and moisture act superficially, but pressure from lying on bony prominences causes deeper lesions which emerge to the surface. The mainstay of management is prevention: pressure relief with frequent turning, appropriate surfaces with the ability to change shape or location to relieve pressure in vulnerable areas, management of incontinence, maintenance of appropriate skin moisture and nutritional support. Treatment if necessary includes dressings, debridement and surgery (20-22).

Intertrigo

This simply means erythema located in opposing skin surfaces. This is prevalent in those with IDD especially if associated with obesity in conditions such as the Down or Prader-Willi syndrome. The lesions may be only secondary to rubbing, but due to moisture accumulation may also contain bacteria or fungal elements

Inflicted lesions

Dermatologic manifestations or repetitive trauma are common in patients with IDD for several reasons. Some conditions are inherently associated with developmental delay and self-mutilation such as congenital indifference to pain and the Lesch-Nyhan and Smith-Magenis syndromes. Often because of lack of impulse control, more severe excoriations can occur over a pruritic medical condition such as eczema. Individuals may have repetitive behavior causing dermatologic findings in a given area due to persistent banging or scratching. Sadly, because of the increased incidence of abuse in this group, suspicion for this should be raised if the lesions are too symmetrical, too streaky, have very sharp borders, perfectly round, are loop-shaped or are located over facial areas such as the nose, lips and ears.

Medication-related dermatologic conditions

Patients with IDD are likely to be taking multiple medications and may suffer dermatologic consequences of that. Common medications include corticosteroids, anticonvulsants and psychotropic drugs. Specifically, oral corticosteroids as associated with acne. In addition, sometimes they could be masking some other inflammatory condition that may have dermatologic manifestations, and that condition will appear during a taper. Drug eruptions from just about any medication are most frequently of the morbiliform nature (about 50%). About 25% of drug eruptions are IgE-mediated (urticarial) and are more likely to be associated with antibiotic administration, particular intravenous or intramuscular. Fixed drug eruptions are erythematous, variable in size and recover slowly over several months. Rarer typs of drug eruptions include vasculitis, erythema nodosum, photosensitivity and lichenoid eruptions. It is important for the clinician to be mindful of bullous eruptions (Stevens-Johnson, Toxic Epidermal Necrolysis) and to be prepared to discontinue the drug (often an anticonvulsant) quickly and administer supportive intensive care (1,19).

Miscellaneous common conditions

Individuals with IDD are also subject to warts and acne.

Warts (HPV)

The causative agent for warts is human papilloma virus (HPV). Most cases of common warts, verruca vulgaris result from direct contact or auto-inoculation, prevalent more in groups of individuals with IDD. Moreover, it is often forgotten that those with IDD are sexual beings and are subject to venereal warts. Sadly, as in physical abuse, sexual abuse must always be considered in this group of patients who may have venereal warts. It is known that Types 6 and 11 predispose to cervical cancer. Ideally HPV vaccine should be administered as soon as possible starting at age 9 years, 3 doses, one month apart.

There are many treatments for common warts which have demonstrated varying degrees of effectiveness. Most are self-limiting and no treatment is an acceptable alternative if the patient wishes this. Various treatments used have been salicylic acid, cryotherapy, bichloroacetic acid applications and duct tape. Genital warts are often treated with Podophyllin applications; immune modulators such as Imiquamod have been effective (1,19).

Acne

Acne is very common among adolescents in general and is particularly significant in those with IDD because of their tendency toward earlier sexual maturation. Also, acne requires scrupulous and consistent management, which can be challenging in this group.

In brief the pathogenesis of acne consists of four basic elements, plugging of the pilosebaceous unit with abnormal keratinization, androgen-induced sebum production causing further blockage, bacterial infection (Propionibacterium acnes) and subsequent inflammation. Comedones may be (white head) or open (black head). Most lesions are popular or pustular, but some develop into nodules and cysts which are more disfiguring. Treatment is usually of a "step-up" nature, often pictured as a ladder. First, 10% Benzoyl Peroxide is given, which is often effective. If not, topical retinoids are an option, such as Retin-A or Adapaline. Azalaic acid is also a good anti bacterial and anti inflammatory. Following this, antibiotics may be administered in conjunction with the present regimen, either locally (Tetracycline, Minocycline) or systemically. Oral contraceptives have demonstrated effectiveness in females through androgen reduction. As a last measure, Isotretinoin may be given orally, but because of severe side effects including abnormal liver function, lipid profiles, pseudotumor cerebri and teratogenic potential, these medications must be used with a dermatology consultation (1,19).

Some iillustrative cases

You are called to the newborn nursery to consult on B, a 16 hour-old infant female who is noted to have "blisters all over. "Past obstetrical history reveals the mother has lost two pregnancies during the first trimester, but this one has gone well to term. She states she has a cousin who has "skin problems" and thought she was "slower", but has no knowledge of further detail. There is no history of herpes infection in the mother, either oral or genital. On exam the baby appears alert, active and generally quite well. There are diffuse blisters all over and they appear to be in a whorl-like pattern. The overall distribution pattern vaguely reminds you of the pictures of dermatomes that you learned in Neuroanatomy during the first year of medical school. With further research you conclude this is a case of incontinentia pigmenti following Blaschko's lines. On the next office visit to your office Mr. and Mrs. L have already consulted the internet and have several questions about the outcomes of their baby regarding neurodevelopment and the skin lesions.

Mrs. F. has been bringing her 4 year old son Jeremy to your office for his entire life. He was diagnosed immediately at birth with Down syndrome. Features at birth arousing suspicion for this diagnosis included hypotonia, low-set ears, flattened occiput, single palmar creases and widened spaces between this 1st and 2nd toes. Although the remainder of his neonatal examination was unremarkable routine echocardiogram indicated an endocardial cushion defect. He underwent successful corrective surgery at two months of age and has been doing well since then. He attends the local pre-school program for children with developmental delay and has been progressing nicely. He now appears to be developmentally at age 2 ½ with appropriate physical, occupational and speech therapy. Of late, Mrs. F has been concerned about his skin. Although she cannot describe it well, it seems to her that it appears a lot "rougher" than that of his peers and seems to have more peeling and flaking. She is wondering if she is not caring for Jeremy's skin properly.

You are seeing David, a 6 month old at his well-child exam. His parents have expressed a concern that he has been having episodes of "too much startling, even more so than he did as a newborn." Further developmental history reveals attainment of normal landmarks for this age. You are contemplating either ordering magnetic resonance imaging of his brain or consulting a neurologist, but since he had no observable abnormal movements during this visit you are leaning more toward reassurance of the parents. However, on examination of the skin you observe a patch of loss of skin pigment, albeit subtle which is slightly ovoid in shape. You now order an MRI scan which reveals a few waxy-looking subependymal nodules. You are now reasonably certain of the diagnosis of tubrerous sclerosis and have prepared for the next meeting with the family to discuss what the future holds. When you meet them, they ask first about skin changes in the future, since this was the area in which the case first manifested inself.

Conclusion

We hope to have instilled in the clinician the ability to recognize that many conditions involving people with IDD have dermatologic manifestations, either in and of themselves, or as secondary occurrences. We have outlined a scheme for identifying these conditions and manifestations and have distilled the information to make it accessible for the clinician to use for diagnosis, management and anticipatory guidance.

References

[1] Pollack BP, Hadley JC and Arbiser, JL. Dermatology. In: Rubin IL, Crocker AC, eds. Medical care for children and adults with developmental disabilities, second edition. Baltimore, MD: Paul H Brookes, 2006:399-418.

[2] Feinberg AN. The integument system: Skin, hair, nails. In: Greydanus DE, Feinberg AN, Patel DR, Homnick DN, eds. The pediatric diagnostic examination. New York: McGraw-Hill, 2008:541-98.

[3] Jones KL, ed. Smith's recognizable patterns of human malformation. Philadelphia PA: Elsevier-Saunders, 2006.

[4] Summar K, Lee B. Cytogenetics. In: Kliegman RM, Stanton BF, Schor NF, St Geme III JW, Behrman RE, eds. Nelson's Textbook of Pediatrics 19th edition. Philadelphia PA: Elsevier-Saunders, 2011:399-404.

[5] Marsh DJ, Kum JB, Lunetta KL, Bennett MJ, Gorlin RJ, Ahmed SF, et al. PTEN mutation spectrum and genotype-phenotype correlations in Bannayan-Riley-Ruvalcaba syndrome suggest a single entity with Cowden syndrome. Hum Mol Genet 1999;8:1461-72.

[6] Shovlin CL. Hereditary haemorrhagic telangiectasia: pathophysiology, diagnosis and treatment. Blood Rev 2010;24(6):203-19.

[7] Shanley S, Ratcliffe J, Hockey A, Haan E, Oley C, Ravine D, et al. Nevoid basal cell carcinoma syndrome: review of 118 affected individuals. Am J Med Genet 1994; 50(3):282-90.

[8] Paller AS, Mancini AJ, eds. Hurwitz clinical pediatric dermatology. Philadelphia, PA: Elsevier-Saunders, 2006:101-102
[9] Quezada E, Gripp KW. Costello syndrome and related disorders. Curr Opin Pediatr 2007;19(6):636-44.
[10] Kent L, Bowdin S, Kirby GA, Cooper WN, Maher ER. Beckwith Weidemann syndrome: a behavioral phenotype-genotype study. Am J Med Genet B Neuropsychiatr Genet 2008;147B(7):1295-7.
[11] Pasquier L, Laugel V, Lazaro L, Dollfus H, Journel H, Edery P, et al. Wide clinical variability among 13 new Cockayne syndrome cases confirmed by biochemical assays. Arch Dis Child 2006;91(2):178-82.
[12] Rosemberg S, Marie SK, Kliemann S. Congenital insensitivity to pain with anhidrosis (hereditary sensory and autonomic neuropathy type IV). Pediatr Neurol 1994;11(1):50-6.
[13] Bloom Syndrome Registry.URL: http://weill.cornell.edu/bsr/
[14] Rezvani I. Tryptophan, Hartnup Disorder, In: Kliegman RM, Stanton BF, Schor NF, St Geme III JW, Behrman RE, eds. Nelson's Textbook of Pediatrics 19th edition. Philadelphia PA: Elsevier-Saunders, 2011:429-30.
[15] Willemsen MA, IJlst L, Steijlen PM, Rotteveel JJ, de Jong JG, van Domburg PH, et al. Clinical, biochemical and molecular genetic characteristics of 19 patients with the Sjögren-Larsson syndrome. Brain 2001;124(Pt 7):1426-37.
[16] McGovern MM, Desnick RJ. Lipidoses (lysosomal storage disorders). In: Kliegman RM, Stanton BF, Schor NF, St Geme III JW, Behrman RE, eds. Nelson's Textbook of Pediatrics 19th edition. Philadelphia PA: Elsevier-Saunders, 2011:482-4.
[17] Tian XL, Kadaba R, You SA, Liu M, Timur AA, Yang L, et al. Identification of an angiogenic factor that when mutated causes susceptibility to Klippel-Trenaunay syndrome. Nature 2004; 427(6975):640-5.
[18] Solomon LM, Esterly NB. Epidermal and other congenital organoid nevi. Curr Probl Pediatr 1975;6(1):1-56.
[19] Feinberg AN, Shwayder TA, Tareen R, Tempark T. Adolescence and dermatology. Int J Child Health Hum Dev 2012;5(4):391-436.
[20] Reuler JB, Cooney TB. The pressure sore. Pathophysiology and principles of management. Ann Intern Med 1981; 94(5):661-6
[21] Berlowitz D. Prevention of pressure ulcers. URL: www.uptodate.com
[22] Berlowitz D. Treatment of pressure ulcers. URL: www.uptodate.com

In: Pediatric and Adolescent Dermatology
Editors: D Greydanus, A Feinberg and J Merrick
ISBN: 978-1-63321-853-6

Chapter 9

Dermatology: Quality of life issues

Mohammad KA Basra*
Department of Dermatology and Wound Healing,
Cardiff University School of Medicine, Cardiff, United Kingdom

Skin conditions are very common in children with almost one child in every four having some kind of skin-related problem. Even though the majority of skin conditions are not life threatening, they can have a major impact on the child. This impact may be physical caused by distressing symptoms, psychosocial due to the disfiguring nature of some skin conditions as well as financial due to direct and indirect costs associated with them. Due to differences in biological and cognitive development, children and adolescents may have some differences in the way their quality of life is affected by skin diseases. This requires age-specific measurement tools for quality of life assessment in children and adolescents. The impact of skin disease has been shown to extend beyond the patients to their immediate caregivers such as parents and family members whose own quality of life may be affected due to patient's skin condition. The family impact could be influenced by different factors such as the nature of child's skin condition and its severity. For optimal management of children's skin condition it is important to gauge the impact on parents and family care givers and provide them with appropriate educational, psychological, and social support to enable them to better cope with their children's skin disease and which has been found to result in better medical and social outcomes. Childhood skin conditions such as eczema impose a substantial financial burden on the society that could arise from direct treatment costs to the health care system and indirect costs such as days lost from work by parents. Unfortunately, most of the research to date on the impact of childhood skin diseases on children and families and in particular their financial implications, has been focused on atopic eczema and there is a need to study the impact of other skin diseases to have a broader idea of the overall burden of childhood skin diseases.

* Corresponding author: Mohammad KA Basra, MBBS, DDSc, MD, Department of Dermatology and Wound Healing, Cardiff University School of Medicine, Heath Park, Cardiff, CF14 4NQ, United Kingdom. E-mail: drkhurshid69@hotmail.com.

Introduction

Changing epidemiology of paediatric diseases, from acute to chronic and from incurable to palliative or curable, has resulted in a growing interest in assessing children's quality of life (QOL). Nowadays, evaluation of QOL is considered a central element of paediatric practice and important for all children i.e., the healthy and the ill (1). In order to understand the QOL issues in children with particular reference to dermatology and the issues surrounding the assessment of QOL in paediatric populations, it important to first understand the concept of QOL. The life time of an individual consists of two fundamental components- quantity of life and quality of life (2). The "Quantity of life" is the number of years from the time of birth to the time of death; the "Quality of life" is the quality of each point in the time between the time of birth and the time of death. Quality of life is an amorphous term and has different meanings for every individual and culture and differs by context, place and time (i.e., it may vary within an individual at different points in time). A number of different concepts have been associated with this term including health-related quality of life, health status, and functional status. Although related and many times used interchangeably, these terms have separate definitions. According to one of the most frequently used definitions, "Quality of life is an individual's perception of their position in life in the context of the cultural and value systems in which they live and in relation to their goals, expectations, and standards and concerns" (3).

In the context of pediatrics, this term refers to: "a child's perception and evaluation of performance in relevant life areas and its feelings related to problems in functioning" (4). It has also been described as: "A measure of how a child views his/her life in relationship to how they could reasonably expect or desire it to be" (5). Health-related quality of life (HRQOL) could be considered a component of overall QOL that is determined by the individual's health and which can be influenced by clinical interventions (6,7). Health status, a related term, indicates a child's level of wellness versus illness (8) and includes the presence of biological dysfunction with or without the level of illness control (9). Finally, functional status could be defined as "a child's ability to perform daily activities that are essential to meet his/her basic needs, fulfil roles and maintain health and well-being" (9).

Since QOL is a purely subjective concept, as expressed by the patient, it is in contrast to other traditional clinical, biological, and radiological measures evaluated by the observers objectively and it depends on the individual needs as perceived by the patients themselves and not the treating physicians (10). Moreover, being subjective in nature, it can be influenced by a number of factors such as the severity of disease, patient's gender, age, ethnic background, social class, personality type, level of anxiety, education, lifestyle, past experiences as well as family functioning (11-13). Irrespective of contextual differences in their meanings, the terms QOL and HRQOL have frequently been used synonymously in the medical literature and for the sake of simplicity and because of it wider application, the umbrella term QOL will be used in this chapter to denote HRQOL.

Paediatric quality of life and its assessment

Children constitute a large proportion of health care consumers and paediatrics represents a major medical speciality. Assessment of QOL in children is as important as in adults. However, compared to adults, the assessment of QOL in young children is believed to be associated with unique problems and challenges (14). Factors such as age and cognitive and emotional development may compromise children's ability to understand their disease or health in general and the questions asked in a QOL questionnaire in specific. Therefore, there is a concern that children may misinterpret the questions. They may also have time perception problems as well as difficulty in using rating scales and lengthy questionnaires. This conception led to some researchers using proxy data provided by parents to measure children's QOL as their own responses were often considered unreliable or inaccurate (15).

However, the evidence suggests that young children can provide reliable and consistent reports on their QOL using structured questionnaires (16). Moreover, significant areas of discordance exist between children and parents about children's health status, the impact of illness, and QOL (17,18). Based on these observations, it seems important to involve children in management decisions related to their care and equally importantly to rate their own QOL, except in situations where they are either incapacitated or too young to complete the questionnaire themselves. Under these circumstances parents or caregivers may provide valuable information based on their judgment of child's health status and QOL (19). In general, there is better correlation between parental proxy data and child's own response for physical parameters compared with psychological ones (15).

Skin disease and quality of life

Skin diseases, although not generally life-threatening, frequently have a major impact on patient's psychological and social life as well as everyday activities, which makes QOL and its measurement particularly important in dermatology (20). Herd et al. hold the view that QOL seems to be more relevant to dermatology than other diseases due to the reasons that many skin disease patients have chronic and incurable diseases and the impact of skin disorders on QoL is subjective as well as related to individual circumstances (21). This view is further strengthened by the fact that many skin diseases are more obvious visibly than many chronic systemic diseases. They have the potential to cause direct impact on children's psyche resulting from having negative childhood experiences such as being bullied at school due to their skin appearance. It is, therefore, not surprising to find that some skin diseases in children can have a greater impact on overall QOL than other chronic systemic conditions. For example, using a generic QOL measure, children with generalised eczema were found to have greater QOL impairment than children with cystic fibrosis, asthma, diabetes, epilepsy, and renal disease (22).

Impact of skin diseases on children's quality of life

Childhood is a stage of life characterised by rapid psychosocial development and emotional vulnerability. Any negative experience during this stage may have an impact on an individual's development and QOL impairment in adulthood. Chronic and disfiguring skin conditions in childhood (i.e., eczema, psoriasis, vitiligo, and acne) have the potential to induce negative experiences and problems in social development (23). Although, there does not seem to be a great deal of difference in children's QOL based on their gender, younger children seem to have greater impairment of QOL (24).

Most of the research on QOL impact of skin diseases in children has been focused on atopic eczema possibly due to its high prevalence among children, its chronic and distressing nature, and its economic implications for the family as well as the health care system. Atopic eczema is one of the most common skin conditions affecting young children and has substantial impact on their QOL and the QOL of their parents. The impact on children could be both physiological and psychological. Physical symptoms and psychological problems have been shown to be common issues for children and infants; the physical symptoms include itching and scratching while the psychological issues include mood changes, feeling sad or upset, embarrassed, and self-conscious, as well sleep disturbance (24,25).

Having eczema can result in lack of self-confidence that could be related to poor self-image and which can ultimately compromise the social development of children (26). In one study, the rate of psychological disturbance was found to be more in children with atopic eczema compared with the control group and there was a linear relationship with the severity of eczema and the resulting psychological disturbance (27). Moreover, compared with controls, pre-school children with eczema were found to show greater dependency on their parents as well as greater fearfulness (28). An important aspect of childhood is playing games and sports. However, having eczema can adversely impact on their leisure activities such as playing and swimming which may be either due to the disease exacerbation or related to its psychosocial consequences such as peer rejection and embarrassment (29).

Pruritus is the predominant physical symptom of eczema and has been shown to result in increased crying, fussiness, and irritability in these children (30). Sleep disturbance is a major issue for children with atopic eczema which is associated with itching and scratching (27). The abnormalities in sleep pattern not only lead to daytime discipline and behaviour problems and impaired performance at school in children but also result in sleep deprivation and exhaustion in parents as will be discussed later in this chapter (31,32).

Psoriasis is another disfiguring skin condition that can have a devastating impact on the QOL of children and their parents. Physical symptoms of itching and scratching, problems with treatment, and the feeling of embarrassment as well as self-consciousness were found to be the three worst aspects in children suffering from psoriasis (33). The same study showed that the QOL impairment was even greater when psoriasis was accompanied by joint problems.

Another study about the impact of juvenile psoriasis also has shown negative effects of the disease on children's physical, social, and emotional functioning with the majority of children reporting feelings of stigmatisation and being bullied (34). Interestingly, in a comparative study from children's perspectives, among various skin diseases, psoriasis followed by atopic eczema caused the greatest QOL impairment while from parents' perspective, the highest score was for atopic eczema followed by urticaria and psoriasis (22).

Quality of life assessment in children with dermatological conditions

Quality of life in children can be assessed using generic and disease-specific measures. Generic measures are applicable to any population subgroup with any condition and are thus, useful for comparing the QOL impact among different conditions. On the other hand, disease-specific measures are applicable to individuals suffering from a particular disease. These measures are useful for detecting change in the condition over time and are more sensitive to change than generic measures. In between these two types of QOL measures there is a third category that could be labelled as speciality-specific measures e.g., dermatology-specific measures.

These measures, although less sensitive to change than condition-specific measure, are useful in comparing the QOL impact of different conditions within that speciality e.g., dermatology. A number of QOL instruments exist to assess the QOL of adults with skin diseases. However, these instruments may not be appropriate for use in children because of the fundamental differences between the conceptualization of children's and adults' QOL. For example, items such as impact of a condition on employment, income and sexuality will not be applicable to children (19). Therefore, in order to be applied successfully, QOL questionnaires should be developed that have domains specific to different age groups with emphasis on the cognitive, psychological, functional, social, and behavioural characteristics of that age group.

In dermatology, children's quality of life has mostly been assessed using a dermatology-specific QOL measure called the Children's Dermatology Life Quality Index (29); also, for infants suffering from atopic eczema, the Infant's Dermatitis Quality of Life Index has been utilized (25). These two commonly used measures are briefly described below. Adolescents have traditionally been categorized with children and their QOL, at least in dermatology, has been assessed either by using the CDLQI (for patients younger than 16 years of age) or the Dermatology Life Quality Index (DLQI, for patients 16 years of age and older) (35). However, as it will be discussed later, there are some differences between children and adolescents that warrant separate QOL assessments. It has only been recently that this important difference is acknowledged and two dermatology-specific measures have been developed specifically for adolescents between the ages of 12 and 19 years and these will be described later in this chapter.

Children's Dermatology Life Quality Index (CDLQI)

Lewis-Jones and Finlay developed this simple instrument for use in daily clinical practice and clinical trials to assess the impact of skin diseases on the quality of life of school-age (4-16 years) children (29). The CDLQI is usually self-completed, however, and children who are unable to complete themselves may require help from their parents or it can even be administered as a proxy measure (36). Being a dermatology-specific measure, the CDLQI has the potential to measure the QOL impact of different skin diseases relative to each other and can therefore be used to compare their impact.

The CDLQI has 10 items covering aspects such as symptoms and feelings, school, holidays, leisure, personal relationships, treatment, and sleep. The total scale score ranges from 0-30; a higher score indicates greater QOL impairment. The scores can also be expressed as the percentage of the maximum score. In the original study, the CDLQI scores were highest in scabies patients (mean CDLQI score=9.5) followed by eczema (mean score=7.7) and lowest in patients with nevi (mean score=2.3). The highest scoring individual question was about symptoms and feelings while the lowest scoring was about friendship.

Test-retest reliability was acceptable and the validity was confirmed by the instrument's ability to differentiate QOL impact between patients and normal controls as well as between inflammatory and non-inflammatory skin diseases. The measure has also shown sensitivity to change following inpatient treatment for atopic eczema and psoriasis and outpatient treatment of acne (37) and following change in clinical severity of the children's eczema (38). The CDLQI has shown strong correlation with both generic QoL measures for children such as the Children's Life Quality Index (CLQI) (22) as well as with disease-specific QoL measures such as Cardiff Acne Disability Index (39).

Recently a set of bands has been proposed to facilitate the clinical interpretation of the CDLQI scores (40). According to this banding system a CDLQI score of 0-1=no effect on child's life; 2-6=small effect; 7-12=moderate effect; 13-18=very large effect; and 19-30=extremely large effect on child's life. A cartoon version of the CDLQI was developed in 2003, which was found to be more easily and more quickly completed (90 seconds vs. 120 seconds for text version); thus it was favoured by children as well as by their parents (41). This version of the CDLQI has been used in a number of studies including study of QoL of children with erythropoietic protoporphyria (42).

Infant's Dermatitis Quality of Life index (IDQOL)

This is a simple proxy-generated disease-specific instrument to measure the impact of atopic eczema on infants (0-4 years old) in the clinical setting and to be used in conjunction with a clinical severity assessment tool (25). The content of the IDQOL was based on parents' views about the QoL impairment of their children caused by atopic eczema. It contains 10 items each with a choice of answers ranging from 0 to 3; 0 = no effect, 3 = very much effect. The questions encompass aspects such as symptoms, sleep, mood, meal-times, family activities, treatment, and dressing and bathing the child. All questions pertain to QOL impact over the previous week. There is an additional question that asks for the parent's assessment of the severity of the child's eczema and it is scored separately on a 0-4 scale where 0 indicates none and 4 indicates extremely severe. The highest scoring IDQOL items related to the physical symptoms of itching and scratching, mood changes, and sleep disruption (25).

Test-retest reliability and sensitivity to change in a small sample of infants post-treatment was found to be good. In a recent study Beattie and Lewis-Jones have shown the usefulness of the IDQOL in routine clinical practice as well as its sensitivity to change after a consultation with a paediatric dermatologist (43). This study also provided further evidence of the validity of the IDQOL on the basis of a high correlation with the clinical severity of the disease and with the Dermatitis Family Impact (DFI) questionnaire (44).

Impact of skin disease on the quality of life of adolescents

Adolescence may be considered to represent individuals in the age range of 13-18 years of age. Adolescence is a transitional period between childhood and adulthood and has unique physical, psychological, and social characteristics that makes this period of life different from children and adults (45). Some of its differentiating aspects include increasing need for autonomy, intimacy, and sexuality as well as the importance of peers. However, as mentioned earlier, adolescents' QOL has been assessed traditionally together with children or adults neglecting these specific aspects of this age group.

Thus far, most of the QOL-related research in adolescents has been carried out in the area of chronic illness and the resulting increased incidence of behavioural, psychiatric, academic, and psychosocial difficulties for adolescents (46). As mentioned above some of the dominant characteristics of this age include preoccupation with self-image, influence of peers, and the need for intimacy. Consequently any illness that affects their physical appearance and body image can have a direct impact on social interaction including relationships with peers and with the opposite sex (47). Furthermore, a negative body image may be associated with a number of psychiatric disorders such as depression and eating disorders among adolescents (48-50).

Skin conditions due to their visible nature can have devastating effects on individuals and in particular adolescents who may develop negative body image leading to an adverse impact on QOL. Unfortunately the QOL research in this important age group in general and specifically in dermatology has been quite disproportionate to the magnitude of general population that this group represents (i.e., 20%). Few studies have empirically investigated the impact that various skin diseases can have on adolescents' QOL (51). Some of the common skin conditions in children and adolescents (such as acne, eczema, and psoriasis) can cause significant QOL impairment (29).

Acne, the commonest skin condition in adolescents, can result in significant morbidity and impairment of QOL in the form of interpersonal difficulties, embarrassment, increased anxiety, shame, and social isolation (20,52). In fact the emotional and social impact of acne has been shown to be comparable with severe disabling conditions like epilepsy and arthritis (53). A skin condition does not have to be physically distressing to affect QOL. Symptomless but highly visible conditions such as vitiligo may induce negative experiences in adolescents in the form of feelings of shame towards peers, avoidance of intimacy, and social as well as sport activities, conflicts with parents, and tendency to do things alone (23).

One of the recent studies with a clear focus on adolescents has identified a number of specific aspects of QOL affecting adolescents with different skin diseases (54). According to the findings of this study psychological impact of skin disease came up as the most frequently mentioned theme (mentioned by 91% of study subjects) and included different aspects of negative emotions such as feeling of anger, frustration, embarrassment, decreased self-confidence, and self-image, being more self-conscious, feeling of being judged, and feeling lonely.

The second most common theme mentioned by study subjects was the physical impact of skin diseases (75%) in the form of itchiness, soreness, pain etc. that resulted in sleep disturbance in as many as one third of subjects. The other common themes affecting adolescents included impact on socializing, making friends, choice of clothing, avoiding public places, effect on sporting, and other leisure activities including swimming. Almost one quarter of adolescents felt that their relationships with the opposite sex were affected due to their skin conditions while 16% felt that their career plans and future aspirations were affected.

Assessment of adolescents' quality of life in dermatology

The assessment of QOL of teenagers or adolescents using age-specific measures is a recent development in dermatology. There are only two QOL measures so far developed for adolescents: Teenager's QOL (T-QOL) questionnaire (55) and Skindex-Teen (56).

Teenager's QOL questionnaire (T-QOL)

T-QoL is a simple 18-item dermatology-specific QOL measure for adolescents recently developed in Cardiff, United Kingdom (55). The initial 32 items of the measure were based on the content analysis of semi-structured interviews with a cohort of 50 adolescents suffering from various skin diseases. Content validity was established by carrying out a pilot study on another sample of 20 adolescents. The revised 30-item version was subjected to field testing in a new sample of 153 subjects. Further 12 items, which had suboptimal psychometric properties, were reduced following application of item response and classical test theory models.

Application of Rasch analysis did not support unidimensionality of the measure and factor analysis identified three domains within the scale. The final 18-item version of T-QoL has 3 response categories: Never=0; Sometimes=1; and Always=3. All questions ask the respondent about the impact of their skin disease on specific QOL aspects at the moment. The score can be presented as an overall summary score (score range=0-36 with the higher score indicating greater QoL impairment) or as score of individual domains: Domain 1 represents self image (score range=0-16); Domain 2 represents physical well-being, and future aspirations (score range=0-8); and Domain 3 represents psychosocial impact and relationships (score range=0-12).

The final validation of T-QOL was carried out in a new cohort of adolescents and the results have demonstrated promising psychometric properties of the measure in terms of construct validity, internal consistency, and test-retest reliability as well as sensitivity to change. The authors of the measure see it as a potentially useful measure in routine clinical practice and in research setting.

Skindex-teen

This is another recently developed "hypothesis-based" 21-item self-administered dermatology-specific QOL measure for teenagers that was developed in the United States (56). The items in the questionnaire inquire about the patients' perception about the impact of their skin condition on various aspects of QOL during the previous four weeks. Each item is scored on a 5 response category: never=0, rarely=1; sometimes=2; often=3; all the time=4. The first draft of the questionnaire having 22 items was formulated based on Skindex, a dermatology-specific measure for adults (57,58). The questionnaire was later revised based on the feedback from 11 dermatology professionals and 20 teenagers.

In the final validation stage, Skindex-Teen was administered to 200 adolescents suffering from various skin conditions. Rasch analysis confirmed the instrument to be multi-dimensional having two factors or domains that were named physical symptoms and psychosocial functioning. The scale can be reported as a total overall score (score range=0-84; higher score=greater QoL impairment) or by the scores of two individual domains: psychosocial functioning (score range=0-64) and physical symptoms (score range=0-20). The final scale has demonstrated good psychometric properties including construct, face, and content validity as well as internal consistency, reliability, and sensitivity to change. The authors of Skindex-Teen believe that the instrument will prove useful for research and clinical applications (56).

Impact of skin disease on family quality of life: The greater patient concept

QoL of individuals is closely related to the QOL of those around them. The relatively new concept of Family Quality of Life (FQOL) has originally emerged as an important outcome of services delivery for individuals with disabilities and their families (59,60). Family Quality of Life (FQOL) refers to "conditions where the family needs are met and family members enjoy their life together as a family and have the chance to do things which are important to them" (61). Like patients' QOL, family's QoL can be influenced by different factors such as the nature of patient's illness, its severity as well as personal and socio-economic and cultural factors.

The studies on care-giving for mentally ill patients have found the impact on family life in the form of disruption of family routine, leisure and social life, financial difficulties, emotional overload, and the stresses on the mental and physical health of other family members (62). Goldstein and Kenet argue that any disease or illness has the potential to disrupt the family life and breaks the family routine especially when the disease is chronic in nature (63). Therefore, it has been suggested that any attempt to estimate the burden of a disease must also take into account the impact of that disease on the family functioning and the family's QOL must be analysed independently and additionally to the patient's QOL (64).

In some specialities, paediatrics for example, the family QOL is regarded as a part of the patient's health (65). However, in dermatology, the awareness of the importance of family QOL is still in its infancy. Due to the chronic nature of many skin diseases, and the way treatment is applied, family members are frequently involved in care-giving especially in case of young children. This could result in parents and other close family members being affected by the patient's skin condition (66-68). There is evidence to show that parent's QOL is not only related to the severity of patient's skin condition (69) but also to the QOL of children (24). In fact parent's QOL can actually improve following successful intervention and improvement in children's skin condition (70).

The impact of a patient's skin disease on family members has been studied in only a small number of dermatological conditions (67,71-75) with most attention focused on atopic eczema (72,76). The families of children with eczema have been reported to have lower QOL than families of healthy children (44,77) and taking care of a child with moderate to severe atopic eczema has been found to be more stressful than caring for a child with insulin-dependent diabetes mellitus (78). This is easy to understand when we know that on an average, parents spent 3 hours per day for treatment of children with moderate to severe eczema (78).

Parents of children with atopic eczema experience a wide range of detrimental effects on their lives (e.g., psychological, social, lifestyle modifications, interpersonal relationships, financial, family activities, sleep, and issues related to the practical care of the patient) (44). According to one study, three of the most common aspects of parents QOL affected by their children's eczema included: helping with the child's treatment, tiredness or exhaustion, and additional expenditure related to treatment and clothes (24). Not surprisingly the same three aspects were seen as most significant in parents of children suffering from psoriasis (33).

Other common aspects affecting psoriasis patients' families have been reported including: treatment- related issues, psychological pressures, social disruption, and limitations of leisure as well as daily activities (67). In a wider cross section of skin conditions, Basra and Finlay demonstrated that skin diseases can significantly impair the QOL of patients' families in a number of diverse ways such as: emotional distress (98% of the family members), burden of care (54%), effect on housework (42%), social life (48%), holidays (46%), financial difficulties (30%), impact on physical well-being (22%), effect on job/study (40%), restriction of leisure activities (26%), sleep disturbance (20%), effect on sex life (8%), and perceived need for support (12%) (66). In order to highlight the significance of this underestimated and often overlooked aspect of skin diseases (i.e., their impact on patient's family), the term "Greater Patient" has been proposed that describes the immediate close social group affected by a patient's skin disease (66).

Emotional impact of a child's skin condition on parents is an important issue that can manifest itself in the form of worry, crying, feeling of guilt and self-blame, anger, sadness, helplessness, and frustration (79). The reaction of people to the patient's skin appearance is a stressful experience for parents and family members and causes a feeling of embarrassment, anger, and frustration (79). Consequently, parents can experience a feeling of social isolation that is mainly due to avoiding people for the fear of having negative and unfriendly interactions with strangers, friends, and family alike (30). The social isolation that family members may experience highlights the need for social and emotional support for these individuals (80). Lewis et al. (81) stressed that social support for families with a member with chronic illness is of great importance in influencing how the family copes with the situation.

Disruption of sleep is another major issue particularly for the parents of children suffering from eczema due to frequent scratching and crying of the children in the night. Su et al. (78) found that between one and two hours of sleep was lost by parents of children with eczema. Sleep was also shown to be a major problem for parents of children with atopic eczema in Lawson's study (44), while Carroll et al. (72) have shown that sleep deprivation can affect all family members and that it is a major stress-causing factor for the families. The implications for parents can be huge; they may need to miss work or avoid outside work altogether; their social functioning can be damaged; and their relationships with their spouse and other family members can be affected along with their parenting behaviour (77,78).

Financial impact on parents is another consequence of skin conditions in children and in particular eczema that has been demonstrated to have a negative effect on the family's financial resources and causes strain on family's budget (44,72). Many parents feel the need to make changes to their lifestyles to adjust with their children's needs, for example, restricting certain diets, making changes in the home, buying special items (i.e., products, clothing, and linens) for the child and even holiday plans as well as outdoor activities sometimes need additional expenditures (30). The direct financial cost of care of a child having moderate to severe eczema was found to similar to type 1 diabetes but substantially higher than for a child with asthma (78).

In addition to the direct financial impact due to extra expenditure, the household may also be affected indirectly through decreased productivity of family caregivers who require time away from work in pursuit of medical attention for their relative patients. Loss of productivity is an important component of overall burden of atopic eczema and is directly related to the severity of disease. For example, the cost in the form of loss of productivity, to families of patients with moderate and severe eczema has been found to be Australian$ 894 and 1,290 respectively (78). Moreover, the mean days lost from work per patient are higher for parents of younger children than parents of older children (82). Bickers et al. (83) have estimated an annual loss of US$ 986 million due to caregivers' lost workdays.

Assessment of family quality in dermatology

A number of disease-specific instruments to measure the secondary impact on the family have been described for atopic eczema (44,84,85). However, there is only one psoriasis-specific (86) and one "generic" dermatology-specific QOL measure that could be used to measure the "secondary" impact on QoL of families across different skin diseases (87). These tools are briefly described below.

Family Dermatology Life Quality Index (FDLQI)

The FDLQI was developed in Cardiff in 2007 as the first dermatology specific self-administered QOL measure to quantify the impact of patients' skin diseases on their family members (87).The content of the FDLQI was based on family members' reports of how their related patients' skin diseases affected their QOL. It has 10 items covering different aspects of family members' QOL such as emotional distress, burden of care, effect on relationships, social and leisure activities, and extra house work due to patient's skin disease. Each question asks family member's perception of the impact on their QOL over the last month and is scored on a 4-point scale with a score range of 0-30; higher scores indicating greater QoL impairment.

The measure was shown to be sensitive to change and demonstrated high internal consistency as well as test-retest reliability. The construct validity of the FDLQI was established by its high correlation with patients' DLQI (35) scores and patients' self-assessed disease severity global question scores. Moreover, the measure was able to discriminate between family members based on the nature of patients' skin diseases; family members of patients with inflammatory skin diseases showing significantly higher FDLQI scores compared with family members of patients with non-inflammatory skin diseases. Within-group analysis of FDLQI scores showed that family members of patients with eczema had greatest QOL impairment followed by acne and psoriasis. The measure has further been cross-validated against generic and disease-specific family QOL tools (86,88,89). The brief and simple design of the FDLQI can make it a practical measure for routine clinical use and an additional outcome measure in clinical research.

Dermatitis Family Impact questionnaire (DFI)

The Dermatitis Family Impact (DFI) questionnaire was the first instrument of its kind in dermatology aimed to measure the secondary impact of atopic eczema on the quality of life of parents of children with eczema (44). It was meant to be used as an additional measure in clinical studies and in clinical practice to guide management decisions.

The 10 items of the DFI were derived from intensive qualitative interviews with families of children suffering from atopic eczema and include areas of family life such as sleep, tiredness, distress, practical difficulties with treatment, and effects on shopping, leisure, housework, family relationships, expenditure, and food. Each question has four possible answers and measures the family impact over the last week only. The total scale score (0-30) is achieved by summing the scores of individual items (0-3); higher score means greater family QoL impairment.

Although the instrument was shown to discriminate between affected families and control families, it was not compared with any other valid QOL instrument for validation purposes; also, neither its reliability nor responsiveness to change was assessed during the initial development process. However, in a recent study, sensitivity of the DFI to change was demonstrated in parents of children with atopic eczema before and after consultation with a paediatric dermatology team (43). The sensitivity of the DFI to change after a dermatology consultation has also been documented by Balkrishnan et al. (70), while Ben-Gashir et al. (69) showed its sensitivity to change after a change in clinical severity of a child's eczema. Further studies have demonstrated good correlation of the measure with other dermatology-specific and disease-specific measures (25,69,90).

Parents' Index of Quality of Life in Atopic Dermatitis (PIQOL-AD)

This is a family/parent oriented QOL measure that was developed simultaneously in several European countries and the United States that adopted a "needs-based" approach (85). This instrument is designed to be completed by parents of children with atopic eczema to assess the impact that their children's eczema and its treatment has on their QOL. The content of the

PIQOL-AD was derived from unstructured interviews with parents of children having atopic eczema.

Rasch analysis was applied to reduce the number of items and prove its unidimensionality. The final questionnaire has 28 items in the form of statements and a dichotomous response system. This scoring system was thought to be less burdensome for respondents and also facilitated equivalence of translation. The dichotomous response choices, however, can limit the responsiveness of the instrument. The measure covers a range of affected parents' needs e.g., need for rest, relaxation, self-respect, independence, personal time and space, control, and also the need for their child to have a safe future.

The test-retest reliability and internal consistency of the PIQOL-AD was demonstrated to be good and construct validity was established by correlating it with the General Wellbeing Index (GWBI) and by the scale's ability to differentiate groups based on parent-perceived eczema severity (85). In a later study of children with atopic eczema treated with pimecrolimus, the PIQOL-AD was shown to be responsive to improvement in children's condition with a 10% reduction in PIQOL-AD scores at baseline and 6 months after using the treatment (91).

A secondary analysis of the data from this and other clinical trials incorporating this measure was used to describe the clinical meaningfulness of the PIQOL-AD scores, which suggests that a change of 2-3 points on the measure should be considered meaningful (92). Although the original measure was intended to be used by parents of children up to the age of 8 years, the authors believe that it could also be used with parents of children up to 12 years.

Childhood Atopic Dermatitis Impact Scale (CADIS)

This is another self-administered "hypothesis-based" instrument to measure the impact of atopic eczema on the QOL of young children and their families (84). The initial 62-item content was derived from published work as well as interviews with affected families and medical professionals. Item reduction was performed by qualitative judgment and psychometric analysis including Rasch analysis. The final 45 items can be explained by a five-scale framework including three parent-related scales (family and social function, emotions, sleep) and two child-related scales (symptoms and activity limitations and behaviour). Each item is scored on a 0-4 scale (0=never, 4=all the time) and inquires about the parent's perception of a particular aspect during the last four weeks. The internal consistency of all the five scales was acceptable and preliminary evidence of content and construct validity was documented. However, test-retest reliability and responsiveness to change was not assessed at the time of questionnaire development.

Psoriasis Family Index (PFI)

This is a self-administered psoriasis-specific measure to assess the impact of the patient's psoriasis on family members and partners (86). It has 15 items and a 4-point response format from not at all (score=0) to very much (score=3); higher scores indicate greater QOL impairment. The items cover different aspects of family members QOL such as psychological impact, extra house work, social and leisure activities, treatment related burden, effect on daily activities, sleep, choice of clothes, holidays, and family relationships. The preliminary results of psychometric analysis of the measure including internal consistency, test-retest reliability, and construct validity are promising. However, further evidence of scale's performance is required in particular its factor structure and sensitivity to change.

Societal impact of childhood dermatological conditions

Skin diseases are very common in the community. The prevalence in school children and adolescents has been found to be between 26% and 31% (93,94). Two of the commonest skin conditions in this age group are atopic eczema and acne; the former being more common in primary school children and latter in secondary school children and adolescents (93). Both these conditions are known to be chronic in nature and carry substantial morbidity for patients and a significant QoL impact on patients as well as their parents.

Generally, chronic skin conditions and some malignant skin cancers drain considerable health service financial resources in the society. The direct costs of treating skin conditions vary from country to country depending on the local healthcare systems. So far most of the research on cost estimation of skin diseases has been focused on atopic eczema. It appears that in addition to direct medical costs, atopic eczema may incur indirect costs in the form of days lost from work, purchase of special household products, clothes and linen, over the counter products, special diets, and cleaning agents, as well as additional transport and parking costs to and from hospital and surgery (95).

In the United Kingdom, the annual cost per child was estimated to be £79.59 and included direct and indirect costs such as the cost of prescriptions, NHS consultations, private consultations, purchase of over the counter products, and income loss (96). According to an Australian study, the annual cost of just medical consultations for a child with moderate and severe eczema was estimated at 389 and 642 Australian dollars respectively while the annual hospitalization cost for a child with severe eczema was 2,912 Australian dollars (78). The mean direct annual cost of treatment of a child with mild, moderate, severe eczema was calculated to be 330, 818 and 1,255 Australian dollars and included costs of special diet, medication, dressings, and medical consultations (78). In fact, the same study found that the cost of treating severe eczema in children has been found to be even higher than treating diabetes and asthma (78).

In the United States, the mean annual per patient total costs including both direct and indirect costs have been estimated to be approximately $609 (82). Also in the United States, according to a conservative estimate 364 million dollars are spent annually for the treatment of childhood atopic eczema (97). Finally, in another study comparing the international costs of treatment of eczema the annual per patient treatment costs ranged from $71 in Netherlands to $2,559 in Germany (98).

Conclusion

Recent advances in medicine have shifted the focus of attention from mortality issues due to acute illnesses such as infectious diseases to long term morbidity issues related to chronic illnesses. The increased survival rates have been accompanied by greater recognition of quality of life of patients as a major outcome. Assessment of quality of life has potential value in evaluating interventions, assessing the outcomes of new therapies, comparing outcomes in clinical trials, and facilitating communication between patients, their family caregivers, and health care professionals. It has also been used as a tool to identify hidden health problems and in monitoring changes in patients' health status and prioritising health issues for individual patients (99). Equally importantly, it helps in commissioning care programmes and in audit work and can also be used as an effective political tool to argue for limited vital resources in a competitive environment in which skin diseases due to their non-life threatening nature, are not viewed as "important" as other medical conditions.

There is a risk that important information will be missed if clinical measures of disease severity are used alone neglecting the QOL impact of the disease. Therefore, it is recommended to use simple QOL measures in clinical practice in conjunction with clinical measures when assessing patients with various skin diseases to have an idea of the overall severity. Quality of life assessment is as important in paediatric population as in adult population. In situations where it is not possible to cure the disease but to control the symptoms, it is important to determine how the disease and/or its treatment impact on the child's QOL. This can aid in making more appropriate management decisions.

Based on the fact that parent's and children's views differ in their perception of illness and treatment and that parents' views about their children's QOL may be affected by their own emotions and mental health, it is recommended that wherever possible, children should rate their own QOL (100). Nevertheless, in certain situations it would be quite acceptable to use proxy rating by parents or carers such as when children are too small or incapable to understand and/or respond to questions in the measure.

When measuring the QOL in a paediatric population, it is important to consider the developmental stage of the respondents as particular dimensions may not be equally important in different age groups (e.g., early childhood vs. late childhood or adolescence). Adolescents have some specific aspects related to their QOL that are different from adults and children's QOL; these include physical maturation, autonomy, peer relationship, sexuality, and body image. It is therefore not appropriate to regard this age group as either children or adults and QOL related research tools should be developed separately for these age groups.

Family members of patients with various skin diseases may be affected in a number of ways by their related patients' conditions and the assessment of QOL of parents and family members of children is an integral component of comprehensive assessment of burden of skin disease in the community. It has been suggested that the optimal management of children's skin conditions should also include interventions to reduce the impact on parents and family members if better medical outcomes are to be achieved. Unfortunately, the current health care systems in many countries including many developed countries, do not provide adequate psychological, social, and financial support to children with various skin conditions and their families.

In order to decrease the burden on this population there is a need for more structured education programmes and specialist care from health care professionals including dermatologists, general practitioners, and paediatricians with special interest in dermatology, psychologists, as well as nurses with special training in dermatology.

In fact the level of care provided by trained nurse practitioners has been found to be as effective as by dermatologists in improving the severity of eczema as well as QOL outcomes (101).

Having a secure support network with good knowledge of the disease can enable the patients and their families to feel more comfortable and less alone. There is evidence that parent education and psychosocial support can go a long way in reducing illness-related stress among parents, increasing parents' confidence in managing their children's eczema, and ultimately in reducing the severity of eczema (102,103). Moreover, patient advocacy groups, wherever available can be useful in improving patient education and decreasing resource utilization (104).

Finally, most of the research on the impact of childhood skin diseases and especially their impact on family and financial implications, has been focused on atopic eczema and there is a need to study the impact of other skin diseases (such as acne, psoriasis, and genodermatoses), to have a broader idea of the burden of skin disease in this population.

Acknowledgments

This paper is a revised and adapted version of an earlier publication: Basra MKA. Quality of life issues in children and adolescents with dermatological conditions and their wider impact on the family and society. In: Tareen RS, Greydanus DE, Jafferany M, Patel DR, Merrick J, eds. Pediatric psycho-dermatology. A clinical manual of child and adolescent psychocutaneous disorders. Berlin: De Gruyter, 2013:95-116.

References

[1] Harding L. Children's quality of life assessments: A review of generic and health related quality of life measures completed by children and adolescents. Clin Psychol Psychother 2001;8:79-96.

[2] Torrance GW. Utility approach to measuring health related quality of life. J Chron Dis 1987;40:593-600.

[3] World Health Organisation. Measuring quality of life: the development of the World Health Organisation Quality of Life Instrument (WHOQOL). Geneva 1993.

[4] Maes S, Bruil J. Assessing the quality of life in children with a chronic illness. In: Rodriguez-Martin J, ed. Health Psychology and Quality of Life Research. Alicante, Spain: Health Psychology Department, University of Alicante, 1995:637-52.

[5] Collier J, MacKinlay D, Phillips D. Norm values for the generic children's quality of life measure (GCQ). Qual Life Res 2000;9:617-23.

[6] Juniper EF. How important is quality of life in pediatric asthma? Paediatr Pulmonol 1997;15:17-21.

[7] Mishoe SC, Baker RR, Poole S, Harrell LM, Arant CB, Rupp NT. Development of an instrument to assess stress levels and quality of life in children with asthma. J Asthma 1998;35:553-63.

[8] Davis E, Mackinnon A, Reddihough D, Graham HK, Mehmet-Radji O, Boyd R. Paediatric quality of life instruments: a review of the impact of the conceptual framework on outcomes. Dev Med and Child Neurol 2006;48:311-18.

[9] Drotar D. Validating measures of pediatric health status, functional status, and health-related quality of life: key methodological challenges and strategies. Amb Paediatr 2004;4:358-64.

[10] Haliousa B, Beumont MG. Lunel F. Quality of life in dermatology. Int J Dermatol 2000;39:801-6.

[11] Eiser C, Morse R. A review of measures of quality of life for children with chronic illness. Arch Dis Child 2001;84:205-11.

[12] Annett RD, Bender BG, Lapidus J et al. Predicting children's quality of life in an asthma clinical trial: what do children's reports tell us? J Pediatr 2001;139:854-61.

[13] Sawyer MG, Spurrier N, Kennedy D, Martin J. The relationship between the quality of life of children with asthma and family functioning. J Asthma 2001;38:279-84.

[14] Mulhurn RK, Horowitz ME, Ochs J, et al. Assessment of quality of life among paediatric patients with cancer. J Consult Clin Psychol 1989;1:130-8.

[15] Eiser C, Morse R. Can parents rate their child's health-related quality of life? Results of a systematic review. Qual Life Res 2001;10:347-57.

[16] Juniper EF, Guyatt GH, Feeny DH et al. Minimum skills required by children to complete health-related quality of life instruments for asthma: comparison of measurement properties. Eur Respir J 1997;10:2285-94.

[17] Eiser C, Kopel SJ. Children's perception of health and illness. In: Petrie KJ, Weinman JA, eds. Perceptions of health and illness: current research and applications. Singapore: Harwood Academic Publishers,1997.

[18] Simeoni M-C, Sapin C, Antonotti S, Auquier P. Health-related quality of life reported by French adolescents: a predictive approach of health status? J Adolesc Health 2001;28:288-94.

[19] Connolly MA, Johnson JA. Measuring quality of life in paediatric patients. Pharmacoeconomics 1999;16:605-25.

[20] Jowett S, Ryan T. Skin disease and handicap: an analysis of the impact of skin conditions. Soc Sci Med 1985;20:425-9.

[21] Herd RM, Tidman MJ, Ruta DA, Hunter JA. Measurement of quality of life in atopic dermatitis: correlation and validation of two different methods. Br J Dermatol 1997;136:502-7.

[22] Beattie PE, Lewis-Jones MS. A comparative study of impairment of quality of life in children with skin disease and children with other chronic childhood diseases. Br J Dermatol 2006;155:145-51.

[23] Linthorst Homan MW, de Korte J, Grootenhuis MA, et al. Impact of childhood vitiligo on adult life. Br J Dermatol 2008;159:915-20.

[24] Ganemo A, Svensson A, Lindberg M, Wahlgren CF. Quality of life in Swedish children with eczema. Acta Derm Venereol 2007;87:345-9.

[25] Lewis-Jones MS, Finlay AY, Dykes PJ. The infants' dermatitis quality of life index. Br J Dermatol 2001;144:104-10.

[26] Cotterill J. Psychiatry and the skin. Br J Hospital Med 1989;42:401-4.

[27] Absolon CM, Cottrell D, Eldridge SM, Glover MT. Psychological disturbance in atopic eczema: the extent of the problem in school-aged children. Br J Dermatol 1997;137:241-5.

[28] Daud L, Garralda M, David TJ. Psychosocial adjustment in preschool children with atopic eczema. Arch Dis Child 1993;69:670-6.

[29] Lewis-Jones MS, Finlay AY. The children's dermatology life quality index (CDLQI): initial validation and practical use. Br J Dermatol 1995;132:942-9.

[30] Chamlin SL, Frieden IJ, Williams ML, Chren MM. The effects of atopic dermatitis on young American children and their families. Paediatrics 2004;114:607-11.

[31] Reid P, Lewis-Jones MS. Sleep difficulties and their management in preschoolers with atopic eczema. Clin Exp Dermatol 1995;20:38-41.

[32] Dahl RE, Bernhisel-Broadbent J, Scanlon-Holdford S, et al. Sleep disturbances in children with atopic dermatitis. Arch Pediatr Adolesc Med 1995;149:856-60.

[33] Ganemo A, Wahlgren CF, Svensson A. Quality of life and clinical features in Swedish children with psoriasis. Pediatr Dermatol 2011;28:375-9.

[34] De Jager MEA, de Jong EM, Evers AW, et al. The burden of childhood psoriasis. Pediatr Dermatol 2011; early online publication (DOI: 10.1111/j.1525-1470.2011.01489.x)
[35] Finlay AY, Khan GK. Dermatology Life Quality Index (DLQI) – a simple practical measure for routine clinical use. Clin Exp Dermatol 1994;19:210-6.
[36] Lewis-Jones S. Quality of life and childhood atopic dermatitis: the misery of living with childhood eczema. Int J Clin Pract 2006;60:984-92.
[37] Lewis-Jones MS, Lawson V, Hill G, Finlay AY. Monitoring childhood skin disease handicap. Br J Dermatol 1996;135(suppl 45):52.
[38] Ben-Gashir MA, Seed PT, Hay RJ. Quality of life and disease severity are correlated in children with atopic dermatitis. Br J Dermatol 2004;150:284-90.
[39] Walker N, Lewis-Jones MS. Quality of life and acne in Scottish adolescent school children: use of the Children's Dermatology Life Quality Index (CDLQI) and the Cardiff Acne Disability Index (CADI). J Eur Acad Dermatol Venereol 2006;20:45-50.
[40] Waters A, Sandhu D, Beattie P, et al. Severity stratification of children's dermatology life quality index scores. Br J Dermatol 2010;163(suppl 1):121(abstr PA-8).
[41] Holme AS, Man I, Finlay AY, et al. The Children's Dermatology Life Quality Index: validation of the cartoon version. Br J Dermatol 2003;148:285-90.
[42] Holme AS, Anstey AV, Finlay AY, et al. Erythropoietic protoporphyria in the UK: clinical features and effect on quality of life. Br J Dermatol 2006;155:574-81.
[43] Beattie PE, Lewis-Jones MS. An audit of the impact of a consultation with a paediatric dermatology team on quality of life in infants with atopic eczema and their families: further validation of the Infants' Dermatitis Quality of Life Index and Dermatitis Family Impact score. Br J Dermatol 2006;155:1249-55.
[44] Lawson V, Lewis-Jones MS, Finlay AY, et al. The family impact of childhood atopic dermatitis: the Dermatitis Family Impact questionnaire. Br J Dermatol 1998;138:107-13.
[45] Frisen A. Measuring health-related quality of life in adolescence. Acta Paediatrica 2007;96:963-8.
[46] Beck AL, Nethercut GE, Crittenden MR, Hewins J. Visibility of handicap, self-concept and social maturity among young adult survivors of end-stage renal cancer. J Dev Behav Paed 1986;7:93-6.
[47] La Greca AM. Social consequences of pediatric conditions: fertile area for future investigation and intervention? J Paediatr Psychol 1990;15:285-307.
[48] Kostanski M, Gullone E. Adolescent body image dissatisfaction: relationship with self-esteem, anxiety, and depression controlling for body mass. J Child Psychol Psychiatry 1998;39:255-62.
[49] Halvarsson K, Lunner K, Sjoden P-O. Assessment of eating behaviours and attitudes to eating, dieting and body-image in pre-adolescent Swedish girls: a one-year follow-up. Acta Paediatrica 2000;89:996-1000.
[50] Stice E, Bearman SK. Body-image and eating disturbances prospectively predict increases depressive symptoms in adolescent girls: a growth curve analysis. Dev Psychol 2001;37:597-607.
[51] Smith JA. The impact of skin disease on the quality of life of adolescents. Adolesc Med 2001;12:343-53.
[52] Krowchuk DP, Stancin T, Keskinen R, et al. The psychosocial effects of acne on adolescents. Pediatr Dermatol 1991;8:332-8.
[53] Mallon E, Newton JN, Klassen A, et al. The quality of life in acne: a comparison with general medical conditions using generic questionnaires. Br J Dermatol 1999;140:672-6.
[54] Golics CJ, Basra MKA, Finlay AY, Salek MS. Adolescents with skin disease have specific quality of life issues. Dermatology 2009;218:357-66.
[55] Basra MKA, Salek S, Tanweer Z, et al. Refinement and validation of Teenager's Quality of Life Questionnaire (T-QoL). J Invest Dermatol 2011;131:S50(abstr 295).
[56] Smidt AC, Lai JS, Cella D, et al. Development and validation of Skindex-Teen, a quality of life instrument for adolescents with skin disease. Arch Dermatol 2010;146:865-9.
[57] Chren MM, Lasek RJ, Quinn LM, et al. Skindex, a quality-of-life measure for patients with skin disease: reliability, validity, and responsiveness. J Invest Dermatol 1996;107:707-13.
[58] Chren MM, lasek RJ, Sahay AP, Sands LP. Measurement properties of Skindex-16: a brief quality-of-life measure for patients with skin diseases. J Cutan Med Surg 2001;5:105-10.

[59] Park J, Hoffman L, Marquis J, Turnbull AP, Poston D, et al. Towards assessing family outcomes of service delivery; validation of a family quality of life survey. J Intel Dis Res 2003;47:367-84.
[60] Poston D, Turnbull AP, Park J, et al. Family quality of life: a qualitative inquiry. Mental Retardation 2003;41:313-28.
[61] Turnbull AP, Turnbull HR, Poston D, et al. Enhancing quality of life of families of children and youth with disabilities in the United States. In: Turnbull AP, Brown I, Turnbull HR, American Association on Mental Retardation, eds. Families and people with mental retardation and quality of life: international perspectives. Washington DC, 2004:51-100.
[62] Group for Advancement of Psychiatry. Family affairs: helping families cope with mental illness. Brumer/Mazet, New York 1986.
[63] Goldstein G, Kenet G. The impact of chronic disease on the family. Haemophilia 2002;8:461-70.
[64] Verdugo MA, Cordoba L, Gomez J. Spanish adaptation and validation of the Family Quality of Life Survey. J Intell Dis Res 2005;49:794-8.
[65] Fink R. Issues and problems in measuring children's health status in community health research. Soc Sci Med 1989;29:715-9.
[66] Basra MKA, Finlay AY. The family impact of skin diseases: the greater patient concept. Br J Dermatol 2007;156:929-37.
[67] Eghlileb AM, Davies EEG, Finlay AY. Psoriasis has a major secondary impact on the lives of family members and partners. Br J Dermatol 2007;156:1245-50.
[68] Elliot BE, Luker K. The experiences of mothers caring for a child with severe atopic eczema. J Clin Nurs 1997;6:241-7.
[69] Ben-Gashir MA, Seed PT, Hay RJ. Is family's quality of life and disease severity related in children with atopic dermatitis? J Eur Acad Dermatol Venerol 2002;16:455-62.
[70] Balkrishnan R, Manul J, Clarke J, Caroll CL, Housman TS, Fleisher AB Jr. Effects of an episode of specialist care on the impact of childhood atopic dermatitis on the child's family. J Paediatr Health Care 2003;17:184-9.
[71] Braue A, Ross G, Varigos G, Kelly H. Epidemiology and impact of childhood molluscum contageosum: A case series and critical review of the literature. Paediatr Dermatol 2005;22:287-91.
[72] Carroll CL, Balkrishnan R, Feldman SR, et al. The burden of atopic dermatitis; impact on the patient, family, and society. Pediatr Dermatol 2005;22:192-9.
[73] Fine J-D, Johnson LB, Weiner M, Suchindran C. Impact of inherited epidermolysis bullosa on parental interpersonal relationships, marital status and family size. Br J Dermatol 2005;152:1009-14.
[74] Miller AC, Cate IM, Watson HS, Geronemus RG. Stress and family satisfaction in parents of children with facial port-wine stains. Pediatr Dermatol 1999;16:190-4.
[75] Rakkhit T, Chen S, Lawley L, Freedman S. The impact of Sturge-Weber Syndrome (SWS) on patients and their families. J Am Acad Dermatol 2006;54(3):1414(Abstr:121).
[76] Warschburger P, Buchholz HT, Petermann F. Psychological adjustment in parents of young children with atopic dermatitis: which factors predict parental quality of life. Br J Dermatol 2004;150:304-11.
[77] Lapidus CS, Kerr PE. Social impact of atopic dermatitis. Med Health R I 2001;84:294-5.
[78] Su JC, Kemp AS, VArigos GA, Nolan TM. Atopic eczema: its impact on the family and financial cost. Arch Dis Child 1997;76:159-62.
[79] Chamlin SL. The psychosocial burden of childhood atopic dermatitis. Dermatol Therapy 2006;19:104-7.
[80] Garwick AW, Kohrman C, Wolman C, Blum RW. Families' recommendations for improving services for children with chronic conditions. Arch Pediatr Adolesc Med 1998;152:440-8.
[81] Lewis FM, Woods NF, Hough EE, Bensley LS. The family's functioning with chronic illness in the mother: the spouse's perspective. Soc Sci Med 1989;29:1261–9.
[82] Fivenson D, Arnol RJ, Kaniecki DJ, et al. The effect of atopic dermatitis on total burden of illness and quality of life on adults and children in large managed care organisation. J Manag Care Pharm 2002;8:333-42.
[83] Bickers DR, Lim HW, Margolis D, et al. The burden of skin diseases: 2004: A joint project of the American Academy of Dermatology Association and the Society for Investigative Dermatology. J Am Acad Dermatol 2006;55:490-500.

[84] Chamlin SL, Cella D, Frieden IJ, Williams ML, Mancini AJ, Lai J, Chren MM. Development of the childhood atopic dermatitis impact scale: initial validation of a quality-of-life measure for young children with atopic dermatitis and their families. J Invest Dermatol 2005;125:1106-11.
[85] McKenna SP, Whalley D, Dewar AL, Erdman RAM, Kohlmann T, et al. International development of the Parents' Index of Quality of Life in Atopic Dermatitis (PIQoL-AD). Qual Life Res 2005;14:231-41.
[86] Eghlileb AM, Basra MKA, Finlay AY. The Psoriasis Family Index: preliminary results of validation of a quality of life instrument for family members of patients with psoriasis. Dermatology 2009;219:63-70.
[87] Basra MKA, Sue-Ho R, Finlay AY. The Family Dermatology Life Quality Index: measuring the secondary impact of skin disease. Br J Dermatol 2007;156:528-38.
[88] Basra MKA, Edmunds O, Salek MS, Finlay AY. Measurement of family impact of skin disease: further validation of the Family Dermatology Life Quality Index. J Eur Acad Dermatol Venereol 2008;22:813-21.
[89] Tadros A, Vergou T, Stratigos AJ, et al. Psoriasis: is it the tip of the iceberg for the quality of life of patients and their families? J Eur Acad Dermatol Venereol 2011;25:1282-7.
[90] Chinn DJ, Poyner T, Sibley G. Randomised controlled trial of a single nurse consultation in primary care on the quality of life of children with atopic eczema. Br J Dermatol 2002;146:432-9.
[91] Whalley D, Hules J, McKenna SP, et al. The benefit of pimecrolimus (Elidel, SDZ ASM 981) on parents' quality of life in the treatment of paediatric atopic dermatitis. Pediatr 2002;110:1133-6.
[92] Meads DM, McKenna SP, Kahler K. The quality of life of parents of children with atopic dermatitis: Interpretation of PIQoL-AD scores. Qual Life Res 2005;14:2235-45.
[93] Fung WK, Lo KK. Prevalence of skin disease among school children and adolescents in a student health service in Hong Kong. Paediatr Dermatol 2000;17:440-6.
[94] Bechelli LM, Haddad N, Pimenta WP, et al. Epidemiological survey of skin diseases in school children living in the Porus Valley (Acre state, Amazonia, Brazil). Dermatologica 1981;163:78-93.
[95] Herd RM. In: Williams HC, ed. Morbidity and cost in atopic dermatitis. Cambridge University Press, 2000;88-9.
[96] Emerson RM, Williams HC, Allen BR. What is the cost of atopic dermatitis in preschool children? Br J Dermatol 2001;144:514-22.
[97] Lapidus CS, Schwarz DF, Honig PJ. Atopic dermatitis in children. Who cares? Who pays? J Am Acad Dermatol 1993;28:699-703.
[98] Verboom P, Hakkaart-Van L, Sturkenboom M, et al. The cost of atopic dermatitis in the Netherlands: an international comparison. Br J Dermatol 2002;147:716-24.
[99] Higginson IJ, Carr AJ. Measuring quality of life: using quality of life measures in clinical setting. BMJ 2001;322:1297-300.
[100] Varni JW, Katz ER, Seid M, et al. The Pediatric Cancer Quality of Life Invetory (PCQL). I. Instrument development, descriptive statistics, and cross-informant variance. J Behav Med 1998;21:19-204.
[101] Schuttelaar MLA, Vermeulen KM, Drukker N, Coenraads PJ. A randomized controlled trial in children with eczema: nurse practitioner vs. dermatologist. Br J Dermatol 2010;162:162-70.
[102] Staab D, von Rueden U, Kehrt R, et al. Evaluation of a parental training program for the management of childhood atopic dermatitis. Pediatr Allergy Immunol 2002;13:84-90.
[103] Broberg A, Kalimo K, Lindblad B, et al. Parental education in the treatment of childhood atopic eczema. Acta Derm Venereol 1990;70:495-9.
[104] Kamalpour A, Gammon B, Chen KH, et al. Resource utilization and quality of life associated with congenital ichthyoses. Pediatr Dermatol 2011;28:512-8.

Section two: Acknowledgments

In: Pediatric and Adolescent Dermatology
Editors: D Greydanus, A Feinberg and J Merrick
ISBN: 978-1-63321-853-6

Chapter 10

About the editors

Donald E. Greydanus, MD, Dr. HC (ATHENS), FAAP, FSAM (Emeritus), FIAP (HON) is Professor and Founding Chair of the Department of Pediatric and Adolescent Medicine, as well as Pediatrics Program Director at the Western Michigan University Homer Stryker MD School of Medicine (WMED), Kalamazoo, Michigan, USA. He is also Professor of Pediatrics and Human Development at Michigan State University College of Human Medicine (East Lansing, Michigan, USA) as well as Clinical Professor of Pediatrics at MSU College of Osteopathic Medicine in East Lansing, Michigan, USA. Received the 1995 American Academy of Pediatrics' Adele D. Hofmann Award for "Distinquished Contributions in Adolescent Health", the 2000 Mayo Clinic Pediatrics Honored Alumnus Award for "National Contributions to the field of Pediatrics," and the 2003 William B Weil, Jr., MD Endowed Distinguished Pediatric Faculty Award from Michigan State University College of Medicine for "National and international recognition as well as exemplary scholarship in pediatrics." Received the 2004 Charles R Drew School of Medicine (Los Angeles, CA) Stellar Award for contributions to pediatric resident education and awarded an honorary membership in the Indian Academy of Pediatrics—an honor granted to only a few pediatricians outside of India. Was the 2007-2010 Visiting Professor of Pediatrics at Athens University, Athens, Greece and received the Michigan State University College of Human Medicine Outstanding Community Faculty Award in 2008. In 2010 he received the title of Doctor Honoris Causa from the University of Athens (Greece) as a "distinguished scientist who through outstanding work has bestowed praise and credit on the field of adolescent medicine (Ephebiatrics)." In 2010 he received the Outstanding Achievement in Adolescent Medicine Award from the Society for Adolescent Medicine "as a leading force in the field of adolescent medicine and health." Past Chair of the National Conference and Exhibition Planning Group (Committee on Scientific Meetings) of the American Academy of Pediatrics and member of the Pediatric Academic Societies' (SPR/PAS) Planning Committee (1998 to Present). In 2011 elected to The Alpha Omega Alpha Honor Society (Faculty member) at Michigan State University College of Human Medicine, East Lansing, Michigan. Former member of the Appeals Committee for the Pediatrics' Residency Review Committee (RRC) of the Accreditation Council for Graduate Medical Education (Chicago, IL) in both adolescent medicine and general pediatrics. Numerous publications in adolescent health and lectureships in many countries on adolescent health. E-mail: donald.greydanus@ med.wmich.edu

Arthur N Feinberg, MD, FAAP is professor of Pediatrics and Adolescent Medicine at the Western Michigan University in Kalamazoo, Michigan, United States. He is also Professor of Pediatrics at the Michigan State University College of Human Medicine, Department of Pediatrics and Human Development, East Lansing, Michigan, as well as Clinical Professor of Pediatrics at the Michigan State University College of Osteopathic Medicine. He attended the Albert Einstein College of Medicine at the Yeshiva University in New York and completed pediatric internship and residency at Montefiore Hospital and Medical Center in New York. After serving two years in the US Navy he entered private practice in Kalamazoo in 1975. His strong interest in teaching led him to join the residency program in Kalamazoo in 1993. He has been recipient of six teaching awards since joining the faculty. His research interests have included newborn topics such as hospital discharge and circumcision and have led to several original publications and numerous book chapters. He has been co-editor of three textbooks. E-mail: arthur.feinberg@med.wmich.edu

Joav Merrick, MD, MMedSci, DMSc, is professor of pediatrics, child health and human development, Division of Pediatrics, Hadassah Hebrew University Medical Center, Mt Scopus Campus, Jerusalem, Israel and Kentucky Children's Hospital, University of Kentucky, Lexington, Kentucky United States and professor of public health at the Center for Healthy Development, School of Public Health, Georgia State University, Atlanta, United States, the medical director of the Health Services, Division for Intellectual and Developmental Disabilities, Ministry of Social Affairs and Social Services, Jerusalem, the founder and director of the National Institute of Child Health and Human Development in Israel. Numerous publications in the field of pediatrics, child health and human development, rehabilitation, intellectual disability, disability, health, welfare, abuse, advocacy, quality of life and prevention. Received the Peter Sabroe Child Award for outstanding work on behalf of Danish Children in 1985 and the International LEGO-Prize ("The Children's Nobel Prize") for an extraordinary contribution towards improvement in child welfare and well-being in 1987. E-mail: jmerrick@zahav.net.il

In: Pediatric and Adolescent Dermatology
Editors: D Greydanus, A Feinberg and J Merrick

ISBN: 978-1-63321-853-6

Chapter 11

About the Department of Pediatric and Adolescent Medicine, Western Michigan University Homer Stryker MD School of Medicine (WMED), Kalamazoo, Michigan USA

Mission and service

The Western Michigan University Homer Stryker MD School of Medicine was started in 2012 and its first class of medical students began in 2014. The Department of Pediatric and Adolescent Medicine has a pediatric residency program which is accredited by the Accreditation Council for Graduate Medical Education (ACGME) in Chicago, Illinois, USA and the current residency program in Pediatrics started in 1990.

The WMED Department of Pediatric and Adolescent Medicine has a commitment to a comprehensive approach to the health and development of the child, adolescent, and the family. The Department has a blend of academic general pediatricians and pediatric specialists. Our Pediatric Clinic team provides a broad spectrum of general well and sick child care (birth through 18 years) including immunizations, monitoring general physical and emotional growth, motor skill development, sports medicine (including participation evaluations and evaluation of common sports injuries), child abuse evaluations, and psychosocial or behavioral assessment. WMED Pediatrics believes in immunizations as a protection against preventative disease processes. Our Pediatrics Clinic is undergoing a transformation to a patient-centered medical home (PCMH). A patient-centered medical home is a way to deliver coordinated and comprehensive primary care to our infants, children, adolescents and young adults. It is a partnership between individuals and families within a health care setting, which allows for a more efficient use of resources and time to improve the quality of outcomes for all involved through care provided by a continuity care team.

Research activities

The Department has a variety of research projects in adolescent medicine, neurobehavioral pediatrics, adolescent gynecology, pediatric diabetes mellitus, asthma, and cystic fibrosis. The WMED Department of Pediatric and Adolescent Medicine has published a number of medical textbooks: Essential adolescent medicine (McGraw-Hill Medical Publishers), The pediatric diagnostic examination (McGraw-Hill), Pediatric and adolescent psychopharmacology (Cambridge University Press), Behavioral pediatrics, 2nd edition (iUniverse Publishers in New York and Lincoln, Nebraska), Behavioral pediatrics 3rd edition (New York: Nova Biomedical Books); 4th Edition: In press. Pediatric practice: Sports medicine (McGraw-Hill), Handbook of clinical pediatrics (Singapore: World Scientific), Neurodevelopmental disabilities: Clinical care for children and young adults (Dordrecht: Springer), Adolescent medicine: Pharmacotherapeutics in medical disorders (Berlin/Boston: De Gruyter), Adolescent medicine: Pharmacotherapeutics in general, mental, and sexual health (Berlin/Boston: De Gruyter), Pediatric psychodermatology (Berlin/Boston: De Gruyter), Substance abuse in adolescents and young adults: A manual for pediatric and primary care clinicians (Berlin/Boston: De Gruyter), and tropical pediatrics (New York: Nova); Second edition in press.

The Department has edited a number of journal issues published by Elsevier Publishers covering pulmonology (State of the Art Reviews: Adolescent Medicine—AM:STARS), genetic disorders in adolescents (AM:STARS), neurologic/neurodevelopmental disorders (AM:STARS), behavioral pediatrics (Pediatric Clinics of North America), pediatric psychopharmacology in the 21st century (Pediatric Clinic of North America), nephrologic disorders in adolescents (AM:STARS), college health (Pediatric Clinics of North America), adolescent medicine (Primary Care: Clinics in Office Practice), behavioral pediatrics in children and adolescents (Primary Care: Clinics in Office Practice), adolescents and sports (Pediatric Clinics of North America), and developmental disabilities (Pediatric Clinics of North America). The Department has also edited a journal issue on musculoskeletal disorders in children and adolescents for the American Academy of Pediatrics' AM:STARs; in April of 2013 a Subspecialty Update issue was published in AM:STARs.

The department has developed academic ties with a variety of international medical centers and organizations, including the Queen Elizabeth Hospital in Hong Kong, Indian Academy of Pediatrics (New Delhi, India), the University of Athens Children's Hospital (First and Second Departments of Paediatrics) in Athens, Greece and the National Institute of Child Health and Human Development in Jerusalem, Israel.

Contact

Professor Donald E Greydanus, MD and Professor Dilip R. Patel, MD
Department of Pediatric and Adolescent Medicine
Western Michigan University Homer Stryker MD School of Medicine
1000 Oakland Drive, D48G, Kalamazoo, MI 49008-1284, United States
E-mail: Donald.greydanus@med.wmich.edu and dilip.Patel@med.wmich.edu
Website: http://www.med.wmich.edu

In: Pediatric and Adolescent Dermatology
Editors: D Greydanus, A Feinberg and J Merrick
ISBN: 978-1-63321-853-6

Chapter 12

About the National Institute of Child Health and Human Development in Israel

The National Institute of Child Health and Human Development (NICHD) in Israel was established in 1998 as a virtual institute under the auspicies of the Medical Director, Ministry of Social Affairs and Social Services in order to function as the research arm for the Office of the Medical Director. In 1998 the National Council for Child Health and Pediatrics, Ministry of Health and in 1999 the Director General and Deputy Director General of the Ministry of Health endorsed the establishment of the NICHD.

Mission

The mission of a National Institute for Child Health and Human Development in Israel is to provide an academic focal point for the scholarly interdisciplinary study of child life, health, public health, welfare, disability, rehabilitation, intellectual disability and related aspects of human development. This mission includes research, teaching, clinical work, information and public service activities in the field of child health and human development.

Service and academic activities

Over the years many activities became focused in the south of Israel due to collaboration with various professionals at the Faculty of Health Sciences (FOHS) at the Ben Gurion University of the Negev (BGU). Since 2000 an affiliation with the Zusman Child Development Center at the Pediatric Division of Soroka University Medical Center has resulted in collaboration around the establishment of the Down Syndrome Clinic at that center. In 2002 a full course on "Disability" was established at the Recanati School for Allied Professions in the Community, FOHS, BGU and in 2005 collaboration was started with the Primary Care Unit of the faculty and disability became part of the master of public health course on "Children and society". In the academic year 2005-2006 a one semester course on "Aging with disability" was started as part of the master of science program in gerontology in our collaboration with the Center for Multidisciplinary Research in Aging. In 2010 collaborations with the Division of Pediatrics, Hadassah Hebrew University Medical Center, Jerusalem, Israel around the National Down Syndrome Center and teaching students and residents about intellectual and developmental disabilities as part of their training at this campus.

Research activities

The affiliated staff have over the years published work from projects and research activities in this national and international collaboration. In the year 2000 the International Journal of Adolescent Medicine and Health and in 2005 the International Journal on Disability and Human Development of De Gruyter Publishing House (Berlin and New York) were affiliated with the National Institute of Child Health and Human Development. From 2008 also the International Journal of Child Health and Human Development (Nova Science, New York), the International Journal of Child and Adolescent Health (Nova Science) and the Journal of Pain Management (Nova Science) affiliated and from 2009 the International Public Health Journal (Nova Science) and Journal of Alternative Medicine Research (Nova Science). All peer-reviewed international journals.

National collaborations

Nationally the NICHD works in collaboration with the Faculty of Health Sciences, Ben Gurion University of the Negev; Department of Physical Therapy, Sackler School of Medicine, Tel Aviv University; Autism Center, Assaf HaRofeh Medical Center; National Rett and PKU Centers at Chaim Sheba Medical Center, Tel HaShomer; Department of Physiotherapy, Haifa University; Department of Education, Bar Ilan University, Ramat Gan, Faculty of Social Sciences and Health Sciences; College of Judea and Samaria in Ariel and in 2011 affiliation with Center for Pediatric Chronic Diseases and National Center for Down Syndrome, Department of Pediatrics, Hadassah Hebrew University Medical Center, Mount Scopus Campus, Jerusalem.

International collaborations

Internationally with the Department of Disability and Human Development, College of Applied Health Sciences, University of Illinois at Chicago; Strong Center for Developmental Disabilities, Golisano Children's Hospital at Strong, University of Rochester School of Medicine and Dentistry, New York; Centre on Intellectual Disabilities, University of Albany, New York; Centre for Chronic Disease Prevention and Control, Health Canada, Ottawa; Chandler Medical Center and Children's Hospital, Kentucky Children's Hospital, Section of Adolescent Medicine, University of Kentucky, Lexington; Chronic Disease Prevention and

Control Research Center, Baylor College of Medicine, Houston, Texas; Division of Neuroscience, Department of Psychiatry, Columbia University, New York; Institute for the Study of Disadvantage and Disability, Atlanta; Center for Autism and Related Disorders, Department Psychiatry, Children's Hospital Boston, Boston; Department of Paediatrics, Child Health and Adolescent Medicine, Children's Hospital at Westmead, Westmead, Australia; International Centre for the Study of Occupational and Mental Health, Düsseldorf, Germany; Centre for Advanced Studies in Nursing, Department of General Practice and Primary Care, University of Aberdeen, Aberdeen, United Kingdom; Quality of Life Research Center, Copenhagen, Denmark; Nordic School of Public Health, Gottenburg, Sweden, Scandinavian Institute of Quality of Working Life, Oslo, Norway; The Department of Applied Social Sciences (APSS) of The Hong Kong Polytechnic University Hong Kong.

Targets

Our focus is on research, international collaborations, clinical work, teaching and policy in health, disability and human development and to establish the NICHD as a permanent institute at one of the residential care centers for persons with intellectual disability in Israel in order to conduct model research and together with the four university schools of public health/medicine in Israel establish a national master and doctoral program in disability and human development at the institute to secure the next generation of professionals working in this often non-prestigious/low-status field of work.

Contact

Joav Merrick, MD, MMedSci, DMSc
Professor of Pediatrics, Child Health and Human Development
Medical Director, Health Services, Division for Intellectual and Developmental Disabilities, Ministry of Social Affairs and Social Services, POB 1260, IL-91012 Jerusalem, Israel.
E-mail: jmerrick@zahav.net.il

In: Pediatric and Adolescent Dermatology
Editors: D Greydanus, A Feinberg and J Merrick
ISBN: 978-1-63321-853-6

Chapter 13

About the book series "Pediatrics, child and adolescent health"

Pediatrics, child and adolescent health is a book series with publications from a multidisciplinary group of researchers, practitioners and clinicians for an international professional forum interested in the broad spectrum of pediatric medicine, child health, adolescent health and human development.

- Merrick J, ed. Child and adolescent health yearbook 2011. New York: Nova Science, 2012.
- Merrick J, ed. Child and adolescent health yearbook 2012. New York: Nova Science, 2012.
- Roach RR, Greydanus DE, Patel DR, Homnick DN, Merrick J, eds. Tropical pediatrics: A public health concern of international proportions. New York: Nova Science, 2012.
- Merrick J, ed. Child health and human development yearbook 2011. New York: Nova Science, 2012.
- Merrick J, ed. Child health and human development yearbook 2012. New York: Nova Science, 2012.
- Shek DTL, Sun RCF, Merrick J, eds. Developmental issues in Chinese adolescents. New York: Nova Science, 2012.
- Shek DTL, Sun RCF, Merrick J, eds. Positive youth development: Theory, research and application. New York: Nova Science, 2012.
- Zachor DA, Merrick J, eds. Understanding autism spectrum disorder: Current research aspects. New York: Nova Science, 2012.
- Ma HK, Shek DTL, Merrick J, eds. Positive youth development: A new school curriculum to tackle adolescent developmental issues. New York: Nova Science, 2012.
- Wood D, Reiss JG, Ferris ME, Edwards LR, Merrick J, eds. Transition from pediatric to adult medical care. New York: Nova Science, 2012.
- Isenberg Y. Guidelines for the healthy integration of the ill child in the educational system: Experience from Israel. New York: Nova Science, 2013.

- Shek DTL, Sun RCF, Merrick J, eds. Chinese adolescent development: Economic disadvantages, parents and intrapersonal development. New York: Nova Science, 2013.
- Shek DTL, Sun RCF, Merrick J, eds. University and college students: Health and development issues for the leaders of tomorrow. New York: Nova Science, 2013.
- Shek DTL, Sun RCF, Merrick J, eds. Adolescence and behavior issues in a Chinese context. New York: Nova Science, 2013.
- Sun J, Buys N, Merrick J, eds. Advances in preterm infant research. New York: Nova Science, 2013.
- Tsitsika A, Janikian M, Greydanus DE, Omar HA, Merrick J, eds. Internet addiction: A public health concern in adolescence. New York: Nova Science, 2013.
- Shek DTL, Lee TY, Merrick J, eds. Promotion of holistic development of young people in Hong Kong. New York: Nova Science, 2013.
- Shek DTL, Ma C, Lu Y, Merrick J, eds. Human developmental research: Experience from research in Hong Kong. New York: Nova Science, 2013.
- Merrick J, ed. Chronic disease and disability in childhood. New York: Nova Science, 2013.
- Rubin IL, Merrick J, eds. Break the cycle of environmental health disparities: Maternal and child health aspects. New York: Nova Science, 2013.
- Rubin IL, Merrick J, eds. Environmental health disparities in children: Asthma, obesity and food. New York: Nova Science, 2013.
- Rubin IL, Merrick J, eds. Environmental health: Home, school and community. New York: Nova Science, 2013.
- Rubin IL, Merrick J, eds. Child health and human development: Social, economic and environmental factors. New York: Nova Science, 2013.
- Merrick J, Kandel I, Omar HA, eds. Children, violence and bullying: International perspectives. New York: Nova Science, 2013.
- Omar HA, Bowling CH, Merrick J, eds. Playing with fire: Children, adolescents and firesetting. New York: Nova Science, 2013.
  Merrick J, Tenenbaum A, Omar HA, eds. School, adolescence and health issues. New York: Nova Science, 2013.
- Merrick J, Tenenbaum A, Omar Ha, eds. Adolescence and sexuality: International perspectives. New York: Nova Science, 2014.
- Diamond G, Arbel E. Adoption: The search for a new parenthood. New York: Nova Science, 2014.
- Taylor MF, Pooley JA, Merrick J, eds. Adolescence: Places and spaces. New York: Nova Science, 2014.

Contact

Professor Joav Merrick, MD, MMedSci, DMSc
Medical Director, Medical Services
Division for Intellectual and Developmental Disabilities
Ministry of Social Affairs and Social Services
POBox 1260, IL-91012 Jerusalem, Israel
E-mail: jmerrick@zahav.net.il

Section Three: Index

Index

#

A

B

C

D

E

F

G

H

I

M

N

O

P

Q

R

S

T

U

V

W

Y

Z